CONTENTS

METHODS OF PSYCHIATRIC RESEARCH

AN INTRODUCTION FOR CLINICAL PSYCHIATRISTS

Edited by

PETER SAINSBURY
M.D., M.R.C.P., F.R.C.PSYCH., D.P.M.

Director of Research,
Medical Research Council Clinical Psychiatry Unit,
Graylingwell Hospital, Chichester

AND

NORMAN KREITMAN
M.D., M.R.C.P.(ED.), F.R.C.PSYCH., D.P.M.

Director of Research,
Medical Research Council Unit for Epidemiological Studies in Psychiatry,
Royal Edinburgh Hospital

SECOND EDITION

LONDON
OXFORD UNIVERSITY PRESS
NEW YORK   TORONTO
1975

Oxford University Press, Ely House, London W.1

GLASGOW NEW YORK TORONTO MELBOURNE WELLINGTON
CAPE TOWN IBADAN NAIROBI DAR ES SALAAM LUSAKA ADDIS ABABA
DELHI BOMBAY CALCUTTA MADRAS KARACHI LAHORE DACCA
KUALA LUMPUR SINGAPORE HONG KONG TOKYO

ISBN 0 19 264419 X

© *Oxford University Press, 1963, 1975*

First published 1963

Second Edition 1975

Printed in Great Britain by The Camelot Press Ltd, Southampton

CONTRIBUTORS

JACQUELINE C. GRAD DE ALARCON, Ph.D.
*Member of Scientific Staff,
MRC Clinical Psychiatry Unit,
Graylingwell Hospital,
Chichester, Sussex.*

ANNEMARIE CROCETTI, DR.P.H.
*Assistant Professor,
Department of Community Medicine,
Mount Sinai College of Medicine,
19 East 98th Street,
New York,
U.S.A.*

G. A. FOULDS, M.A., Ph.D.
*Member of Scientific Staff,
MRC Unit for Epidemiological Studies
    in Psychiatry,
Department of Psychiatry,
Royal Edinburgh Hospital,
Morningside Park, Edinburgh.*

FAY FRANSELLA, B.A., Ph.D., Dip.Psych.
*Senior Lecturer in Clinical Psychology,
Royal Free Hospital School of Medicine,
University of London.*

DAVID GOLDBERG, D.M., M.R.C.P., M.R.C.Psych., D.P.M.
*Professor of Psychiatry,
The University Hospital of South
    Manchester,
West Didsbury, Manchester.*

R. E. KENDELL, M.D., F.R.C.P., M.R.C.Psych., D.P.M.
*Professor of Psychiatry,
University of Edinburgh,
Royal Edinburgh Hospital,
Morningside Park, Edinburgh.*

NEIL KESSEL, M.D., F.R.C.P., F.R.C.Psych., D.P.M.
*Professor of Psychiatry,
University of Manchester.*

NORMAN KREITMAN, M.D., M.R.C.P.(Ed.), F.R.C.Psych., D.P.M.
*Director,
MRC Unit for Epidemiological Studies in
    Psychiatry,
Department of Psychiatry,
Royal Edinburgh Hospital,
Morningside Park, Edinburgh.*

M. H. LADER, M.D.,
F.R.C.Psych., D.P.M.

Senior Lecturer, Member of MRC External Scientific Staff,
Institute of Psychiatry,
University of London.

DENIS LEIGH, M.D.,
F.R.C.P., F.R.C.Psych.

Physician to the Bethlem Royal and Maudsley Hospitals,
London.

A. B. LEVEY, M.A., Ph.D.

Member of Scientific Staff,
MRC Clinical Psychiatry Unit,
Graylingwell Hospital,
Chichester, Sussex.

A. E. MAXWELL, M.A.,
M.Ed., Ph.D.

Professor of Psychological Statistics,
Head of Biometrics Unit,
Institute of Psychiatry,
University of London.

L. T. MORTON, F.L.A.

Formerly *Librarian,*
Medical Research Council,
National Institute for Medical Research,
London.

MARY P. PATTEN, B.A.

Lecturer in Extra-Mural Studies,
Queen's University,
Belfast.

D. A. POND, M.D., F.R.C.P.,
F.R.C.Psych., D.P.M.

Professor of Psychiatry,
London Hospital Medical School,
University of London.

JUNE M. PRESS, M.A.

Formerly *Assistant Lecturer,*
Department of Social and Preventive Medicine,
Queen's University,
Belfast.

PETER SAINSBURY, M.D.,
M.R.C.P., F.R.C.Psych.,
D.P.M.

Director,
MRC Clinical Psychiatry Unit,
Graylingwell Hospital,
Chichester, Sussex.

J. C. SHAW, B.Sc., Ph.D.

Physicist,
MRC Clinical Psychiatry Unit,
Graylingwell Hospital,
Chichester, Sussex.

MICHAEL SHEPHERD, D.M., *Professor of Epidemiological Psychiatry,*
    F.R.C.P., F.R.C.Psych.,   *Institute of Psychiatry,*
    D.P.M.   *University of London.*

GLENN D. WILSON, M.A.,   *Lecturer,*
    Ph.D.   *Institute of Psychiatry,*
                                     University of London.

JOHN K. WING, M.D., Ph.D.,   *Director,*
    F.R.C.Psych., D.P.M.   *MRC Social Psychiatry Unit,*
                                 Professor of Social Psychiatry,
                                 Institute of Psychiatry, and London
                                     School of Hygiene,
                                 University of London.

PREFACE TO THE SECOND EDITION

This edition shows a number of changes from the original version. Nine of the contributors to the first edition have kindly supplied an updated chapter, which in almost every instance has been extensively rewritten. In addition nine new chapters have been included. Two of these additional contributions deals with aspects of social psychiatry—a reflection perhaps on the growing interest in this area—but others are concerned with matters such as laboratory techniques applicable to psychophysiological studies. We hope that the balance of the volume has remained such that the inexperienced psychiatrist or behavioural scientist will find in it much to guide him in whichever direction he chooses to travel.

The decade since the first edition has seen the establishment of the Royal College of Psychiatrists, and it is hoped that among the consequences of this major event in British psychiatry will be an improved standard in the training of young psychiatrists and an increasing investment in research. But the provision of facilities does not automatically follow from professional reorganization, and this is particularly true for research guidance. We are keenly aware that many psychiatrists working in settings outside the main university centres still lack advice and encouragement to embark on research. It remains our hope that this volume will help to meet their needs. Though some of the chapters are perhaps a little more advanced than those of the first edition it is still our intention to provide an elementary manual of research techniques for those inexperienced in such matters.

Inevitably contributors have written in the context of the British scene, but we are aware that for psychiatrists in developing countries, access to research expertise may be especially difficult. Their needs have been borne in mind and we would like to think that they too will find the volume relevant to their situation.

Lastly, the editors would like to thank all who have contributed to this book, not only for what they have written, but also for their ununfailing good humour in enduring editorial caveats, obstructions and general harassment. We can only hope that their endurance has not been in vain.

Graylingwell Hospital　　　　　　　　　　　　　　　　　P. S.
Royal Edinburgh Hospital　　　　　　　　　　　　　　　N. K.

August 1974

PREFACE TO THE FIRST EDITION

The contributions to this book are based on a course of seminars given during 1960–1 under the auspices of the Royal Medico-Psychological Association, and were planned by the secretary of the clinical sub-committee of the Research and Clinical Section of the Association. Their first and principal purpose was to introduce psychiatrists working in the mental hospital to the basic procedures, methods and techniques of clinical research, particularly those who had not had the opportunity of a postgraduate academic training. They are therefore primarily directed to those who wish to begin research or to work for a doctorate, but who feel uncertain how to set about it. As the book is intended to be a beginner's guide to the subject, many contributors have not hesitated to give a frankly elementary account of their subject or to give it a strictly practical emphasis.

It was hoped that if the series was planned in this way it might diminish some of the over-rated notions about research which seem to deter or intimidate the potential investigator. For one reason or another, experimentation and systematic inquiry into clinical problems has too often been made to appear an unduly intricate and recondite activity. The notable truth about good clinical research is the almost inevitable way in which it emerges from observations made in the course of the daily work with patients. Also what is often remarkable is its simplicity: the obviousness of the hypothesis, the uncomplicated method, and the conciseness of the findings.

We presumed that many more psychiatrists are concerned to do research than in fact do it, and that given the opportunity to become familiar with its more practical aspects they would be prepared to make a start. The lively comments and response to the suggestion of a course of this kind made it evident that psychiatrists felt a real need for a straightforward and elementary introduction to research methods.

We also hope that these contributions will encourage clinical research in the mental hospital. To say there is an urgent need for more research into mental disorder has, at last, become a commonplace; but the promotion of it is still only beginning. The attitudes, ideas, traditions, and administration which hinder the furthering of psychiatry and research into it remain very much alive. The medical student's introduction to these subjects in many medical schools is still so insufficient that the likelihood of his being attracted to either is far less than it might be. Openings for a postgraduate training in psychiatry which bring the doctor in close contact with research are exceptional; the tradition persists that the psychiatrist can learn his subject while working in the mental hospital with the minimum of formal academic instruction.

As long as the mental hospital and psychiatry remain academically isolated, it will be difficult to foster research. The new chairs in psychiatry in the universities and teaching hospitals will bring psychiatry into close contact with other disciplines—biochemistry, sociology, and so on—and so fertilize and stimulate psychiatric inquiries. Students and doctors will also become more closely acquainted with, and recruited to, the study of the problems of mental illness early in their careers. These academic centres, however, will need to collaborate intimately with the mental hospitals. The mental hospital and its new derivatives—planned and actual—will remain the source and field for clinical research; that is to say, it must originate largely from those to whom this book is addressed.

One of the attractions of psychiatry is the opportunities it offers to an averagely inquisitive and adventurous doctor to make useful and original contributions—especially of a clinical kind. Occasions for clinical research in the course of the day's work—on the description, natural history and outcome of illness, for example—are numerous. Clinical psychiatry though alive with ideas and theories, is starved of quite simple facts; it is rich in hypotheses, but poor in the experimental confirmation of them. We are firmly of the view that what is in short supply is not the ability or inclination to do research, but the knowledge of how to go about it—hence the emphasis of the contributors of this book on methods likely to be helpful to the practising clinician.

We are very indebted to the Royal Medico-Psychological Association and to the committee of the Research and Clinical Section for their active support in organizing the seminars and for encouraging us to publish the contributions.

Graylingwell Hospital   P. S.
Chichester   N. K.

May 1962

ACKNOWLEDGEMENTS

The Editors acknowledge permission to reproduce the following:

In Professor Shepherd's chapter, FIG. 7.1 is from Dr. I. Sutherland's 'Statistical Aspects of Clinical Trials' in *Report of a Symposium on Clinical Trials*, Pfizer Ltd., and FIG. 7.2 is from H. Rashkis and E. Smarr, *Psychiatric Research Reports 9*, American Psychological Association.

1

CHOICE OF A SUBJECT FOR
CLINICAL RESEARCH

D. A. POND

In the ten years or more since Dr. Mayer-Gross wrote this chapter in the first edition, the underlying philosophy of clinical research has remained the same, but there have been tremendous changes in its practice, especially as regards psychiatry. Our subject is no longer a cottage industry when contrasted with the sophisticated means employed in the laboratory and at the bedside by our medical colleagues. We had little more apparatus than laborious handwritten notes that bear the same relationship to modern methods as do the string and sealing wax days of atomic physics to a nuclear reactor.

It is worth reiterating what are the fundamental qualities of clinical research as opposed to what can best be described as non-clinical, since the other words usually contrasted with clinical such as 'pure' or 'experimental' often appear to denigrate our subject, especially in the eyes of the newly-fledged science graduate. By definition clinical research begins, continues and ends with the patient, but on the way may take excursions to any number of basic sciences. The methods with which it is prosecuted as regards the refinement of hypotheses, the methodology, the reliability and validity of results, and so on, should be as rigorous as is possible within the limits of our concern with the patient. The clinical research worker has, in fact, the edge on his other colleagues, since in the end it is he alone who is able and willing to take into account all the possible variables that might affect the observations or experiments that form the substance of his research. He cannot, without jeopardizing the quality of his work, say 'Let us ignore this and this factor, which might be relevant'. It follows from this that though his work may be often imprecise because of the complexity of the relevant factors, yet he does at least recognize the limitation and as far as possible uses a sophisticated test design which will reduce effects which he cannot completely control to an assessable, if not strictly measurable, size.

As far as psychiatry is concerned there have been both great theoretical advances and great methodological advances in the past ten years. The theoretical advances have mainly come from an important flow of ideas from academic non-clinical psychology and sociology. Clinicians are no longer brought up on a mixed diet of a curious subject called 'medical psychology'—a mixture of Freud and water—and crude pseudo-organic concepts of brain function that represent an increasingly fossilized form of associationist psychology fashionable around the beginning of this century. From what used to be the rather academic subject of experimental psychology, there now flows a powerful stream of types of learning theories with appropriate experimental techniques for analysing many situations in terms of stimulus, response, reward, etc. Still newer advances, which are going to make a great impact in the next ten years, stem from information and control theories that form the mathematical basis of the computer technology.

Similarly, from current sociological theory we learn new ways of looking at group interactions, e.g. role-playing as it affects patients' (and doctors') behaviour. So far it is mostly what is often called micro-sociology rather than macro-sociology; that is, small groups (rather than whole societies) the theoretical understanding of which is beginning profoundly to change our way of looking at the origins and treatment of mental illness.

There have also been various significant advances in the neurosciences that are much more closely related to the traditional basic medical sciences. Neuropharmacology, for example, with a whole new range of psychotropic drugs, may have achieved its therapeutic triumphs largely by the well-tried method of serendipity, but the growing knowledge of neuro-transmitters must inevitably slowly change our understanding of mental processes. However, there is no need to dwell quite as much on this aspect of the new theoretical advances as on psychology and sociology, because for most clinicians exposure to these advances occurs more or less automatically in the course of medical and psychiatric training.

Side by side with the theoretical advances one must also briefly refer to the most important methodological changes that have occurred, especially as regards psychological techniques. The standardization of psychological interviews is now an essential part of interview techniques. It is no longer sufficient to rely on the unstructured clinical chat and the unsystematic gathering of clinical information. Similarly, sociological studies about family interactions are being increasingly formalized. The use of special recording techniques, such as closed circuit television, also enable clinical interviews to be recorded as they proceed with little or no interference with the human one-to-one interaction. A primary data-gathering situation is thus amenable to objective reassessment time and time again by other observers. Ethnological principles of recording behaviour are being fruitfully applied to the study of child and family interactions in free situation, even their homes. They are also applicable to the study of non-verbal communication generally, e.g. in group psychotherapy. Telemetric methods are also being refined and made more reliable, so that a few simple neurophysiological variables, such as heart rate or skin resistance, and even brain potentials, can be recorded while the subject is freely moving in an experimental situation or an interview.

All these methodological advances imply, therefore, that the clinical research worker would be well advised at least to find out whether any of these methods could be easily applied to his particular problem. Doctors ought not to rely much longer entirely on unaided observation, laboriously and inaccurately recorded subsequently by handwriting. It is, however, important to stress that no amount of gadgetry and theoretical sophistication can make up for barrenness of ideas and sloppy ways of working. Much clinical research is rightly little more than an extension of first-class but routine clinical work. As Medawar has said, any diagnostic investigation of a patient properly carried out is a scientific exercise; the clinician proceeds to the understanding of the patient not just by indiscriminate amassing of data, nor by pure intuition, but by formulating a hypothesis (a possible diagnosis) and applying the appropriate clinical and perhaps laboratory tests to confirm or deny the hypothesis. If it is disproved, then another is formulated and tested in similar fashion. The hypothetico-deductive method is the corner-stone both of clinical work and scientific research, but to go beyond the study of a single patient as far as his clinical needs are concerned to a definite scientific investigation of him or others like him, is often an arduous task. From the hunch to the protocol is a Pilgrim's Progress in which Giant Despair looms large.

WHO DOES CLINICAL RESEARCH?

Although this book is largely directed to the psychiatrist—the medically qualified specialist in his subject—it is perhaps worth noting that there are about four different types of scientists who are actively interested in our field. The medically qualified psychiatric trainee tends to be the most advanced in age. He has been through a long apprenticeship, and, even if he has not stopped off at one or other points of his training to do some special research or postgraduate special study in, for example, a basic science, he is likely to be around thirty years old before he feels in a position to know enough to do clinical research. The dangers that such a person may suffer are a consequence of the length and intensity of training required to reach high clinical competence. He has become so much part of the team in a hospital that it is difficult for him to keep alive that little streak of nonconformity so essential for the original idea. However, the isolated worker-genius is largely a figment of the imagination and inapplicable to the clinical field. The isolated geniuses in the history of science are young men looking at problems with eyes unblinkered by years of training. It is a well recognized fact that students of human nature tend to make their original contributions when older than, for example, mathematicians, though the capacity for original work has often already shown itself by pieces of often quite unrelated research done by such clinicians as early as when they were students. Freud may not have stumbled on psychoanalysis until he was forty but he had shown original scientific drive before that, and some people still think he did his best work when writing on aphasia!

These points are worth making because the young clinician must increasingly relate to three other groups of workers. The non-medical clinical psychologist is likely to be his most frequent scientific colleague, a man perhaps ten years younger than he is, fresh from the academic rigours of a degree course that includes a lot of statistics, and a suspicion that human nature is best observed in a well-ordered laboratory. In many psychiatric academic departments there will also be laboratory-oriented medical scientists expert in, for example, neurophysiology. They sometimes need convincing that what is so far not measurable may, nevertheless, not only exist but be preponderant in determining human behaviour. Lastly, there will be sociologically-oriented scientists who may well regard the whole concept of psychiatric illness as an extreme and regrettable example of social processes that should be reversible by social means.

Clinical research work in psychiatry is thus becoming surrounded by an exciting new host of colleagues, and in this way the clinical research worker's position increasingly resembles that with which the young medical research worker has long been familiar. It follows from this that at some stage he may need some special training and experience, and to this matter we must now turn.

HOW TO START RESEARCH

Potential research work often starts by chance observation in a particular patient or a group of patients who happen to be seen sufficiently close together for common factors to become apparent. This observation may suggest some possible line of research, and then the long process begins of trying to mould the hunch into the protocol. It is at this point that you should think about the advisability of taking time off to get some special knowledge of a particular field.

Young psychiatrists, in particular, do not sufficiently often try to get away to work in another hospital or a laboratory either part-time or, preferably, whole-time for a year if possible. Even today many trainees have a totally inadequate knowledge of the sciences basic to psychiatry, such as sociology and psychology. They learn far less of these subjects than does the young research worker in medicine of the basic sciences, like biochemistry, relevant to *his* subject. Ideally, of course, a man should become aware of his potential and his senior tutors and advisers sufficiently interested in his potential to get him time off to learn the new subjects, perhaps even before medical qualification. However, a man should not try to dabble in too many fields. If he has become interested in neurophysiology through some patients who had peculiar EEGs, then he should not also try to take some time off to work in a department of sociology.

The opportunity to talk over possible ideas about research must be taken from the beginning. You must never be too proud to take advice and ask assistance from all and sundry. However, you should choose your senior colleague carefully; it is only too easy for disillusioned older workers to make it plain that your ideas are even more half-baked than their own probably were twenty years ago, and that you have quite clearly not read all the literature and in particular omitted that important article in the Zeitschrift für something-or-other in 1890.

When first starting, it is often an advantage to be the junior member of a team—preferably by invitation. In this way, one can learn from watching the interactions of those who are more experienced and discover that most of them make crass mistakes, anyway. Collaboration with a colleague at a more equal level, particularly if he is in a different but related field, for example neuropharmacology or sociology, is very helpful. However, as far as possible, try to participate in the design of the investigation with which you are becoming associated. Beware of becoming just a stooge; and likewise, incidentally, beware of using stooges to do all the data-collecting which you then write up, occasionally without appropriate acknowledgement. That distinguished clinical researcher (and no stooge) Professor Stengel was once heard to say, 'In a paper I once wrote under the pseudonym of . . .'! There is no substitute for doing most of the work yourself, but to expect to be able to do it all quite alone is likely to be as fruitful as parthenogenesis.

Relations with statisticians are particularly difficult to get right. This is the subject of another chapter in this book and all that can be said here is the personal view that they make good servants but bad masters; in particular, of course, never expect them to have any original idea for your clinical research. This is your prerogative if you want to do a piece of work, but please consult them early on before the research is three parts finished and you begin to realize that you need a little bit of help with fiddling the results before they make sense.

The time and the place to do clinical research should be as clearly demarcated as possible from everyday routine. It takes courage and determination to shut the door on the clamant needs of patient care and to put up with the catty comments of your colleagues that you never do any work but leave them to get on with the real job of getting people better. On this side you will be accused of selfish bloody-mindedness, whereas your non-clinical colleagues with whom you are trying to work will doubtless regard your clinical work as dabbling in a trade that (these days, at any rate) will appear to carry the chance of a Distinction Award rather than that plate in Harley Street that has become so tarnished.

WHAT TO STUDY

Trying to give advice on a topic for clinical research is like giving advice on choosing a wife. At first sight it seems as if mate selection is a random process and all things are possible. In practice, choice is limited by personal ability and the availability of suitable clinical material. The subject is rapidly changing as can be observed by reading the topics suggested only ten years ago by Mayer-Gross. Many of these seem quaintly old fashioned, particularly as regards the way they are conceptualized, and the same will doubtless be said of all of the following suggestions.

Some types of clinical research are now fairly well formalized. The drug trial is an outstanding example: the techniques for choosing the right sort of patient, the detailed spelling out of the clinical observations to be made and the protocol to be observed; the statistical management of a double blind trial when this is appropriate; the use of independent observers to validate one's observations, etc., are valuable techniques to learn. Such a trial provides for many people an easy, if not a very inspiring, entrée into clinical research. Comparative beginners can be easily fitted into a trial that is being organized by workers experienced in this field. The tidy formulation of such a project does, however, mean that joining in gives a limited view of the uncertainties and excitements of research into more unknown fields. It is also easy to become seduced by the blandishments of the drug firms anxious to have their wares marketed with the kudos of having been approved by an independent scientific investigator. The assessment of other forms of therapy, for example dynamic psychotherapy, behaviour therapy, etc., is proving far more difficult, though in the end this may perhaps be more rewarding. It is a sad commentary on psychiatry that we try to do so much for so many with so little idea of its effectiveness.

There was a time when the careful description of symptoms was a subject dignified by being called phenomenology. Then it became unfashionable. Symptoms, it was thought, were just the means, the signals, to get the patient to the psychiatrist who was much more interested in interpersonal relationships and intrapersonal dynamics. However, symptoms have suddenly come back, with the current interest in behaviour therapy, and this is an area of research that is likely to keep quite a lot of people busy for several years. It is an outstanding example of the application of theoretical psychological ideas whose origins owe little or nothing to clinical science.

On the other hand, interpersonal interaction in small groups, as an object of study, is a way in which interest in intra-psychic dynamics has been supplemented rather than superseded. The study of the family relations of schizophrenics by questionnaires, tape-recorded interviews, etc., are natural subjects for clinical research. Such studies, in particular, show very well the important way in which a clinical investigation should improve routine clinical work and not just be of academic theoretical interest.

Spreading still further out from the interpersonal, there is much to be done in the field of psychiatry in the community. Some of this may be called 'operational research', which is of special interest to the Department of Health. Topics needing further research are, for example, the effects on mental health of changing social circumstances in New Towns, or of the breadwinner becoming redundant and needing retraining at a relatively late age. The effects of better training in psychiatry for general practitioners so that they become more aware of the pschodynamics of their relationships with their patients have not been properly evaluated. Collaboration with one or more general practices is a particularly fruitful way of initiating research into all sorts of topics—your local branch of the Royal College of General Practitioners will be a good place to start looking for colleagues.

So far, even less exploited are the implications of carrying out the Kilbrandon and Seebohm Reports. When the social services are completely organized with properly trained staff, it is probable that a great deal of psychological disorder that now flows through medical channels may not come our way at all; for example, marriage guidance (and even more important prophylactically, marriage preparation) may well be an area of psychological problems which will come into medical care only if there are obvious somatic complications affecting, for example, choice of contraceptive. The change in social attitudes is best symbolized by people becoming clients, not patients. It may result in all sorts of other changes such as a fall in the demand for maintenance psychoactive drugs 'on the Health'. What are of interest here are common conditions and common practices in which apparently small changes in behaviour could have big social implications. Though much of this research will be done by social scientists without a medical or psychiatric context, yet for the psychiatrist there is, for example, still much useful research to be done on the common psychosomatic disorders that seem mainly connected with adult sexual relationships. Stengel's work on pain, and that of Murray Parkes and others on bereavement, show how much good work can be done on disorders and conditions that seem at first to be commonplace and everyday.

Psychiatry is often one of the last branches of medicine to get started in developing countries. In them the clash of cultures will further sharpen the alert doctor's awareness of sociological factors in mental disorder. In primitive societies, too, there may be so far unknown toxic, metabolic, and infective causes of organic mental disorder. Quite simple methods of systematic data collection may be enough to gather what is needed. In more primitive surroundings it is easy to feel that no research can be done without a large computer to handle complicated data in sophisticated ways, but it has been said more than once that the computer has become the biggest enemy of the best research as it encourages the idea that statistical manipulation will make good silk purse papers out of worthless sows' ears data. It is much better in such situations to take advantage of the special circumstances and not sigh for sophisticated biochemical colleagues to carry on with research into the metabolic causes of schizophrenia.

The alert research worker may be able to take advantage of some occurrence outside his control; for example, a natural disaster such as the Bristol floodings of a few years ago, or the administrative reorganization of a medical or social service. The natural experiment can be utilized to assess the effects on patients' symptoms or behaviour, or the epidemiology of a psychiatric disorder. The main difficulty is to have available an adequate, relevant account of conditions existing before the traumatic event.

Particular opportunities occur in many of the sub-specialties of psychiatry, such as psychogeriatrics, and mental handicap, and especially the grossly neglected area of psychosomatic medicine. The opportunities for collaboration of medical and surgical colleagues will greatly increase over the next few years as the main place of work of in-patient clinical psychiatry is being transferred from the large remote asylum to the psychiatric wards of a busy district general hospital. Daily contacts with medical colleagues will not only suggest various pieces of work, but perhaps also help to convince them that their patients have minds as well as bodies.

Arthritis in all its forms is a particularly fertile field. Psychosomatic medicine here got off to an unfortunate start with an attempt to delineate certain personality factors as common to all patients who suffer from some form of arthritis and the claim was made that psychological factors largely cause the organic disorder in the first place. Nowadays we have less confidence about aetiology and are more concerned about the proper assessment of the patient's personality as it may affect the course of the disease. The pain and stiffness are very largely subjective experiences, and the limitation of movement of a joint is determined more by the patient's tolerance of discomfort than physical disability. The lack of correlation between objective joint changes as seen, for example, in an X-ray, and the patient's complaints about that joint, never ceases to cause surprise. Why there should be such discrepancies certainly involves a psychological factor. Similarly, few disorders in medicine require more active collaboration of the patient in his treatment than physiotherapy exercises that form the most important part of the management of many forms of arthritis.

Almost every other specialty in medicine and surgery await systematic psychiatric investigation. Many simple operations, such as D. & C., are fraught with psychiatric overtones. There is the suspicion that a great many fewer such operations would be done if a routine psychiatric evaluation was carried out prior to all such so-called minor surgery, rather than occasionally afterwards when surgeon and patient have got tired of each other.

Many people feel that appointment at a comparatively early age to a consultant post in a good district hospital means settling down to about thirty years of routine clinical work without the possibility of any stimulus to research, especially if the hospital is geographically remote from a university centre. In fact, such an appointment provides an opportunity for really long-term prospective studies that no one else is in a position to do. The young research worker, anxious to climb the academic ladder, wants to get on with something which will soon produce a higher degree and the quick results that seem necessary for promotion. The higher echelons of the academic world will not start long-term research as they will retire before the end of it is in sight. As a result, very few studies extending into the second generation ever get to the point of being published. J. W. B. Douglas's famous follow-up of 5,000 children born more than twenty-five years ago is an honourable exception. Clearly, a clinician with few research aids cannot expect to do anything as sophisticated and as elaborate as this study, but personal observations of small, selected groups, carried over years, are well worth while.

WHY DO RESEARCH?

To do research mainly to get material for a thesis or a higher degree is a laudable ambition that deserves more encouragement than it usually gets. Many fall by the wayside as writing a thesis is as much a test of perseverance as intelligence. Before embarking on such a work, however, be sure that your topic will be acceptable to a university and that you have proper advice about its scientific quality. Examiners hate having to reject bad theses which they realize must represent years of sweat and toil but carry no other reward except the degree. Others carry out research for the kudos of publication, which is still considerable, though a few good papers are better than many bad ones.

The most important value of research, however, is that it is not only research into the outside world but also research into oneself. It is learning to acquire critical judgement, not only of the works of others, but also in the evaluation of one's own abilities. Through it one should acquire the habit of constant checking on the validity of everyday clinical practice. For example, are your routine drug regimes for depression and other psychiatric illnesses up to date and still effective? Are you making sure that your junior medical and non-medical colleagues carry out your plans for the patients properly? Do you listen to patients carefully and is there a proper feedback to you of your junior's critical comments on your ideas and practices? A little healthy scepticism about one's clinical skill is all the more effective if it results in an investigation to confirm or deny doubts.

There is, however, what might be called the psychopathology of research. The hunch—the original idea—is an autochthonous idea, differing from a psychotic delusion only in being reality testable and tested. Some people nourish it so closely to their own bosoms that it is never allowed to see the light of day for fear of it being ridiculed or destroyed. On the other hand, self-destructive criticism leading to failure to finish anything is worse than no critical ability at all. People are put off starting research more by fear of such ridicule than through failing to have ideas. To finish a piece of research takes considerable determination, and sheer laziness or discouragement by seniors has caused the abandonment of much more research than mere lack of intellectual capacity. Many hours of boredom and routine work are inevitable in any study however exciting in conception it might seem to be at the beginning, and however interesting its final form. But the satisfaction of finishing a piece of work is great indeed, and should be within the grasp of many more people than at present undertake research in psychiatry. The harvest is truly great and the labourers few, so—have a go!

2

APPLYING FOR A GRANT AND ADMINISTERING RESEARCH

PETER SAINSBURY

These contributions are intended to have a strictly practical and do-it-yourself emphasis; accordingly, I shall discuss three rather mundane aspects of research. The first is how to get money to do it. Writers on clinical research have neglected this commonplace problem, although the awkward question of meeting the expenses of an investigation is a major obstacle which has to be overcome if the work is to proceed. Research usually entails expenses of some kind; these may be quite modest when limited to such minor items as stationery, postage, and typing; although they can soon accumulate. Expenses quickly become a problem if travel costs, new apparatus, or specialized technical help are required; they become formidable if a full-time medical or scientific collaborator is needed, or if the project is of a kind which will occupy the workers for two or more years; salaries alone may then entail a grant of some thousands of pounds.

The second common-or-garden problem I would like to discuss concerns the administration of a research project, because, as a matter of practical fact, this is one of the basic hazards of any undertaking. Unless the organization and day-to-day planning of the work is carefully taken into account, it is unlikely to reach a successful conclusion. However important the aims or original the methods, nothing will come of them unless they are feasible and efficiently implemented; either the grant will have run out before the work is completed or the investigator will be left with fragments of data which it is not possible piece together. In addition, not only must the research be practicable but it must also be ethically acceptable.

Thirdly, ways and means of getting a training in research will be considered. This is a common problem facing the young psychiatrist who is either contemplating research as a career or seeking an academic appointment in which some research is mandatory or, at least, encouraged and opportunities for it provided.

OBTAINING A RESEARCH GRANT

The following steps must be taken in making an application for a research grant. After you have chosen your topic, you must crystallize it into the precise question or number of questions you wish to be able to answer. It follows from this that you must also have designed a means for obtaining the answer, and this will be the experimental method and the procedure of your investigation. Next, you will have to commit these ideas to an application form in such a manner that the chances of your request being granted are at a maximum. Lastly, you will also need to know to whom to send your application; and surprisingly enough, there are quite a large number of bodies which are keen to support psychiatric research and have ample funds for this purpose. The current policy of the Medical Research Council, for instance, is to give priority to psychiatric applications. I think it is insufficiently known that worthwhile, carefully thought out, and adequately prepared requests for grants seldom fail to get support; and certainly not from lack of money. These points will now be considered in more detail.

CHOICE OF TOPIC

In the last chapter Professor Pond discussed the essential preliminary of choosing a subject for research. I therefore only need to restrict my comments to the more practical aspects of what research to do.

Many psychiatrists with inclinations to research are too modest about the value of their ideas, though it is perfectly clear when they are informally discussing some clinical problem that they have a fund of interesting notions. Further, their speculations and criticisms about what they read in journals or textbooks, if rephrased as questions, can often be translated into ideas for research. I believe these inquisitive clinicians do not always realize that their reflections and questions are the stuff from which original work derives. Were one therefore habitually to jot down ideas that catch one's interest, or questions as they occur to one, I think one would soon find one had a surfeit of proposals for research. Incidentally, I am surprised how ephemeral many of one's ideas are, and how they elude one unless committed to an envelope or notebook at the time.

I also believe that it is most important, when choosing a topic for research, to go for something which really interests one. There is a tendency to put aside one's real preference, and to defer instead to the opinion of a respected senior or to the dictates of whatever happens to be fashionable to study at the moment. But only those inquiries which are sustained by a genuine interest are likely to prosper.

Quite often, however, some fortunate opportunity can help in the choice of a research, and such opportunities become more evident if a deliberate watch is kept for them. The district in which the psychiatrist is working may have some unique characteristic to exploit. At Graylingwell, for example, we were lucky because the catchment area included a New Town, Crawley; we turned this to our advantage by studying the psychiatric consequences of the common stress of moving house and adjusting to a new social environment.

Not only the district, but the special facilities or departments in the hospital in which the psychiatrist works may also help to determine his choice. The consultant who visits the wards of a general hospital might avail himself of their more specialized laboratories, perhaps to explore the disturbances in blood chemistry in the many toxic-confusional states he is required to advise on—their aetiology is not yet adequately described; while the psychiatrist with access to a cumulative case register can obtain samples of whatever patients interest him; the scope of his inquiries is almost unlimited, ranging from psychiatric rarities such as cannabis psychoses to the long-term outcome of psychopathic personality or the evaluation of mental health services.

The kinds of patients referred to a hospital or service will also be determined by the social and demographic characteristics of the district and by its administrative programme which may include some novel features such as a community psychiatric nursing service or a geriatric assessment unit, in either case some singular possibilities for research may be suggested.

THE APPLICATION

Assuming the subject is chosen, the next task is to transform it into a successful application for a research grant. How may this be done? The pitfalls are numerous. They include all those encountered in the design of any experiment, problems which are discussed in more detail by other contributors. Only some more general observations on preparing the application are described here.

The first point to bear in mind is that the application should be a simple, straightforward description of what you want to do and how you are going to do it. You should have already written this down somewhere, for it is valuable in thinking about any project to describe to yourself its purpose and the method you might use to achieve it. Fortified by this preliminary exercise, you will then need to write to the body whose support you desire to seek for an application form and for their guidance notes—most of them provide notes of this kind— and a cardinal rule is to stick exactly to their instructions. It is also important to remember that the body to whom you apply will usually be composed of laymen as well as scientists and doctors; you should not assume they will be psychiatrists or that they will have a special knowledge of the subject you have selected. It is essential, therefore, that you describe your proposals in plain English without verbosity or unnecessary technical jargon, which confuse the assessors as well as the applicant. Dr. Ffrangcon Roberts (1960) tells how these and other common errors may be avoided in *Good English for Medical Writers*.

AIMS

Most applications have to be drawn up under specified headings. They usually begin by asking what is the aim of the investigation. In the first instance this should, in one or two precise sentences, state the purpose of the research and why it is worth doing. Because it is less stilted, this, in my view, is preferable to the more formal approach of presenting the aim as a 'hypothesis'; though it may with advantage next be restated in that form or later in the following section. Beware of having too many aims; though sometimes necessary, more often it suggests the project is over-ambitious. After the assessor has read the summary of your objectives he should have a very clear idea of what you intend to do, which he can then bear in mind while he proceeds to find out why you think this problem is worthwhile and how you are going to study it. These two items will be the next headings in your formulation.

BACKGROUND OF THE INVESTIGATION

Remember that each assessor has many papers to read and will be endeared to an applicant who can be concise. So, in discussing the background to the proposed aims describe, with the support of only the most relevant reference, the present state of knowledge of the subject and how your investigation will advance it. You should also indicate in what way the work would make an original contribution of scientific or practical value to the problem. This will be done with due modesty; committees distrust boastful claims.

By this time, if this is done, it should be plain to the assessor that this applicant knows what he wants to do and why he thinks it is important to do it. Having established this important attitude of mind in your reader, you can proceed to the next and more thorny subject heading.

THE PLAN AND METHODS OF INVESTIGATION

At this point the applicant describes the plan of his research and the procedures appropriate to realizing his aims. In my experience of reading projects, the plan is commonly inadequate in the following ways:

1. Definitions: If the research is a clinical investigation, clearly describe the characteristics of the cases you intend to examine, in

other words *define* in everyday language the patient population you are going to study; and if the cases are to be selected in some way, indicate the criteria by which this is to be done. If on the other hand, you propose examining a sample of some kind, as in epidemiological studies, indicate the steps you will take to ensure it is representative of the population you are concerned with. In fact, it is important to define your terms whenever this will improve the clarity and precision of your method. Exact definitions are often difficult in psychiatry (psychopathic personalities, for example), in which case a working definition may be used such that another person will be able to recognize the sort of behaviour or case you are dealing with.

2. Assessments: When outlining the experimental procedure it is important to describe exactly the clinical, social, psychological, or other assessments you intend to make of your cases. There will not be sufficient space to go into details, nor will it always be possible to do so at this stage of the inquiry, but enough must be said to let the assessors know you are aware of the need to obtain *reliable* assessments, and that you have thought about the way this will be done. In clinical research, assessments of changes in behaviour are those most often needed; consequently, measurements will often be of a relatively crude order: scores obtained from questionnaires, rating scales, and psychological tests, or simply the agreement between observers whether an event has or has not occurred. Where a new or unfamiliar instrument is to be used sufficient information about its construction, the items it contains, and how it is scaled should be included to show that it is likely to measure what it is meant to. In any case the assessors' understanding of your problem will be increased if it is clear that, despite the limitations of such measures, they are expected to meet the requirements of the research because steps will be taken to ensure that they are both reliable and valid.

Sociological assessments are frequently included in research projects these days when the social causation of illness, the effects on behaviour of social treatments and environment, and the need to evaluate services are increasingly recognized. The methods available for rating attitudes and for categorizing family or social characteristics have similar defects; and these will also have to be frankly dealt with.

Alternatively, the experimental observations may be physiological measures, such as changes in heart rate or a spectral analysis of the EEG. Though a gain in precision can be expected, the technical problems will be correspondingly more difficult; and you must be seen to have recognized what these are. The temptation, by the way, to add in some physiological measures for the sake of scientific respectability must be resisted: they are only acceptable when they are necessary to solve your problem.

3. Technical Problems: At this early stage of the work the applicant is not always able to give details of all the techniques he proposes to use; nevertheless it is essential that he should have carefully considered each of them; and if a technical problem is outside the applicant's competence he should indicate that he has already consulted a physicist, epidemiologist, or whoever the appropriate expert is, and thereby assured himself that his intentions are within the bounds of what is practicable. His position will be even stronger if he can make it clear he has done some successful preliminary testing before applying for the grant. So if some special technical procedure must be used, this should be discussed beforehand with a specialist who will vouch for its feasibility. It would not be enough to say, for instance, that blood pressure will be continuously recorded without making it clear how this will be done.

Where the investigation is on the borderland between psychiatry and some other discipline (and it is in such regions that valuable findings often emerge), it will always be appreciated if the collaboration or supervision of a suitably experienced worker throughout the period of the study has been enlisted.

THE DESIGN

If there are manifest defects in overall design, the application will (or should) fail. Again the plan for carrying out the proposed work should be plainly described; the major variables which will be taken into account should be briefly indicated, distinguishing the experimental or dependent ones from the independent variables. Thus in a clinical trial the new drug will be the dependent, and the patients' outcome the independent variable.

The question the research worker must constantly ask himself is whether his plan will provide a sure test of his hypothesis; and, in particular, whether sources of error are sufficiently controlled. In a well-planned study, biases due to procedures for selecting, recording, and ordering the various observations will also have been recognized and eliminated. Standard designs are available for dealing with all the usual experimental situations; when in clinical trial, for example, it is appropriate to compare the patient with himself, when with a matched control, and when with an independent one; or what designs are best suited to comparing a number of samples. Sufficient it is to say it is important that you should be familiar with those commonly used and with the kind of questions they are able to answer.

Advice on design and statistical procedures must be sought during this preliminary stage of the inquiry, that is while the blueprint is being drawn up. It is only possible to take full advantage of the statistician's skill in ensuring economy of observations and in obtaining the maximum information from the data, or even any useful information at all, if he is consulted while the plan can still be modified. That such advice has been taken and assurances given that the statistical analysis of the findings is both attainable and provided for should be mentioned in the application.

THE SUPPORT REQUESTED

The applicant should be *realistic* about his requirements, and make sure they are essential to the work—an electric typewriter is a welcome acquisition but unlikely to make or mar a project—and accurately estimated; but do not be diffident about asking for what *is* needed. If, for example, you want to employ an assistant, quote a salary attractive enough to induce someone to apply for the job and do not necessarily offer the lowest point of the appropriate scale. (Your hospital's general office can advise you about salary scales for most jobs.) It is also important to remember that each stage of the research (planning it, trying it out, doing it, and writing it up) is likely to take twice as long as you suppose. So do not be carried away by over-optimism when assessing the time it will take to complete the various stages of the project; grant committees are more inclined to be of a pessimistic disposition. Another estimation people are often unrealistic about is the amount of work their assistant will finish within a given time, so be reasonable about his dedication to your cause—he may not be prepared to give you eighteen hours a day and seven days a week.

ETHICS

Where research involves human subjects they must suffer no harm or distress; standards of responsibility and confidentiality, with which it is essential to comply, are set out, for example, in the Medical Research Council's Report (1964) and British Medical Journal (1973). The importance of safeguarding the mentally ill is rightly emphasized; their valid consent to participate in the research, or that of their relatives, should always be sought. Moreover, where the proposed clinical investigations are not a necessary part of their care and treatment, the agreement of the ethical committee of your hospital must have been obtained, and evidence of this should accompany the application.

OTHER CONSIDERATIONS

Grants are normally awarded for up to three years, so the programme of work should relate realistically to the period for which support is requested; an application that neglects this precept can fail, especially if the work can clearly never be completed within the term of the grant.

The reasons for, and details of, the support requested, must be as carefully weighed by the applicant as they will be by the committee.

CMP

A grant may cover: the salaries of graduate or technical assistants, that of the applicant, and clerical needs; expenses for apparatus and other laboratory costs; computing, travel, and other incidentals such as postage when these are clearly essential to the research, as in epidemiological and follow-up surveys.

A grant-holder may be required to report progress annually; a final report is always asked for.

Finally, whoever gives the grant will want to know where the work is to be carried out; and whether the head of the departments and the host institution have agreed to provide accommodation and the other facilities needed to complete it. The grant is usually administered by the hospital or university in which the work will be done.

SOURCES OF GRANTS

The BMA's planning unit publish a valuable booklet *Research Funds Guide* [see APPENDIX] giving the addresses to which inquiries and applications may be made. The United Kingdom Postgraduate Awards published by the Association of Commonwealth Universities [see APPENDIX] lists grants, scholarships, and fellowships tenable at British universities. Sources of grants and fellowships for psychiatric research are of two principal kinds. The first are those in which the money ultimately derives from public funds: the DHSS, the Regional Hospital Boards, and endowment funds of Hospital Group Management Committees, the Research Councils, in particular the MRC and the SSRC, and the quinquennial allocations by the University Grants Committee to departments of psychiatry.

The second are various private foundations, trusts, other voluntary bodies, and the pharmaceutical firms. The Mental Health Research Fund (now the Mental Health Trust and Research Fund) is the one most active in supporting psychiatric research, and the National Society for Mentally Handicapped Children in supporting research into mental subnormality. The Directory of Grant-Making Trusts gives a comprehensive list of charitable organizations and details of fund available for research into mental (and other) disorders, with additional information on the particular charitable purposes for which they can be given, and the address to write to.

Some comments follow on the bodies to whom applications are most commonly made.

THE DEPARTMENT OF HEALTH AND SOCIAL SECURITY

Parliament has accepted the Government's policy for promoting research and development (Her Majesty's Stationery Office, 1972) by commissioning research (the customer/contractor principle). A number of Departments ('customers'), including the DHSS, have appointed a Chief Scientist who will identify areas in which applied research is needed. In the case of the DHSS, he will collaborate with medical and social scientists and the MRC in defining objectives; the latter acting as 'contractor', advise on the feasibility of the objectives, and undertake the work. One consequence of this policy will be that the DHSS (and other Departments such as the Home Office) will have increased funds for applied research; and because clinical investigations necessarily have practical objectives many should qualify for support from this source. In any event, substantial funds will be available from the DHSS's Health Services Research Board for project grants relating to patient care, such as the evaluation of services and needs (McLachlan, 1973); and money will also be transferred to the MRC for applied clinical research.

REGIONAL BOARDS AND HOSPITAL MANAGEMENT COMMITTEES (AND AREA HEALTH BOARDS)

Each Regional Board has an annual allocation for research and a committee that awards grants from it. Psychiatrists wishing to apply for support for clinical investigations in the hospitals administered by the Board or for work which relates to the service needs of the region, but which does not entail costs above, say, the salary of a full-time senior registrar or expensive apparatus, should not hesitate to seek advice from the Senior Administrative Medical Officer. A formal application will be required and if this is successful the grant-holder will be left to carry out the work in the way he finds most convenient subject to an annual progress report if the grant is for two or three years. A Consultant, for example, might apply for the salary of a social worker or the cost of apparatus, or a registrar for clerical or other assistance and expenses.

Hospital Management Committees which have endowment funds are able to make small research grants for assistance and apparatus. So if the requirements are modest you may need to go no further than the hospital secretary's office.

The Regional Health Boards will administer the research allocation after 1974.

THE MEDICAL RESEARCH COUNCIL

The MRC is the principal source of grants for biomedical research in the United Kingdom. In 1971–2 the Council awarded £4·2 million for project grants. The Council regularly reviews its scientific policies about research priorities; currently mental health, drug dependence, and alcoholism are problems in which special efforts are being made to expand research. Furthermore, the office of the grant awards division welcomes inquiries [see their booklet *Research Grants*, APPENDIX]. In these circumstances no applicant should have misgivings about approaching them. Generous support is available to those who adhere to the Council's rules for making an application: a concise statement of objectives, how they relate to existing knowledge and why they are likely to advance it, and how the work will be planned so as to realize the aims within the period of the grant—the usual maximum is three years.

The grants committee of the Council's Clinical Research Board meets regularly, but it is advisable to apply about six months before the date on which work will start. The committee has psychiatric members, and it also seeks the opinions of independent referees.

A grant holder is usually asked to report on his progress about half-way through the period of support and on the termination of the grant. It is possible to apply later for supplementary support if unanticipated costs arise; but extensions of the grant beyond the specified duration will only be approved after the work has been specially reviewed.

The Council, it is often said, set unduly high standards and have a preference for the basic sciences; this view is by no means justified: original work of any kind is very likely to get support, but any committee assessing research has to satisfy itself that its grant holders are able to achieve what they propose.

THE SOCIAL SCIENCE RESEARCH COUNCIL

This scheme for administering grants resembles the MRC's in that each application is sent to a referee with special knowledge of its topic; the project is then assessed by one of the Council's 'subject committees', for example the psychology committee. About £2m of the SSRC's funds are currently available for grants. The Council supports work on social psychiatry and drug dependency for instance. The applicant may discuss his application with the Council's staff and obtain their comments so that it will be more likely to meet the committee's requirements. Their booklet *Research Grant Schemes* should also be consulted [APPENDIX]. The SSRC require an annual and a final progress report; and requests for supplementary grants, should expenses have been underestimated, are treated sympathetically.

OTHER OFFICIAL SOURCES

The Science Research Council also gives grants for short-term research in the basic sciences including psychology [APPENDIX]. Now that pollution is a matter of public concern studies of its medical effects would be supported by the Natural Environment Research

Council; and other Government Departments may be interested in your research if it links with their own needs for information; thus a forensic psychiatrist might address his inquiries to the Home Office.

RESEARCH IN SCOTLAND

Officially supported research may be either by direct application to the MRC or to the Scottish Secretary of State's Chief Scientist Organisation which on the one hand gives project grants for medical, technical and equipment expenses within the NHS, and on the other supports operational research into the functioning of health services. As in England and Wales the research worker may also apply for support from the funds available to Regional Hospital Boards of Management. The relevant address for inquiries and applications in Scotland is given in the APPENDIX to this chapter. Until recently, the Scottish Hospitals Endowment Research Trust was a separate source of research fellowships and short-term project grants, but all applications are now made to the Chief Scientist's Organisation.

PRIVATE FUNDS AND TRUSTS

THE MENTAL HEALTH TRUST AND RESEARCH FUND

This is a voluntary body, and the only one solely concerned to promote research in mental illness. Its members are of the opinion that research into mental illness should not be wholly dependent on public funds. They believe that an independent private fund has a valuable role in providing an alternative body to support research endeavour, and that this is important in psychiatry where expert opinions are divided on fundamental issues. In the last financial year the Fund approved grants and fellowships to the value of nearly £100,000.

The Fund also publish a booklet, *Conditions Applicable to Research Grants*, which provides a useful introduction to how grants are usually applied for and administered. It also includes a helpful guide to the formulation of an application for a research grant [see APPENDIX]. The address for inquiries is given in the APPENDIX.

OTHER TRUSTS AND SOURCES [see APPENDIX]

The Wellcome Trust, for example, will consider applications for equipment and assistance when support is unobtainable from official sources; the Nuffield Provincial Hospitals Trust specifically supports research on hospital and other health services, and on preventive services; and the Smith, Kline, and French Foundation also awards grants to individuals including small sums for projects urgently in need of help because of unanticipated expenses.

Other sources are available for special purposes. The WHO and the National Institute of Mental Health, Bethesda, Maryland, are actively concerned in promoting international studies in psychiatry and instigating research in countries with limited resources in trained scientists and funds.

Within the United Kingdom, there are trusts to further research in specified disorders relating to mental illness: the British Epilepsy Association; the Joseph P. Kennedy Jr. Foundation and the National Society for Mentally Handicapped Children both have ample funds to provide individual grants for projects on mental retardation; the Migraine Trust; the Spastics Society; and the Schizophrenia Research Fund.

Before formally applying inquiries should first be made at the addresses listed in the APPENDIX.

PHARMACEUTICAL FIRMS

A number of manufacturers will give grants to individuals usually for work of interest to the Company; and psychiatry is a speciality in which at least a dozen of them are concerned. Applications are made to the Medical Director, and he will understand your need for assurance that the research will be independent.

Finally, it is likely the Royal College of Psychiatrists will also, before long, begin to support research. So it is evident that an applicant has several choices. Do not despair, therefore, if your application is rejected; if one source of support does not recognize its merits, another may very well do so; particularly if it is on a topic they are sympathetically disposed to. But it is always wise to re-examine the rejected application carefully and to seek the advice of an experienced researcher, especially if it has been criticized on some point of design or method with a hint that a revised application would be considered.

THE ORGANIZATION AND
ADMINISTRATION OF RESEARCH

A second important, but little considered, aspect of clinical research is the day-to-day administration of a project. So many excellent schemes end disappointingly, not because they were badly designed, but simply because they were incompetently executed. As much care and thought needs to be directed to the organization of the project, such as the instruction and preparation of all those taking part, and the precise arranging of schedules and so on, as was given to the application.

So besides formulating the purpose and method of his research, the research worker should draw up a detailed programme of the procedure he intends to follow. This will set out exactly what everyone in the project does and when they do it. It will remind him with whom the project must be discussed and make clear just what their instructions are. Everyone taking part, as well as receiving a copy of the overall plan, should also be given a typewritten account of what they personally are being asked to do. This account should include definitions of the terms and criteria being used, so that your collaborators may accurately identify the cases to be examined or recognize the behaviour to be recorded. The place and times at which the observations are required must be explicit; and the rules for completing the records, making ratings, etc. must also be stated, with clarifying examples where there is room for doubt.

Trial runs and pilot studies are often an indispensable prelude to the main project. They not only allow the reliability of observations and the accuracy of apparatus to be assessed, but also provide a dress rehearsal which often reveals crucial flaws in the organization of the inquiry. Where some novel procedure or new area of study is proposed, a preliminary grant may be sought just to examine its feasibility.

It is one thing to provide one's collaborators with guidance notes of the kind I have been discussing, another to obtain and then maintain their active interest and support. The first steps are usually straightforward; permission to use the facilities of most institutions is, as a rule, readily granted, whether it be to interview patients, borrow equipment, or use records. It is the clerk, technician, sister, or doctor whose normal routine is actually disturbed, or demands on whose time are made, that presents a problem. Most people when approached express a genuine wish to be helpful; but this initial readiness must be nourished, if necessary by repeated explanations of the purpose not only of the project as a whole, but also why tiresome details are required in the way they are, at the time that they are, and as often as they are. Their difficulties should be discussed with them and their criticisms invited; the investigator must then be prepared to meet these as far as is possible. As the project proceeds explanations, encouragement, and signs of appreciation are important aids to sustaining their interest and co-operation. The nursing staff, for example, participate more readily when they fully comprehend the investigation and feel they are usefully contributing to it. On the other hand, they are also able to effect a campaign of working to rule—not yours, but somebody else's rules—if they are not well disposed to the inquiry; in which event it is more likely to be your fault than theirs. And once a negative attitude has been engendered the whole operation will be in serious danger: records are not completed, the needed patient is away on leave, or the duty doctor instead of the research worker was called to adjust the doses of the drug, thereby disorganizing a carefully prepared design. So regular meetings with key colleagues to discuss difficulties and unload irritations are just as important as calibrating the apparatus or standardizing conditions.

Efficient organization is vital in studies that require visits to patients' homes or to their relatives, appointments with healthy controls, the examination of cases at strictly prescribed intervals, and when it is crucial to the design to be certain that cases are not missed. In all these situations a reliable system which ensures appointments are arranged in good time and which unfailingly locates the appropriate cases is absolutely essential. Making these arrangements is very time-consuming, so it may be necessary to delegate the work to someone recruited and trained for the purpose.

The reason for not doing research commonly given by psychiatrists is that thay already have more to do than they can cope with. I do not believe this is always the main difficulty hindering them; though finding time is a real problem. But there are ways of planning research to overcome this. I refer to the sort of investigation which, once devised and properly organized, runs itself. The material used is the clinical observations unavoidably made in the daily routine. It is the method of recording these observations and it is the care given to ensuring that the rules for doing so are accurately observed that translates them into the data of research. Little extra work is involved to effect this, only some initial skill in planning and administration. Even the tabulating and statistical calculations may be effortlessly done if the inquiry is planned so as to take advantage of punched cards and other computing devices.

I will give two examples of the kind of investigations which might prove to be worthwhile without involving the busy clinician in much extra work. First, let us suppose a psychiatric consultant's engagements include a weekly psychosomatic clinic in the local general hospital, and that he is interested in low back pain. A view he holds (his hypothesis) is that patients with backache can be classified into four types: anxiety states with muscular tension; depressive disorders (with hypochondriacal preoccupation); conversion hysterics, and purely organic ones. His routine clinical questioning and examination of each patient will provide much of the data needed to elucidate his problem. But to complete this comparatively undemanding research he must ensure that the backache patients recruited to the study are recognizable by precise criteria; and that certain observations, carefully defined beforehand, are consistently recorded on all of the patients on prepared case sheets. Moreover, the patients can also become willing research assistants. While waiting to see the doctor, they can keep themselves interested adding further psychological data by completing some appropriate self-administered questionnaires such as the Goldberg's General Health Questionnaire or the Middlesex Hospital Questionnaire. Finally, a clerk can obtain much of the routine, identifying data; she can also transcribe the categorized and itemized data from the clinician's records and from the psychological tests to punch cards. In a year or two, enough patients will have been accumulated for the cards to be analysed.

Secondly, there are now Cumulative Case Registers in three or four regional centres on which uniform data on all patients referred to the psychiatric services are systematically recorded, and subsequent events, such as admission to hospital, discharge, contacts with outpatients, or other selected data are added. Registers of this kind provide the psychiatrist with almost unlimited material for research ready to hand. He can investigate the natural history of mental disorders; their causes; their relation to the social environment; the effects of services on their outcome and so on. The publications of Wing (1972) on the Camberwell, and of Birtchnell (1973) on the Aberdeen Registers aptly illustrate their application to clinical and health service research.

FELLOWSHIPS AND TRAINING IN RESEARCH

Psychiatrists in training have less opportunity to participate in research than do trainees in the other major specialities; furthermore, the associations that medical students and newly qualified doctors have with psychiatric research workers are also very meagre. If research is to prosper and more recruits to it are to be found these contacts need to be developed. However, most universities with a medical faculty now have academic departments of pyschiatry; and in some research is being actively promoted. Nevertheless, in only a few centres are trainee psychiatrists offered courses in methods of psychiatric research and the necessary technical skills, such as statistics, or given the option to undertake original work, such as a dissertation, as part of their specialists' examination. What is worse, is the paucity of research appointments in the academic departments from which to train and embark upon a career in research. Though favourable attitudes to, and an informed curiosity about, research may be fostered by closer contact with it, something more is needed once interest has been excited: the opportunity to learn by assisting an experienced research worker and by putting one's own ideas to the experimental test.

At present this need for training in research is, for the most part, met by the Scholarships and Fellowships awarded by the Research Councils and the private Foundations.

The Medical Research Council not only provides assistance in various ways to those wishing to prepare themselves for careers in psychiatric research, but is keen to have more applications from mental health workers. Their awards range from intercalated courses during the initial medical training to postdoctoral fellowships to major research centres abroad.

Those most likely to concern readers of this book are:

1. Scholarships for training in research methods. These are awarded to recent medical graduates who wish to be trained in and pursue a career in research. They are granted for one year to work under direction in recognized institutions and are renewable. Applications are made through the Heads of the University Departments or of other Institutions.

2. Junior Research Fellowships are intended for post-registration medical graduates, and may be held in the departments in which they are already working or at other suitable centres. Their purpose is to prepare the graduate for a career in clinical research and to enable him to study research methods. The fellowships are normally tenable for three years.

3. Clinical Research Fellowships make similar provisions to enable graduates of Registrar or Senior Registrar status to study research methods in the basic subjects appropriate to their speciality. Information and application forms for Fellowships can be obtained from the MRC's Training and Awards Division.

4. Other Fellowships awarded by the Council include travelling fellowships, United States Public Health Service Fellowships, and Anglo-French Clinical Research Scholarships. They are for medical graduates who already have experience in research, and are usually for one year. The Mapother Bequest Research Fellowship in Psychiatry is also awarded by the Council.

The Social Science Research Council supports postgraduate training in medical sociology and psychology; and it also offers a few Fellowships [see APPENDIX].

PRIVATE FOUNDATIONS AND VOLUNTARY BODIES

Those which provide research training fellowships are listed in the Directory of Grant-making Trusts already referred to. Of particular importance to psychiatrists are: the whole-time Junior and Senior Fellowships awarded by the Mental Health Trust and Research Fund; the Beit Memorial Fellowships and the Smith and Nephew Fellowships which are open to Commonwealth students to carry out research in Great Britain; the Wellcome Trust awards research fellowships in Clinical Science and Clinical Pharmacology; the five Sir Henry

Wellcome Travelling Fellowships are annually administered by the MRC; and the Ciba Foundation offers medical exchange bursaries in experimental medicine to allow young British and French doctors to visit medical research institutes in one anothers countries over a period of 2–4 months.

REFERENCES

BIRTCHNELL, J. (1973) The use of a psychiatric case register to study social and familial aspects of mental illness, *Soc. Sci. Med.*, **7**, 145.

BRITISH MEDICAL JOURNAL (1973) Ethical criteria (Editorial), *Brit. med. J.*, **i**, 187.

BRITISH MEDICAL ASSOCIATION (1968) *Research Funds Guide*, BMA Planning Unit Publication, London.

HER MAJESTY'S STATIONERY OFFICE (1972) *Framework for Government Research and Development*, Cmnd. 5046.

MCLACHLAN, G. (1973) *Portfolio for Health: 2. The Developing Programme of the DHSS in Health Services Research*, Nuffield Provincial Hospitals Trust, London.

MEDICAL RESEARCH COUNCIL (1964) *Responsibility in Investigations on Human Subjects in Report of the Medical Research Council 1962–1963*, H.M.S.O., London.

NATIONAL COUNCIL OF SOCIAL SERVICES (1971) *Directory of Grant-Making Trusts*, London.

ROBERTS, FFRANGCON (1960) *Good English for Medical Writers*, London.

WING, J. K. and HAILEY, A. M. (1972) *Evaluating a Community Psychiatric Service*, Nuffield Provincial Hospitals Trust, London.

APPENDIX

Addresses to which to write for information and Application Forms:

ASSOCIATION OF COMMONWEALTH UNIVERSITIES, 36, Gordon Square, London, W.C.1.
A booklet: *United Kingdom Postgraduate Awards.*

BEIT MEMORIAL FELLOWSHIPS FOR MEDICAL RESEARCH, Francis House, Francis Street, S.W.1.

BRITISH MEDICAL ASSOCIATION, Tavistock House, Tavistock Square, London, WC1H 9JP.
A booklet: *Research Funds Guide.*

BRITISH EPILEPSY ASSOCIATION, 3, Alfred Place, London, W.C.1.

THE CIBA FELLOWSHIP TRUST, 96, Piccadilly, London, W.1.

JOSEPH P. KENNEDY JR. FOUNDATION, Suite 510, 719, Thirteenth Street, Washington, D.C., 20005, U.S.A.

MEDICAL RESEARCH COUNCIL, GRANTS AND TRAINING AWARDS DIVISION, 20, Park Crescent, London, W1N 4AL.
Booklets: *Research Grants,* and *Fellowships and Scholarships awarded by the Medical Research Council.*

MENTAL HEALTH TRUST AND RESEARCH FUND, 8, Wimpole Street, London, W1M 8HY.
A booklet: *Conditions Applicable to Research Grants,* also issued is *A Guide to the Formulation of an Application.*

MIGRAINE TRUST, 33, Queen Square, London, W.C.1.

NATIONAL INSTITUTE OF MENTAL HEALTH, DIVISION OF RESEARCH GRANTS, Bethesda, Maryland, 20014, U.S.A.

NATIONAL SOCIETY FOR MENTALLY HANDICAPPED CHILDREN, 86, Newman Street, London, W.1.

NUFFIELD PROVINCIAL HOSPITALS TRUST, 3, Prince Albert Road, London, N.W.1.

ROYAL COLLEGE OF PSYCHIATRISTS, Chandos House, 2, Queen Anne Street, London, W1M 9LE.

SMITH AND NEPHEW FELLOWSHIPS, SMITH AND NEPHEW ASSOCIATED COMPANIES LTD., 2, Temple Place, Victoria Embankment, London, W.C.2.

SMITH, KLINE, AND FRENCH FOUNDATION, Mundells, Welwyn Garden City, Herts.

SCHIZOPHRENIA RESEARCH FUND, Tile Hatch, Bishops Down Park Road, Tunbridge Wells, Kent.

SCIENCE RESEARCH COUNCIL, State House, High Holborn, London, WC1R 4TH.
A booklet: *SRC Research Grants.*

SOCIAL SCIENCE RESEARCH COUNCIL, State House, High Holborn, London, WC1R 4TH.
A booklet: *Research Grant Scheme.*
SPASTICS SOCIETY, 12, Park Crescent, London, W.1.
WELLCOME TRUST, The Secretary, 52, Queen Anne Street, London, W.1.
(For Sir Henry Wellcome Travelling Fellowships, see Medical Research Council.)
WORLD HEALTH ORGANIZATION, Office of Mental Health, 1211 Geneva 27, Switzerland.

SCOTLAND

CHIEF SCIENTIST ORGANISATION, St. Andrew's House, Edinburgh, EH1 3DE.

3

THE LIBRARY AND THE RESEARCH WORKER

L. T. MORTON

It may be said that medical research begins and ends in the library. Having chosen a subject for research and found means of pursuing it, the research worker must next turn to the library to discover what, if anything, has already been done on the subject. When his research is completed, or at certain stages in it, he must publish his findings in the literature if they are to be of any value to others.

It is hardly necessary to emphasize how important it is for the researcher to keep abreast of the literature on subjects with which he is concerned. He should regularly set aside a certain amount of time for study in the library and should work out a system of monitoring the relevant current literature and keeping personal records and indexes of material that are likely to be of future use.

ARRANGEMENT WITHIN THE LIBRARY

As soon as he joins a scientific institute the research worker should acquaint himself with its library facilities, with the periodicals and abstracting journals dealing with his own and related subjects, and with the classification scheme in use. In some institutions instruction in the use of the library is offered to users.

The most important section of a research library is that devoted to periodicals. These are usually kept together, the unbound parts within easy access of the bound volumes. Journals may be arranged in a subject grouping or in alphabetical order of title. Recently-received issues are often displayed in a special place to facilitate monitoring.

The *catalogue* may be on cards, in book form, or loose-leaf (sheaf catalogue). It may be (1) an author catalogue, in which entries are arranged under the names of authors; (2) a subject catalogue, where books on the same subjects are grouped together but in which there are no author entries; (3) a dictionary catalogue, with author and subject entries arranged in one alphabet. Most libraries have at least author and subject catalogues. Periodical publications are usually recorded in a separate section of the catalogue.

The *classification scheme* may be one designed for general use, such as the Dewey decimal classification (much favoured by public libraries) or its expansion, the Universal Decimal Classification (used at the Royal Society of Medicine library). Some schemes such as the Barnard classification and the scheme developed by the National Library of Medicine at Bethesda, Maryland, have been designed specially for medical libraries. Most libraries classify their material in accordance with one of the recognized schemes, although in some cases individual schemes have been devised to meet the special needs of particular libraries.

PERIODICALS

As already mentioned, periodicals form the most important part of a live scientific library. Many journals on the fringe of medicine are consulted by medical researchers. Biology, genetics, biochemistry, pharmacology, and psychology are a few of the subjects that impinge on medicine. The use of radioisotopes has brought physics journals into the medical library; the electrocardiograph and the electro-encephalograph have introduced journals on electronics; developments in the study of antibiotics have produced demands for botanical and mycological literature; and there are many other examples to show the wide field in which the medical research worker has to seek his information.

Scientific journals came into being in the mid-seventeenth century following the establishment of scientific societies. Both were due to the desire of those concerned to disseminate the discoveries being made at a time of significant scientific advancement. The first journals were the transactions of the scientific societies, and the *Philosophical Transactions of the Royal Society*, founded in 1665, is one of the oldest of these. Some medical papers appeared in its first volume.

From purely scientific journals it was only a short step to journals devoted more specifically to medicine and later to medical specialties. It is of interest that the first British specialist journal in the medical field was the *Asylum Journal of Mental Science* which was begun in 1855, shortened its title to *Journal of Mental Science* in 1858 and adopted its present name, the *British Journal of Psychiatry*, in 1963. Psychiatry was therefore the first specialty in this country to maintain its own journal. *Brain*, a journal of the highest standing and concerned with experimental and clinical neurology, first appeared in 1878. The *Journal of Neurology, Neurosurgery and Psychiatry* started life under a slightly different name in 1920.

In the seventeenth century ten medical journals are known to have been published. Today the number is difficult to determine but it must be about 6,000, of which 2,200 are considered of sufficient importance to be indexed in *Index Medicus* and abstracted in the appropriate publications. These journals between them publish about a quarter of a million papers a year.

CATALOGUES AND FINDING LISTS

The most up-to-date list of current medical journals is probably the one listing the periodicals indexed in *Index Medicus*. It is revised each year and published in the January issue of the *Index*. (It contains about 2,200 titles.) It has two sections, an alphabetical listing in abbreviated form followed by full title, and an alphabetical listing under full title followed by the abbreviated form. The list is also published separately and in this form has two more sections, giving listings under subjects and countries.

Another important list is *World Medical Periodicals* (3rd edition, 1961, with supplement, 1968). It includes current and important discontinued journals dealing with medicine, dentistry, pharmacy, and veterinary science and gives title, publisher, frequency, and an abbreviated form of title. It includes a subject index divided by countries, and a country index.

Biochemical Serials 1950–1960 is an extensive list of periodicals held at the National Library of Medicine. There are 8,939 titles in the list, all current at some time between 1950 and 1960. It is particularly useful because it gives volumes and dates, frequency, change of title, and cross references from oriental language titles to their English equivalents.

Excerpta Medica, the abstracting service described elsewhere in this chapter, has published (1964) a list of the periodicals abstracted in its publications. This contains 2,728 titles. A much smaller catalogue is *British Medical Periodicals* (3rd edition, 1973), a select and annotated list of 235 journals published in Britain. The information provided for each entry includes the types of papers published, frequency of issue, subscription rate, and policy with regard to book reviews, summaries, etc.

The British Library (Lending Division) and the Science Reference Library have published lists of their periodicals but the first does not include details of holdings (volumes, dates, etc.).

One of the most comprehensive catalogues of journals is the *World List of Scientific Periodicals* (4th edition, 3 vols., 1963–5) which records many thousands of scientific (including medical) periodicals in existence between 1900 and 1960, even if no longer current. It indicates their location in nearly 300 libraries in Britain. It also gives a standardized form of title abbreviation which has been adopted by a number of journal and book editors throughout the world.

An even more extensive finding list is the *British Union-Catalogue of Periodicals*. This provides 'a record of the periodicals of the world, from the seventeenth century to the present day, in British libraries'. It appeared in four volumes, 1955–8, with a supplement in 1962, bringing the coverage up to 1960. It is being continued in a quarterly supplement, *New Periodical Titles*, cumulated annually, compiled by the British Library (Lending Division).

INDEXES TO THE LITERATURE

Almost all the important printed medical literature ever published has been indexed. The first indexes appeared in the sixteenth century but it is not necessary to go back further than 1880 for the commencement of the most comprehensive index to medical literature extant. The *Index-Catalogue of the Library of the Surgeon General's Office*, Washington, is the first essential tool to be used for a thorough review of the literature. Its parent library, now the National Library of Medicine, is the largest medical library in the world. In 1962 it was moved from Washington to new purpose-built premises at Bethesda, Maryland, near the National Institutes of Health.

The *Index-Catalogue* is an author and subject catalogue in dictionary form. Its object was to record all books, pamphlets, and most papers in the thousands of journals on its shelves. The catalogue began to appear in 1880 at the rate of about a volume a year, each volume covering a letter or two of the alphabet. On the completion of the alphabet a new series was started, again working through the alphabet and indexing the material that had accrued in the interim. A third series followed the second and a fourth was begun in 1936. Unfortunately, however, the catalogue proved incapable of coping with the rapidly increasing volume of literature. Its alphabetical arrangement led to large accumulations of material that might have to wait as long as twenty years before appearing in it. Publication of the catalogue ceased in the middle of the fourth series in 1955, when it had reached the letter M. Even so, it provides a vast index of books and papers published from the earliest times to the middle of the twentieth century.

Although the *Index-Catalogue* deals only with the literature in the library it represents, it is so comprehensive that some users have come to regard it as a bibliography of all medical literature. In fact the early volumes were published when the library still lacked many of the older books and journals, and it is sometimes necessary to consult later series to find items published before 1880.

The *Index-Catalogue* has been supplemented and superseded as far as books are concerned by other catalogues from the National Library of Medicine. The latest is the *National Library of Medicine Current Catalog*, which records material as soon as it is received in the library. This is issued monthly, with quarterly and annual cumulations. It contains entries both under authors and under subject headings.

The next important index is the *Index Medicus*, also published by the National Library of Medicine. This was begun in 1879 and continued until 1927, each year being represented by one volume. It was then combined with a similar but smaller publication of the American Medical Association and continued as the *Quarterly Cumulative Index Medicus* until 1956. Each volume has, in one alphabet, author and subject entries for the papers indexed in it and includes a list of the journals from which they are taken and an index of recently-published books.

Wartime difficulties caused delay in the publication of the *Quarterly Cumulative Index Medicus* until it eventually appeared three years late. A more punctual but less conveniently arranged index, the *Current List of Medical Literature*, was launched in the United States in 1941 and continued until 1959. Nowadays the early volumes are of little use except to librarians, being to a large extent duplicated by the *Quarterly Cumulative Index Medicus*, but the last three years (1957–9) are of importance because the volumes of the *Q.C.I.M.* for 1956 did not appear until 1959, by which time a new *Index Medicus* was planned to commence in 1960. The three-year gap is thus filled by the *Current List*.

The year 1960 marked an important advance in medical indexing, with the appearance of a new *Index Medicus* compiled at the National Library of Medicine. This is published monthly, with an annual *Cumulated Index Medicus*. Over a quarter of a million papers are indexed in it each year under author and subject entries. The list of subject headings used is published separately each January under the title *Medical Subject Headings (MeSH)* and is also included in the annual cumulation. The list of journals whose papers are indexed is published in the January issue each year and also in the annual cumulation. A section included in each issue is the Bibliography of Medical Reviews, which repeats entries from the main index concerning review articles. This is very useful as a short cut to this type of paper; each entry includes the number of references quoted in the review.

Since January 1970 the National Library of Medicine has also been responsible for the publication of an *Abridged Index Medicus*, also issued monthly, modelled on the *Index Medicus* and containing citations to the papers in just over 100 English-language journals. The low cost of this smaller index justifies its purchase by small libraries taking comparatively few journals although it has unfortunately a noticeable American bias in its selection of journals.

Another useful index is *Current Contents, Life Sciences.* This is published weekly. It reproduces the contents pages of nearly 1,000 journals sometimes in advance of publication. An alphabetical index of journals and the addresses of first authors is included in each issue and a weekly subject index is also available. A cumulative index of the journals covered is published three times a year. *Current Contents* is particularly useful for checking the contents of journals not easily available at first hand. Two recent additions to the *Current Contents* series are: *Current Contents, Behaviorai, Social and Educational Sciences,* and *Current Contents, Clinical Practice.*

ABSTRACTING SERVICES

Abstracting services may be divided into two types:

1. Those giving *complete cover*, in which an attempt is made to include an abstract of every paper published on a particular subject.
2. Those giving a *selective coverage*, in which only the more important papers are chosen for abstracting. Such abstracts are usually more discursive, informative, and critical than those in complete-cover journals.

Abstracts may also be divided into two types, informative and indicative. An informative abstract gives all the essential details contained in the paper abstracted and provides all the basic information given by the original writer, making it unnecessary for the reader to consult the original unless he needs details of techniques or methods, or requires further information on case records, etc. An informative abstract is particularly useful where an original paper is published in a periodical difficult to obtain or written in a foreign language. An *indicative* abstract is one that merely outlines the scope of a paper, helping the reader to decide whether it is worth while to read the original.

The principal abstracting journals concerned with neurology and psychiatry are:

Excerpta Medica. Section 8: Neurology and Neurosurgery. Amsterdam, in publication since 1948. This appears monthly and attempts complete coverage of the literature. Abstracts are in English, of reasonable length.

Excerpta Medica. Section 32. Psychiatry. Amsterdam, in publication
since 1966. Monthly. Complete cover of the literature. Abstracts
are in English of reasonable length. From 1948–65 appeared as
part of *Excerpta Medica, Section 8.*

Psychopharmacology Abstracts. Bethesda, Maryland, in publication
since 1961. Monthly. Complete cover. Abstracts in English, about
3,600 a year.

Zentralblatt für die gesamte Neurologie und Psychiatrie. Berlin, in
publication since 1910. 18 issues a year. Complete cover. Abstracts
in German, about 5,500 a year. Suspended for several years
during and after the last war.

The *Neurologisches Centralblatt* covers literature published during the
years 1882–1921. *Psychological Abstracts*, which began as the *Psychological Bulletin* in 1921, deals not only with psychology but also includes
neurophysiology, psychiatry, psychoanalysis, hypnosis, etc.

Turning to more general abstracting journals, mention may be made
of *Chemical Abstracts*, which covers a wide field including such subjects as neuropsychopharmacology. *Biological Abstracts* also has a wide
range, as does *International Abstracts of Biological Sciences*, which is
particularly useful for papers on physiology.

LITERATURE SEARCHES

The principal indexes to medical literature have been described and
we can now see how they work in practice. If, as an example, we wished
to compile a bibliography on 'disorders of memory' we would first
consult the appropriate volumes of the *Index-Catalogue* under 'Memory,
disordered', with the following result:

	Books	Papers
1st series, Vol. 9 (1888)	3	39
2nd series, Vol. 10 (1905)	18	191
3rd series, Vol. 7 (1928)	3	27
4th series, Vol. 10 (1948)	7	55
	31	312

and thirteen cross-references to related subjects. Next, the *Quarterly
Cumulative Index Medicus* would be examined from 1948 to 1956,
the *Current Index to Medical Literature* from 1957 to 1959, and the new
Index Medicus from 1960 to date. We would also look at the National
Library of Medicine book catalogues that have partially replaced the

Index-Catalogue. From all these a very extensive list of references would be obtained.

Nowadays, with the vast amount of literature involved, it is more usual to work back from the present time until a good review or monograph is found that summarizes or includes references to earlier important work. In this connexion the Bibliography of Medical Reviews that appears in *Index Medicus* and has already been described should prove useful. Another publication, *Current Medical References,* edited by M. J. Chatton and P. J. Sanazarow, might be consulted. It is an annotated list of representative references covering most branches of medicine and includes citations to both books and journals. It does not claim to give the 'best' references but it does provide a good representative list covering a wide range of sources. It is a good starting point when one is embarking on a new subject. It is revised about every two years.

In searching the literature the abstracting journals should not be overlooked. Besides providing references to original sources they may help the reader to decide which papers should be read in the original and which could be discarded.

COMPUTERIZED INFORMATION SERVICES

Several computerized information retrieval services covering the medical sciences are now available. Two may be mentioned here.

When the new *Index Medicus* was planned a computerized system was developed to reduce the time required for composition and printing. This system also made possible the manipulation of the store of information thus accumulated so that requests for references on specific topics could be met rapidly and mechanically, avoiding the tedious manual search. The system is called the Medical Literature Analysis and Retrieval System (MEDLARS). It may be used for retrospective searches of the periodical literature back to 1964, and for current-awareness searches which provide a regular up-dating supply of references. The latter are also called SDI (selective dissemination of information) searches. The National Library of Medicine, which operates MEDLARS, regularly supplies the British Library (Lending Division) (BLL) with MEDLARS tapes. The BLL therefore deals with users in this country through their libraries. The results of MEDLARS searches are provided in the form of computer print-out. A charge is now made for these searches. Further information about the MEDLARS service may be obtained from the BLL at Boston Spa, Yorkshire, or from any medical library.

The Excerpta Medica Foundation in Amsterdam operates a computerized information retrieval service based on its abstracting service.

Both retrospective and SDI searches are available and the print-out for the latter includes an abstract when one is available. A charge is made for the service.

LIBRARIES

Britain is well served with medical libraries. Members of the Medical Section of the Library Association have compiled a *Directory of Medical Libraries in the British Isles*, the third edition of which, published in 1969, gives details of about 400 libraries, large and small, general and special. It has a subject index and may be consulted for information dealing with neurology and psychiatry. A much larger and more general reference book to sources of information is the *Aslib Directory*. It is published in two volumes: Vol. 1, science, technology and commerce, 1968; Vol. 2, medicine, social sciences, humanities, 1970. It gives details of several thousand libraries and it is available for consultation in most large libraries.

The most important medical library in Britain is that of the Royal Society of Medicine. It possesses some 350,000 volumes, and takes more than 2,500 current journals, all the important ones in duplicate. It offers other bibliographical services to its members, including facilities to use MEDLARS. The library of the British Medical Association has about 80,000 volumes and takes 2,000 current periodicals. It also offers other bibliographical services. Both these libraries have postal facilities, both are available only to their members.

The principal library of psychiatric literature is that maintained at the Institute of Psychiatry, an institute of the British Postgraduate Medical Federation, attached to the Maudsley Hospital. This specialist library takes about 300 periodicals; it is intended for research. The Institute of Neurology at Queen Square, London, another postgraduate institute, has a library with about 200 periodicals and is specially strong in material on clinical neurology. Other collections include the small but valuable library of the Royal College of Psychiatrists. Until 1971 this was the Royal Medico-Psychological Association. Its library was formed in 1895 with the collection of Daniel Hack Tuke as its nucleus. The Tavistock Institute of Human Relations and the Tavistock Clinic maintain a joint library at Belsize Lane, London, NW3, which includes about 200 journals.

The principal medical research library in Britain is that maintained by the Medical Research Council at the National Institute for Medical Research, Mill Hill, London. With a stock of 35,000 volumes and about 700 sets of current periodicals, it not only serves the scientific staff at the Institute but is also available to those working in MRC Units elsewhere. A number of these Units have their own specialized collections, usually made available within the Council by interlibrary lending. A recent addition is the Council's Clinical Research Centre at Northwick Park, Harrow; as its title suggests, it is well stocked with clinical material (5,000 books, 600 sets of current journals).

Messrs. H. K. Lewis, the medical and scientific publishers and booksellers at 136 Gower St., London, WC1, maintain a first-class subscription lending library of 130,000 volumes. It includes almost all modern works in the English language. There is a good catalogue to 1963, with supplements for 1964–6 and 1967–9, including subject indexes. Incidentally this catalogue is very useful in tracing or selecting books. Paperbacks are not included in Lewis's Library. Cost of subscription is modest and a reduced rate is available to undergraduates. A similar type of library is maintained by Donal Ferrier, the Edinburgh medical and scientific booksellers. This has a stock of over 30,000 volumes.

In London the public libraries, by agreement, collect between them all books published in Britain and such foreign publications as they can afford. They also take a selection of periodicals. Under this scheme Westminster City Libraries maintain a medical collection at the Public Library, Marylebone Rd., London, NW1, appropriately near Harley Street.

Nowadays no live scientific library can hope to be completely self-sufficient; it must engage in interlibrary borrowing and lending if it is to function properly. One of the most useful developments in this connexion in recent years is the establishment of the National Lending Library for Science and Technology, now reorganized as the British Library (Lending Division), at Boston Spa, Yorkshire. This library takes about 40,000 current periodicals, including all important medical and scientific titles. It also has a large and growing collection of books. Its journals are kept in unbound parts to facilitate borrowing. Multiple copies of the most frequently used journals are taken. Service is rapid: 'same-day service' is usual. There is also a photocopying service and facilities for translation from Russian. Borrowing from the BLL is through accredited libraries which must purchase and use borrowers' vouchers. The BLL has published a catalogue of its periodical holdings and also issues a useful monthly index of conference proceedings available in the library.

The National Central Library, formerly in London, has become part of the British Library. Its stock and union-catalogues have been incorporated in the BLL. It was the recognized national centre for the loan between libraries of all kinds, both in Britain and abroad, of books not easily obtainable otherwise. It was in fact a central clearing house with a large collection of its own and the ability to call on many other libraries throughout the world.

THE LITERATURE OF
NEUROLOGY AND PSYCHIATRY

A selection of journals concerned with neurology, psychiatry, and psychology is given at the end of this chapter. Some abstracting journals are described on pages 35–6. For a comprehensive list of journals on these subjects the reader is referred to the List of Journals Indexed in Index Medicus, included in the January issue of the *Index Medicus* and in the annual *Cumulated Index Medicus*. This list is also published separately.

An up-to-date account of the literature of psychiatry is given by Helen Marshall (1974), librarian of the Institute of Psychiatry, who describes current journals, abstracting services, reviews, monographs, books, and reference works. Ennis (1971) and Menninger (1972) have published guides to the literature, and an excellent Reading List in Psychiatry, compiled by B. M. Barraclough and B. E. Heine for the Royal College of Psychiatrists Clinical Tutors' Sub-Committee, was published in a second edition in 1972 by the *British Journal of Psychiatry*.

A useful guide for the compilation of a basic list of books and journals in a particular branch of medicine is *Books and Periodicals for Medical Libraries in Hospitals* (Library Association, 1973).

More detailed information on most of the topics discussed in this chapter will be found in the writer's *How to Use a Medical Library* (1971).

REFERENCES

ENNIS, B. (1971) *Guide to the Literature in Psychiatry*, Los Angeles.

LIBRARY ASSOCIATION (1973) *Books and Periodicals for Medical Libraries in Hospitals*, 4th ed., London.

MARSHALL, H. (1974) Psychiatry, in *The Use of Medical Literature*, ed. Morton, L.T., pp. 287–308, London.

MENNINGER, K. (1972) *A Guide to Psychiatric Books*, 3rd ed., New York.

MORTON, L. T. (1971) *How to Use a Medical Library*, 5th ed., London.

APPENDIX

SOME JOURNALS DEVOTED TO NEUROLOGY,
PSYCHIATRY, AND PSYCHOLOGY

Acta Neurologica Scandinavica, Copenhagen.
Acta Psychiatrica Scandinavica, Copenhagen.
Acta Psychologica: European Journal of Psychology, Amsterdam.

American Journal of Orthopsychiatry, New York.
American Journal of Psychiatry, Hanover, N.H.
American Journal of Psychology, Austin.
American Journal of Psychotherapy, Lancaster.
Annales Médico-Psychologiques, Paris.
Année Psychologique, Paris.
Archiv für Psychiatrie und Nervenkrankheiten, Berlin.
Archives of General Psychiatry, Chicago.
Archives of Neurology, Chicago.
Australian and New Zealand Journal of Psychiatry, Melbourne.
Behavioral Neuropsychiatry, New York.
Biological Psychiatry, New York.
Brain, a Journal of Neurology, London.
Brain Research, Amsterdam.
British Journal of Addiction, London.
British Journal of Medical Psychology, London.
British Journal of Psychiatry, London.
British Journal of Psychology, London.
British Journal of Social and Clinical Psychology, Cambridge.
Canadian Psychiatric Association Journal, Ottawa.
Comprehensive Psychiatry, New York.
Confinia Neurologica, Basel.
Confinia Psychiatrica, Basel.
Developmental Medicine and Child Neurology, London.
Diseases of the Nervous System, Galveston.
Electroencephalography and Clinical Neurophysiology, Amsterdam.
Encéphale, Paris.
Evolution Psychiatrique, Paris.
Fortschrifte der Neurologie, Psychiatrie und ihre Grenzgebiete, Stuttgart.
Hygiène Mentale, Paris.
International Journal of the Addictions, New York.
International Journal of Psychiatry, New York.
International Journal of Psycho-analysis, London.
International Journal of Social Psychiatry, London.
Journal of Child Psychology and Psychiatry, London.
Journal of Clinical Psychology, Brandon, Vt.
Journal of Comparative and Physiological Psychology, Washington.
Journal of Experimental Psychology, Washington.
Journal of Nervous and Mental Disease, Baltimore.
Journal of Neurology, Neurosurgery and Psychiatry, London.
Journal of Neuropathology and Experimental Neurology, Baltimore.
Journal of Psychiatric Research, Oxford.
Journal of Psychosomatic Research, London.
Mental Hygiene, Albany.

Monographien aus dem Gesamtgebiete der Psychiatrie, Berlin.
Nervenarzt, Berlin.
Neurology, Minneapolis.
Progress in Neurology and Psychiatry, New York.
Psychiatria Clinica, Basel.
Psychiatria, Neurologia, Neurochirurgia, Amsterdam.
Psychiatric Quarterly, Utica.
Psychiatrie, Neurologie und medizinische Psychologie, Leipzig.
Psychiatry, Washington.
Psychological Bulletin, Washington.
Psychological Medicine, London.
Psychological Review, Washington.
Psychosomatic Medicine, New York.
Psychotherapy and Psychosomatics, Basel.
Quarterly Journal of Experimental Psychology, Cambridge.
Revue Neurologique, Paris.
Schweizer Archiv für Neurologie, Neurochirurgie und Psychiatrie, Zurich.
Seminars in Psychiatry, New York.
Social Psychiatry, Berlin.
Zeitschrift für Psychotherapie und medizinische Psychologie, Stuttgart.
Zeitschrift für Neurologie, Berlin.

4

THE DESIGN OF EXPERIMENTS IN PSYCHIATRY

G. A. FOULDS

INTRODUCTION

To argue that psychological experiments should not ape too slavishly physical experiments is not to argue that they should be any the less rigorous, though we would do well to heed the warning of William James that at a certain stage in the development of any science 'a degree of vagueness is what best consists with fertility'. It is a sobering thought that some of the most illuminating work in psychology has been initiated by men who were poor formal theorists and indifferent experimenters; but such men are dangerous. The vast majority of us will do less harm if we try to learn the trade.

The aim of this chapter is to discuss and illustrate various types of design which are appropriate for answering different types of questions. We will consider studies which make comparisons between groups, within groups, or within individuals. Each in turn may be handled cross-sectionally or longitudinally. This gives rise to six types of question, for which examples might be as follows:

Between-group cross-sectional: 'Are men more extraverted than women?', when the question is answered by taking samples of men and women at one particular point in time.

Between-group longitudinal: 'Is the decline in intelligence with age greater among men than among women?', when the question is answered by following up men and women over a period of time.

Within-group cross-sectional: 'Are depressives more X than Y?', when the question is answered by taking a sample of depressives at one particular point in time.

Within-group longitudinal: 'Do depressives become less X and/or Y after treatment?', when the question is answered by following up a group of depressives over a period of time.

Within-individual cross-sectional: 'What psychiatric symptoms has Mr. X?', when the question is answered by studying Mr. X on one occasion.

Within-individual longitudinal: 'Which symptoms of Mr. X change most, and most quickly, without formal treatment?', when the question is answered by following Mr. X up over a period of time.

The type of design adopted is, of course, determined by the type of question we wish to answer. Thus, in a between-group cross-sectional study—such as that determined by the question: 'Are men more extraverted than women ?'—the original sample will have been selected in such a way that the two groups differ in respect, ideally, of only one variable, sex. The same thing will then be done to each group—say, administering an Extraversion Questionnaire. Any differences that we may find we hope will be attributable to that variable which enabled us to distinguish between the groups in the first place, namely sex and not, say, intelligence, social class, or educational level.

For the between-group longitudinal question 'Is the decline in intelligence with age greater among men than among women ?', we would, of course, require equally good random samples of men and women. Further, if it transpired that there was a significant difference between the groups on first testing, we would have to match the two groups in this respect before looking at the re-test results, since duller people might decline more rapidly with age than brighter people.

For the question 'Are depressives more X than Y ?', we require two standardized measures and one group. We might take successive admissions to a hospital or clinic of those cases who receive a diagnosis of depression. We would require to know in advance what percentage of a sample of the general population obtained each possible score on both measures. From these data the means and standard deviations could be equated so that direct comparison could be made between the two scores. We might then find that the mean scores of depressives on X and Y were respectively a half, and one and a half, standard deviations above the normal mean. The significance of this difference could be tested by a t test for correlated scores.

Given these two standardized measures of X and Y and our sample of depressives, we could answer the question 'Do depressives become less X and/or Y after treatment?' by randomly assigning half of the depressives to placebo and half to anti-depressant drug treatment. We could then re-measure each group at an appropriate time after the end of treatment. It should be noted that if the prior standardization of the test did not include re-test data at an interval comparable with the one in the study, it would be necessary to re-test a group at the appropriate time interval to control for practice effect. The placebo group would not be a suitable control group, since many people are known to be placebo-reactors. We might find that the active treatment group declined in X from means of 20 to 15 and in Y from means of 20 to 18; whereas the placebo group scored 20 and 18 on both. If normals also had means of 20 on the first occasion and 18 on the second, we could then conclude that this particular anti-depressant drug produced a decrease in X in depressives newly admitted to hospital. We might, of course, obtain other results, such as that both groups declined in X, but not in Y. We would than conclude that X is a less enduring characteristic than Y, but one which is unaffected by therapy.

For the question 'What psychiatric symptoms has Mr. X ?', we would take a sample of those experiences which we regarded as constituting psychiatric symptoms or signs. This might be done by administering a wide-ranging symptom inventory or by eliciting from the individual all his complaints.

Having obtained a list of symptoms by either of the above methods, we could keep the patient off treatment for a period of time and then re-examine him to determine which symptoms change most without formal treatment. If we re-examined him on several occasions, we could determine which symptoms changed most quickly and with fewest fluctuations.

In order to allow for more detailed discussion we will limit attention to between-group cross-sectional studies, within-group longitudinal studies, and within-individual longitudinal studies. We will then conclude with a section on prospective longitudinal studies which range over a period of years rather than weeks or months, since these have their own specific problems.

BETWEEN-GROUP CROSS-SECTIONAL STUDIES

Students first coming to psychiatric textbooks—whether they be psychiatrists, clinical psychologists, psychiatric social workers, or occupational therapists—complain that all the syndromes seem to have the same symptoms. This frequently leads to the view, from which many never recover, that taxonomy has no place in psychiatry. The view to which it should lead is that we need to know a great deal more about the generality and specificity of symptoms. Applying a symptom-sign inventory to different diagnostic groups constitutes a straightforward example of the between-group study. The accompanying six histograms [FIG. 4.1] represent the number out of twenty hysterics; anxiety states; neurotic depressives; psychotic depressives; paranoid schizophrenics; and non-paranoid schizophrenics who complained of (1) a tendency to cry rather easily; (2) life no longer being worth living because of some loss or disappointment; (3) palpitations and breathlessness; (4) having said things that have injured others; (5) hearing voices without knowing where they come from; (6) being a condemned person because of their sins. These are six of the eighty items in the symptom-sign inventory.

A tendency to cry rather easily is complained of by at least half of five out of six groups. This symptom, therefore, is common, but

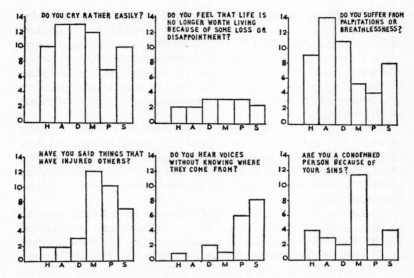

FIG. 4.1. Distribution of symptoms in six diagnostic groups.
H = Hysteria; A = Anxiety; D = Neurotic depression; M = Psychotic depression;
P = Paranoid schizophrenia; S = Non-paranoid schizophrenia.

relatively non-discriminative. Its only value would seem to be in differentiating paranoid schizophrenics from anxiety states, neurotic and psychotic depressives.

Life is no longer worth living because of some loss is very uncommon and non-discriminative. It therefore has no diagnostic value.

Palpitations and breathlessness is a fairly common complaint and is relatively specific to neurotics as opposed to psychotics, although non-paranoid schizophrenics rather spoil this differentiation.

Having said things that have injured others is rather common amongst psychotics, but not amongst neurotics. Within these two classes it is not very discriminative, although non-paranoid schizophrenics may be significantly lower than psychotic depressives.

Hearing voices is not a common symptom in general; but it does differentiate schizophrenics from all other groups. Within schizophrenia it is not discriminative.

Feeling condemned for one's sins is rare in all groups except for psychotic depressives.

In writing descriptions of syndromes these distinctions should be borne in mind. Quite naturally the clinician cannot keep in his head complex frequency tables. He is, therefore, often reduced in practice to dichotomizing his information, so that a symptom is attached to a particular syndrome and excluded from others. Relative weights which could be given to items are not given and, therefore, information is lost which would be useful. Weighting has not always been ignored by clinicians, particularly where schizophrenics have been concerned. The primary symptoms or signs of schizophrenia, as suggested by Bleuler and others—thought disorder, flattening or incongruity of affect and disturbance of the relationship with the external world, can probably be viewed, in the terminology used here, as symptoms or signs of very high specificity. Without these symptoms or signs one would hesitate to diagnose schizophrenia; with them one would hesitate not to do so. A more systematic collecting of symptom or sign frequencies in all psychiatric groups would then be the best way of ascertaining what are the primary or essential symptoms or signs of each of the diagnostic categories. Armed with such tables, it would be possible to say what the odds were on a particular patient falling into a particular category.

Between-group cross-sectional studies then are concerned with the frequency with which attributes are to be found in different groups, if they be of an all-or-none type; or with quantitative differences in some variable between two or more groups. They are concerned with increasing the accuracy of our description and identification of individuals as members of groups or with ascertaining something more about the attribute. An example of the quantitative difference on a single variable would be differences between melancholic and paranoid subjects in respect of scatter of dots, when such subjects are asked to tap as fast as possible for 10 seconds on a quarto sheet of plain paper. Here again we are giving the same task to different groups. In an experiment this scatter was measured by placing a transparent template marked off into half-inch squares over the tapping paper. The median score for melancholics was three squares entered and for paranoids twenty-one squares.[1] Scattered tapping was thus found to be an attribute which distinguished paranoids from melancholics. We cannot say that it is specific to paranoids until we have tested other groups—nor is it of much theoretical interest until we know more about it. Since, in psychiatry, it would be very rare indeed to find any symptom that pertained exclusively to one particular group, especial care is needed in interpreting any relationships that are found.

[1] Since the range of scores gave a markedly skewed distribution, a non-parametric test (the Mann Whitney U test) was used. The difference was, of course, highly significant, p being < 0.002.

The formula for this procedure, when the larger group is between 9 and 20, is:

$$U = n_1 n_2 + \frac{n_1(n_1 + 1)}{2} - R_1,$$

where R_1 is the sum of ranks assigned to the group whose sample size is n_1 (see Siegel, 1956).

A particular association between a symptom and a diagnostic category may be due to the association of each with a third variable. For example, in psychiatry one such variable which is likely to be obtrusive is age, since the usually accepted diagnostic categories are themselves related to age. Thus it is claimed that early waking is associated with psychotic depression. Some of my colleagues and I have asked about 150 patients whether or not they tend to wake early and the percentages saying they did were as follows: schizophrenics (non-paranoid) 25; paranoid schizophrenics 25; anxiety states 44; neurotic depressives 50; hysterics 60; psychotic depressives 75. Psychotic depressives tend to be the oldest of the functional groups and common experience suggests that we need, or at any rate get, less sleep as we grow older. Within the psychotic depressive group only 50 per cent under the age of 60 complain of early waking as against 85 per cent over the age of 60. So we find, in so far as our method of collecting the information can be accepted, that early waking is associated with age rather than with psychotic depression. When the groups are more clearly equated for age, the percentage of psychotic depressives complaining of early waking is not significantly greater than the percentage of neurotic depressives, anxiety states, or hysterics.

There are two main ways in which we can get rid of age—one is by matching the groups for age and the other is by the use of the partial correlation technique. Matching for age is a feasible technique only if we can do this without grossly distorting the representative nature of the sample. Thus we could probably use this method when comparing groups of involutional depressives and paraphrenics, since they would naturally tend to be somewhat similarly distributed for age. On the other hand, paranoid schizophrenics and hebephrenics would differ in respect of age by so much that equating these two groups for age would mean that we would finish up with quite atypical cases in at least one of our groups. In such a case statistical correction would be more appropriate. This will be dealt with in the next section.

WITHIN-GROUP LONGITUDINAL STUDIES

Psychomotor retardation, projection, or intellectual impairment may be attributes in the main associated respectively with psychotic depression, paranoid states, and schizophrenia. When we wish to account for the appearance and disappearance of these attributes, when we want to study processes, we turn to the within-group method.

The group we examine need not, of course, be a diagnostic group. In fact it is unlikely to be unless the process we are investigating is highly specific. Thus, we might wish to study psychomotor retardation, which may to some extent cut across diagnostic categories. In such an instance we might work with a group of patients who complained of, or who showed definite evidence of, psychomotor retardation.

The illustrative study which follows is defective in that, when wishing to investigate psychomotor retardation, a group of depressives was taken, certainly predominantly psychotic, without in fact ascertaining that the particular members of the group were retarded. Though psychomotor retardation is relatively specific to psychotic depression, not all psychotic depressives are retarded. The results obtained are likely, therefore, to be less clearcut than they might have been had retarded patients only been used.

It was hypothesized that the slowness of depressives in doing the Porteus Mazes might be due in part to their attention being divided between the test and preoccupation with feelings of unworthiness, wickedness, and so forth.

In order to test this 'divided-attention' hypothesis, a technique of distraction was used. On some performances of the test, subjects had to repeat numbers after the tester. Assuming that they would be unable to attend to three activities concurrently, one or more must be excluded from awareness. If attention to the maze tracing or to the counting be sacrificed, the subject has withdrawn from the field. Only two out of thirty-two, in fact, did this. In the thirty who did the test, attention to the counting and to the maze tracing was, of course, sufficient to keep them in the field. This does not imply complete obliteration of awareness of affective disturbance throughout the test. Inter-individual differences in the effect of counting may relate to differences in the ability to alternate rapidly between the tasks. However, it was predicted that counting would, at least partially, blot out irrelevant preoccupations and would result in a speeding up of performance.

Two groups matched for age, sex, intelligence, psychosis, and neurosis were used. Group A did the mazes without counting, then twice with counting and finally again without counting. Group B started with counting, then did two runs without counting and finally with counting. In order to eliminate initial speed differences between subjects, for each subject the time score at each administration was taken as a percentage of his total time for all four runs.

On the first run, on which A subjects did not count, whilst B subjects did, B subjects were significantly quicker ($p < 0.01$). On the second and third runs, on which A subjects counted and B subjects did not, A subjects were significantly quicker ($p < 0.05$ and < 0.01 respectively). On the final run, on which A subjects did not count, whilst B subjects did, B subjects were quicker, but not significantly so. In the main, therefore, the prediction was confirmed that distraction in the form of simultaneous counting would result in the speeding up of the tracing

EMP

of mazes by depressed patients. Concern here is not with the generality of the results, but only with the method of approaching the problem.

One can, of course, test more than one process at a time. Another study aimed at showing that if one deliberately preoccupied normal subjects, they would slow up on maze performance. One could then apply distraction as with the depressives. For preoccupation, subjects were asked to learn a stanza of poetry, which they had to repeat to themselves as they traced the mazes.

The design of this experiment was as follows:

Let O = ordinary administration (i.e., without counting or repeating poem).
Let P = mazes with distraction but not poem.
Let Pd = poem with distraction.

Then Group A does :   O;   Od;   Pd;   P.
      Group B does :   Od;   P;   O;   Pd.
      Group C does :   Pd;   O;   P;   Od.
      Group D does :   P;   Pd;   Od;   O.

Examination of both rows and columns will show that, with this design, there is never any repetition of sequence. If Groups A, B, C, and D are random subsamples of a homogeneous population, we can sum all O, all Od, all P and all Pd. The effect of order of performance (i.e. of practice) will have been controlled, since each appears in each position. We can then test for the significance of the differences between O and Od; O and P; O and Pd; Od and P; Od and Pd; P and Pd. With a group of university students, what happened was that the P and Pd times exceeded all others.[1]

This type of design would also be appropriate for assessing the action of several drugs of short-term effect. Thus if we are assessing the effect of *Sodium Amytal* on catatonic stupor, which we will suppose we can measure on a quantitative scale, we might do this: subject A would be measured for stupor, then given *Sodium Amytal*, again measured for stupor, allowed time for the effects to wear off, measured for stupor again, given a placebo, measured for stupor. Let us suppose that Mr. A was deeply in stupor with a score of, say, 15. After *Sodium Amytal* he comes right out and scores 1. After the effect of *Sodium Amytal* has worn off, he goes back into deep stupor and scores 15; after the placebo, he remains at 15. We would hesitate to attribute this clear-cut result to the effect of *Sodium Amytal* because he might have been just about to come out of stupor spontaneously. Our conviction that this recovery

_____

[1] Unfortunately, subjects on Pd were 'set' to return to the poem as soon as they had said a number. Depressives have no such set and the analog therefore does not hold.

really was due to *Sodium Amytal* could be strengthened in two ways. The intra-individual way would be by repeating the experiment several times with Mr. A. The intra-group way would be by doing the same experiment with several other people as like as possible to Mr. A and by doing a similar experiment, except that the *Sodium Amytal*–placebo order would be reversed, with several more people like Mr. A. If the results were fairly consistent, the explanation in terms of spontaneous remission would be untenable. We could conclude that *Sodium Amytal* brings catatonic schizophrenics out of stupor. There might be the odd one or two who did not come out of stupor or who came out of stupor with the placebo. For these anomalous cases we would have to seek for further explanations. The former might for some reason require higher dosage and the latter be hysterics who had been misdiagnosed.

In the preceding examples variables whose effects we wished to eliminate have been controlled by the experimental design—groups were matched for age, sex, intelligence and so forth, or the design was such as to control for practice effect. Such experimental controls are not always possible. In these instances statistical control is appropriate. The following problem typifies this usage.

A large number of schizophrenic patients were tested on the Progressive Matrices test [FIG. 4.2]. The length of time patients had spent in hospital varied from a few days to over twenty years. Ages ranged from about 17 to 62. Scores on Progressive Matrices ranged from about 8 to 57. There were thus three sets of quantitative measures. Clearly age and length of time in hospital must be positively related and probably highly related (0·66). We know, from studies with normals, that Progressive Matrices scores are, in the age range in question, negatively related to age (roughly − 0·3). This will, therefore, probably be the case with schizophrenics. The question which interests us most, of course, is the remaining one—the relationship between Progressive Matrices and length of stay in hospital. Length of stay in hospital incidentally was so highly correlated with illness (0·91) as defined by time since first admission, that they can be used interchangeably. So the question is, do schizophrenics show a progressive decline with length of illness over and above that to be expected from the normal ageing process? To answer this question we require three correlation coefficients. In the present instance these were: matrices and age $xz - 0·32$; matrices and length of illness $zy - 0·24$; age and length of illness $yz + 0·66$.[1]

---

[1] The formula for partial correlation is:

$$rxy.z = \frac{rxy - rxz.ryz}{\sqrt{1-r^2xz}\ \sqrt{1-r^2yz}}$$

The symbol $rxy.z$ is to mean 'the correlation between x and y holding z constant' (Cannon, 1955).

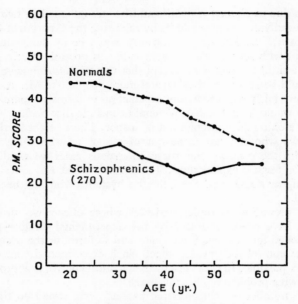

FIG. 4.2. Progressive Matrices against age.

In the present example, we find that Progressive Matrices score correlates -0.24 with length of illness; but that, when age is held constant, the correlation between Progressive Matrices and length of illness falls to -0.02 PM. There is some reason to believe that schizophrenic performance drops sharply at the beginning of the illness; but thereafter it would appear that the progressive decline in Matrices scores is due to normal ageing and not to any schizophrenic process.

To summarize thus far: in between-group cross-sectional studies, we try to answer questions about the relative frequencies of attributes, such as 'does psychomotor retardation occur more frequently in depressed patients than in schizophrenics? In within-group longitudinal studies, we are concerned with the *process* 'psychomotor retardation' and we try to answer questions such as 'what causes retardation?' or 'under what conditions does retardation appear or disappear?'

The distinction between within-group and within-individual studies is not very clear cut. Often, when we are mainly concerned with answering a question about a particular individual, we make at least implicit reference to norms of behaviour. Sometimes we do not make such reference. An attempt will now be made to deal with these two types of study.

WITHIN-INDIVIDUAL LONGITUDINAL STUDIES

Is Mr. B intellectually deteriorated since he sustained a head injury or is he manifesting a hysterical reaction? To avoid certain of the complex and controversial problems involved in answering this question, let us suppose that we were fortunate enough to have given Mr. B certain intelligence tests prior to his head injury. We re-test him subsequent to his head injury and find that his score has dropped by 8. He has solved eight fewer items correctly. We cannot, on this evidence alone, conclude that he is showing signs of intellectual deterioration. It might be, though of course it is extremely unlikely, that most people do much worse when taking our particular test for the second time. People might be more bored and careless and thus make more mistakes. Obviously we need to refer to what most normal people do in these circumstances. Let us suppose that on the average, people get three more problems right on retest. Not everyone will, of course, have got three more right. Some may have got six more right, some two more wrong, and so on. In our particular example, we want to know how many normal people get eight more wrong. Let us suppose that only 2 per cent of normal people and 10 per cent of hysterics do this; whereas 60 per cent of people who have had head injuries with prolonged unconsciousness do so. We can then state that, since Mr. B's performance shows a more marked falling off than 98 per cent of the normal population and than 90 per cent of hysterics, he is *probably* showing intellectual deterioration.

Intra-individual studies without reference to outside norms may be exemplified by the *Sodium Amytal* study to which reference has already been made. Let us again suppose we wish to know whether or not *Sodium Amytal* will bring Mr. C out of stupor. We could measure his degree of stupor, give him so much *Sodium Amytal*, remeasure degree of stupor, allow a rest period, measure for stupor, give a placebo, remeasure. If we got positive results in favour of *Sodium Amytal*, we might repeat the experiment, except for reversing the *Sodium Amytal*–placebo order. After a number of such trials we could compute the mean difference between measures taken after *Sodium Amytal* and after the placebo and test for the significance of the difference of this mean from zero.[1] This example would only hold as it stands if the pretreatment measures remained constant. We would, therefore, only

[1] The formula for this procedure would be:

$$t = \frac{\overline{X}\sqrt{N}}{\sigma}$$

that is, the mean times the square root of the number of measures divided by the standard deviation. The significance of 't' is found by entering the appropriate table at $n - 1$, the number of measures minus 1 (see Chambers, 1946a).

give the treatment to patients scoring the maximum for stupor. If these conditions did not hold, the procedure would require some modification.

Often in treatment studies we wish to examine each patient on several occasions by means of rating scales. Since the rating scores are unlikely to approximate a normal distribution on all occasions, we need a trend analysis which does not require this assumption. Ferguson's (1965) Nonparametric Trend Analysis takes account of the non-independence of scores when the subject is rated a number of times with the same scale and enables one to evaluate non-linear trends in the data. This method has been described and illustrated in detail by Philip (1969).

LONG-TERM FOLLOW-UP STUDIES

Unique and invaluable information can be obtained from longitudinal studies; but prospective studies which range over a period of years rather than weeks or months are difficult to carry out. Little more can be done here than to allude to some of the difficulties and to some ways of overcoming them. What can most readily be done is to advise anyone who contemplates embarking on such a project to seek the aid of someone experienced in this type of work and to seek that aid at the earliest possible moment.

Obviously one has to be assured of a reasonable degree of staff continuity. This can most easily be achieved by a Research Unit or a University Department committed to the project. Given this, the major difficulties concern sampling and measurement.

The initial sampling of the population with which one is concerned is not basically different from any other type of study. The main problem is that of drop-outs from the original sample at follow up.

Let us take the problem of the decline of intellectual ability with increasing age in the general population. If one seeks to recruit a group of subjects for a cross-sectional study one is likely to find that able people tend to volunteer oftener than less able and more young people than old. The interaction of these two variables will result in greater under-representation of the less able in the older than in the younger groups, so that the decline in ability with age is underestimated. If one attempts to keep up the numbers in the older groups by using institutionalized subjects, this may result in overestimating the decline in ability.

In a longitudinal study one may largely overcome the problem of a low volunteer rate in the aged by starting with a group of young people; but problems will emerge at follow-up, say, twenty years later. Those who feel that their abilities are declining may be less willing to cooperate at that stage. Thus, again the decline may be underestimated. One would, however, be able to look at the original scores of those who subsequently volunteered for re-testing and those who did not to determine whether or not they differed from the beginning. This is not a complete safeguard, since, even if they did not differ originally, one cannot assume that decline in ability will be uniform for all subjects.

Where one is concerned with life data about which one can turn to other sources of information, these difficulties are somewhat lessened. Kish (1970) studied the relationship between post-hospital drinking status and source of information at follow-up. Mail follow-up produced only 50 per cent returns; but, by various other means, it was possible to obtain information for another 47 per cent. His study used 3 reporting intervals—3, 6 and 12 months post-discharge; 3 drinking status levels—much improved, improved and unimproved; and 2 information sources—the subject and other information sources. By means of two 2×3 tables he was able to estimate the differences between co-operative and non-cooperative subjects. He concluded that one should assign 60 per cent of the latter to the unimproved group, 25 per cent to the improved group and 15 per cent to the much improved group. These figures were much more adverse than those obtained from the co-operative group. Here again the original information could be used to determine whether or not the two groups differed initially in respect of variables such as drinking pattern, age of onset of excessive drinking, personality traits and attitudes, sex, social class, chronological age, intelligence, civil status, etc.

If tasks involving skills are harder to handle than life data, studies concerned with attitudes are even more difficult. This is so because the problem of cultural change may play a much greater part.

Let us suppose that between 1960 and 1970 a particular society had moved towards a more liberal attitude to mental illness. A cross-sectional study carried out in 1970 might demonstrate that older people were less liberal than younger people; but a longitudinal study might show that people became more liberal with age. Or again, a cross-sectional study carried out in 1970 might have shown that younger men wore their hair longer than older men; but a longitudinal study might have shown that men in general wore their hair longer in 1970 than in 1960. By 1980 the fashion may have changed to short hair. If the young are more immediately and whole-heartedly responsive to changing fashions, older men may find themselves wearing longer hair than the young. Then presumably short hair will become the sign of degeneracy. Here, as in the final examples, the advantages of a combined cross-sectional and longitudinal approach are shown.

Let us now suppose that we wish to determine whether or not the amount of psychological disturbance in a community has increased between the years 1960 and 1970. We will assume that we have a reasonably valid and reliable measure of psychological disturbance. In 1960 we may have sampled groups of subjects at ages 20, 30, and 40. These groups we re-test in 1970, when the groups are then aged 30, 40, and 50 respectively. In 1970 we take a cross-sectional sample of persons aged 20, 30, and 40 for comparison with the groups of that age in 1960. We might obtain the results in TABLE 4.1 (with the second cross-sectional sample coming last).

TABLE 4.1

1960		1970		1970	
AGE	MEAN SCORE	AGE	MEAN SCORE	AGE	MEAN SCORE
20	10			20	10
30	6	30	6	30	6
40	2	40	2	40	2
		50	1		
Total mean 6		Total mean 3		Total mean 6	

Given near perfect sampling at all stages, we could conclude that individuals had become less psychologically disturbed with increasing age, but that the amount of psychological disturbance in the community had not changed between the years 1960 and 1970.

An alternative set of results might be as in TABLE 4.2.

TABLE 4.2

1960		1970		1970	
AGE	MEAN SCORE	AGE	MEAN SCORE	AGE	MEAN SCORE
20	10			20	14
30	6	30	10	30	10
40	2	40	6	40	6
		50	2		
Overall mean 6		Overall mean 6		Overall mean 10	

Here individuals had become neither more nor less psychologically disturbed with increasing age; but the amount of psychological disturbance in the community increased in the decade from 1960 to 1970.

To sum up, the sampling problem in extended longitudinal studies is mainly one of retaining the representativeness of the sample, hopefully achieved at the beginning of the study, at all subsequent stages. The measurement problem is least acute when one is concerned with life data, where sources of information external to the subject are obtainable. It is somewhat more acute when one is concerned with estimating abilities or skills, when experimental or statistical controls for practice effects may be necessary. Such controls are often of great importance in short-term follow-up studies and these have been discussed in the section on 'Within-individual longitudinal studies'. Where the intervals between occasions are very long, practice effects are often negligible.

The more responses to the tasks call forth learned skills or attitudes rather than innate abilities the more the possibility that cultural or educational changes during the period of study will occur. These will need to be separated out from development changes within the individual. These cultural factors will be most influential in studies of attitude change. A sophisticated handling of some of these issues can be seen in, for example, Himmelweit *et al.* (1958) or Kuhlen (1964).

REFERENCES

CHAMBERS, E. G. (1946) *Statistical Calculations for Beginners*, (a) 32–6; (b) 116–27.

FERGUSON, G. A. (1965) *Nonparametric Trend Analysis*, Montreal.

HIMMELWEIT, H. T., OPPENHEIM, A. M., and VINCE, P. (1958) *Television and the Child*, London.

KISH, G. B. (1970) The relationship between post-hospital drinking status and source of information upon follow-up, *Newsletter for Research in Psychology*, Veterans Administration Center, Bay Pines, Florida, xii, 2, May.

KUHLEN, R. G. (1964) Personality change with age, in *Personality Change*, Worchel, P., and Byrne, D., eds., New York.

PHILIP, A. E. (1971) A method for analysing assessments of symptom change, *Brit. J. Psychiat.*, **115**, 1379–82.

FURTHER READING

ANDREWS, T. G., ed. (1948) *Methods of Psychology*, New York.

BROWN, C. W., and GHISELLI, E. E. (1955) *Scientific Method in Psychology*, New York.

FISHER, R. A. (1942) *The Design of Experiments*, London.

JAHODA, M., DEUTSCH, M., and COOK, S. W. (1951) *Research Methods in Social Relations*, Vol. 1, Chapters 2 and 3, New York.

KLINE, N. S. (1953) Samples and controls in psychiatric research *Psychiat. Quart.*, **27**, 474.

MAXWELL, A. E. (1958) *Experimental Design in Psychology and the Medical Sciences*, p. 147, London.

MEEHL, P. E. (1954) *Clinical versus Statistical Prediction*, Minneapolis.

MEEHL, P. E., and ROSEN, A. (1955) Antecedent probability and psychometric signs, *Psychol. Bull.*, **52**, 194–216.

NORTHROP, F. S. C. (1947) *The Logic of the Sciences and Humanities*, Chapters 1 and 2, London.

O'NEIL, W. M. (1957) *Introduction to Method in Psychology*, p. 155, London.

STAUDT, V. M., and ZUBIN, J. (1957) *Psychol. Bull.*, **54**, 171–96.

5

CO-OPERATION WITH A STATISTICIAN

A. E. MAXWELL

INTRODUCTION

To some readers it may well appear that the title of this chapter is a contradiction in terms. The brand-image of a statistician, in common with that of a surgeon, tends to be one of a gruff, unapproachable fellow with lethal skills. If you are unfortunate enough to have to see him professionally he generally administers an anaesthetic which renders you oblivious for some time of what is going on. But the results, though painful, are generally beneficial, for the fact is that in any branch of research where the *counts* taken or the *measurements* made are subject to error a knowledge of statistical methodology is indispensable for a proper assessment of the results obtained. Aware of this, some research workers have equipped themselves with sufficient statistical knowledge to deal with their own problems, but in general such is not the case and co-operation with a statistician is then advisable. My task is to consider how such co-operation can be utilized to the best advantage.

As a beginning it will be helpful to outline in a broad way the scope of our discussion. Statistics, though still a young science, already has many facets so that even a specialist in the subject can hope to keep up to date only with relatively circumscribed aspects of it. In my case this rules out reference to large-scale field studies of an epidemiological and sociological nature. My everyday work is concerned more with (1) the analysis and assessment of data collected mainly by psychiatrists and pyschologists when interviewing and testing patients, and with (2) the design of experiments. It is appropriate to deal with the latter first.

A few decades ago when statistical methods consisted largely of descriptive techniques—for summarizing, in a more or less concise way, the information in a body of data—it was natural enough for a research worker, *after* he had made his observations, to approach a statistician for help in analysing them. Under these conditions difficulties of interpretation often arose, but everybody hoped for better luck next time. Today a different procedure is advisable, for there now exists a very powerful body of knowledge about statistical experimentation, subsumed under the title *design of experiments*, of which every research worker should be aware. The new approach stems largely from the work of the late Sir Ronald Fisher (1935), and—though initiated in the field of agricultural experimentation—is of very general application. For reasons of space only a few aspects of it can be considered here.

COMPARATIVE STUDIES INVOLVING TWO GROUPS

In research work in psychiatry, as in other fields, many of the investigations carried out and experiments performed are comparative in nature. For instance, a new method of therapy is suggested, say, the treatment of schizophrenics with barbiturates as an alternative to an established procedure such as insulin-coma treatment, and it is required to compare the new method with the old. Now it stands to reason that if you wished to compare these two treatments on two groups of patients it would be essential for the groups to be alike in all respects other than their treatments. If this were not so any differences in recovery observed between the groups could not be attributed unambiguously to the differential effects of the treatments alone. But how are the groups to be equated? The problems which arise here are many and varied. Indeed, I mention this comparison between barbiturates and insulin-coma treatment intentionally, for the difficulties which arise in comparing them are well discussed in a paper by Ackner *et al.* (1957), to which you may wish to refer.

In experiments such as the one just mentioned we are dealing with the familiar situation where you have an experimental group (the barbiturate group) and a control group (the insulin-coma group). Now the notion of a control group has been widely misunderstood. Too often it has been taken to mean that results exist for a group, external to the experiment in hand, which can be used as a standard with which to compare the results obtained in the experiment. This erroneous notion must be eradicated for it has led in the past to a lot of bad experimentation and gratuitous argument (Armitage, 1960). A control group, if it is to provide an unbiased standard of comparison for an experimental group, must not be external to the experiment; on the contrary, it must be part and parcel of it.

When comparing two treatments the *first* problem then is to arrange matters so that two groups are obtained which may safely be taken to be alike before the experiment begins—while the *second* problem is to ensure that during the experiment the environmental conditions of the groups are similar. The statistician's way of obtaining groups which are alike is to allot the subjects available for the experiment to the separate groups in a random way, say by the toss of a coin or by drawing names from a hat. In addition, if all the subjects to be included are known fairly well in advance it improves the chances of getting similar groups, for the allocation can be made in a stratified random way—the randomization of females, for instance, can be done separately from that of males, of older patients separately from that of younger patients, of more severely ill patients separately from that of less severely ill patients, and so on. This act of objective randomization, while it cannot ensure that the two groups will be identical in all respects, does eliminate the possibilities of conscious or unconscious bias in allocation. Moreover, it enables one to calculate the probability that any observed discrepancy between the groups could have arisen by chance.

Another point in the conduct of an experiment to which careful attention must be given concerns the measurements and observations which are to be made. These must be such as are likely to reflect, directly or indirectly, the differential effects, if any, of the treatments. If truly objective measures of these effects are not known and you are dependent on subjective assessments and ratings by a nurse or doctor, then care should be taken to avoid observer bias. In the latter case it is advisable that the person making the assessments should not know, in the case of any individual patient, the group to which he belongs or the treatment involved. In the case of barbiturates versus insulin-coma treatment of schizophrenics, the numerous questions, of immediate and long-term interest, which arise in assessing the results of that comparison, are well discussed in the paper referred to and are instructive to read.

MORE ELABORATE DESIGNS

From the above discussion of a straightforward experimental design, involving just two groups, it might appear that the statistician's role is a relatively minor one—even if we grant him credit for showing how the results can be analysed and the necessary tests of significance carried out. But to dismiss him at this stage would be premature. Those of you who have looked at a modern book (Cochran and Cox, 1958) on the design of experiments, will be aware of the great variety of designs which now exists. These designs may be thought of as precision instruments of great ingenuity, each applicable in more or less specific situations, and each constructed to make possible specific comparisons in a precise and efficient way. It is impossible for me to mention more than one or two of them here but you should try to find out what you can about them and if you think they are relevant to the solution of problems you have, you should consult a statistician for further information.

Now you have all heard it said that if a statistician is to be called in to give advice on an experiment then he should be called in right at the beginning. This is especially true where the designs already referred to are concerned, for their use implies that right from the beginning of the investigation certain rules of experimental procedure have to be obeyed. If these rules are not obeyed then the results of the investigation may be ambiguous, or it may be impossible to answer the specific questions being asked. An example will help to make the point clear. Suppose a surgeon wishes to assess the effect of some brain operation on, say, the cognitive ability of those who have to undergo it. In this situation it might appear reasonable to the layman to administer a battery of standardized tests to the subjects before the operation, and again after they had recovered from the physical effects of it, and then to compare the results. But there is a snag here for there is evidence to show that subjects, unsophisticated in the test situation, improve somewhat in their test performance on successive occasions of testing: moreover, if the same tests have to be employed on each occasion then practice effects may be present. To see how these possibilities complicate matters let us suppose that a group of subjects had an average intelligence quotient of, say, 110 points before the operation, and an average quotient of the same size after it. The investigator would now be in a dilemma, for while he might expect the average value to drop as a result of such a major operation he might equally well expect it to increase due to practice effect and increased sophistication in the test situation. Having collected his data in the way he did he would be unable to disentangle these different effects. Luckily the dilemma can be avoided for there are special experimental designs (Cox, 1955) which can be adapted for dealing with the situation (Maxwell, 1958). Had the investigator seen a statistician before doing his testing the latter could have shown him how to conduct the investigation so that an estimate of the effect of the operation, uncontaminated by the other effects mentioned, could be obtained and tested for significance. But to achieve the desired result the investigator would be required to follow slavishly certain rules which the statistician would lay down and this would call for close co-operation between the two. To assure you that the effort is worth while it is worth noting that doing an experiment the statistician's way has other, less obvious but very important, advantages, for it invariably means that the amount of information obtained from it is a maximum for the amount of work involved. This is one of the statistician's aims when constructing a design. To underline the point let us consider in some detail a specific investigation in which one of the classic experimental designs was employed.

THE SIMULTANEOUS COMPARISON OF A NUMBER OF TREATMENTS

Many of you will be aware that some uncertainty exists about the relative merits of different barbiturate preparations—and different doses of these preparations—as hypnotics, and Professor J. Hinton, while still at the Institute of Psychiatry, did an experiment to clarify the matter. This experiment involved eight 'treatments' in all, including a placebo. These were adminstered to hospital patients at bed-time in the form of tablets which were indistinguishable in every way so that the patients were unaware that different treatments were involved. The statistical problem was one of designing an experiment which would make possible an unbiased comparison of the effectiveness of the treatments for inducing and maintaining sleep.

One way of doing this experiment, which might come to mind, would be to try out each treatment on a separate group of patients and then compare the results obtained. But the possibility of being able to set up as many as eight similar groups simultaneously would be remote, for an adequate number of patients suitable for inclusion in the experiment would hardly ever be available. Moreover, since one of the treatments is a placebo, an ethical problem might arise if it were proposed to keep one group of patients on it for any considerable length of time. To circumvent these difficulties a latin square design was employed and the advantages of using it in the situation in question are now considered.

A latin square is a square array of letters in which any given letter occurs once in each row and once in each column of the array. Examples of such arrays, and an explanation of how to choose one on any particular occasion, are given in Fisher and Yates's book of statistical tables (1957). Here is an example of an eight by eight square. This size of square is relevant in the present discussion since we wish to compare eight different treatments.

An 8 × 8 Latin Square

D	C	A	G	H	F	B	E
B	E	H	F	G	A	D	C
F	G	E	H	C	D	A	B
E	H	G	B	D	C	F	A
C	A	B	D	E	G	H	F
A	B	C	E	F	H	G	D
G	D	F	C	A	B	E	H
H	F	D	A	B	E	C	G

If each of the eight letters, A to H, is now assigned—preferably at random—to one of the eight treatments then we can refer to the treatment by the letter which denotes it. Now if the successive columns of the square are taken to refer to eight consecutive nights, and eight patients for inclusion in the experiment are allotted at random to the eight rows of the square, we have a balanced design in which each patient on each consecutive night gets a different treatment. Moreover, for every batch of eight patients each treatment is administered an equal number of times.

This arrangement has certain obvious advantages—and certain, less obvious, disadvantages. One advantage is that the placebo, which has been included in the design to provide us with control data, is administered only once to each patient and this eases our consciences where ethical questions are concerned. Another advantage is that since each treatment is administered once on the first night of the experiment, once on the second night, and so on, no single treatment can on the average be deemed to have an advantage over another should it be the case—as might well be—that the patients' conditions were gradually improving as the experiment proceeded. Of course, should it so happen that the patients' conditions were changing in a differential way then some bias in the subsequent comparisons of the treatments would probably be present, but this can to some extent be guarded against by the choice of patients to be included in the experiment in the first instance. There is the possibility, too, that different patients might react differently to different treatments, but this is unlikely with drugs bearing a strong family resemblance. Disrupting effects of the kind just mentioned certainly have to be borne in mind, but if they may be considered to be relatively unimportant the final and outstanding advantage of the design can be utilized. This advantage is a mathematical one for it so happens that when the experiment is conducted in the manner indicated three different sets of comparisons can be made—independently and with a minimum of calculation. One is the comparison of the treatments themselves, in which we are especially interested: another is the comparison of patients' progress on the successive nights, while a third is the comparison between patients themselves, and this will tell us how homogeneous they are as a group. This seems to be a fair return for the amount of effort expended.

A final and important aspect of the experiment has, of course, still to be considered, for though the relative effects of the treatments have been mentioned, no reference has yet been made to the measurements and assessments on which the comparisons are to be based. The first of these was an objective measure, for the beds which the patients occupied were fitted with a mechanical device which gave a continuous record of their movements during the night. Supplementary evidence was also obtained by the nurses, who kept a record of the total time the patients slept within specified hours of the night, and who also noted the time taken by each patient to get to sleep after the administration of the drugs, and any breaks in sleep which occurred. In addition the patients were seen each morning by a doctor who obtained reports from them about the quality of their sleep, and noted any hangover effects. Neither the nurses nor the doctor were aware at any time of the particular treatment which the patient had had on a particular night.

As a full account of the experiment and a discussion of the results (Hinton, 1961) has appeared in print we shall rest content with this description of the statistical aspects of it. It would be easy to follow it up with reference to many other types of statistical design and to demonstrate their relative merits in different situations, but perhaps enough has been said to convince the reader that co-operation with a statistician is likely to be to his advantage should he have an investigation in mind. While plain common sense plays a leading part in the conduct of an experiment, common sense combined with statistical 'know-how' is better.

STATISTICAL COMPUTATIONS

In the past one of the greatest deterrents to the use of experimental designs, other than the most simple, was the thought of being involved in laborious calculations. With the advent of electronic computers this disagreeable aspect of the work has been removed and computer programs are now readily available for most of the better known designs as well as for handling large bodies of data, or files, frequently required in operational studies. But this new facility brings with it an added responsibility for the experimenter since he now has to acquire a more profound understanding of the basic principles of statistics if he is to use intelligently the programs available. This means that co-operation with a statistician has assumed an even greater importance than heretofore.

The computer too has called for a readjustment on the part of statisticians in their approach to their subject. For one thing it enables them to be more realistic about basic assumptions commonly made for the purpose of simplifying their models. For example it is possible to check the common assumption that the error terms in a model are normally distributed, and so on. It is also possible now to analyse more efficiently serial data which are a feature of much experimental work in the medical and behaviour sciences. But the most immediate effects which computers have had is seen in the greatly increased use of multivariate techniques. These should prove to be of considerable value to research workers in pyschiatry since their investigations tend to be multivariate by nature and, in general, the variates are correlated. The danger here, as elsewhere with computers, is that available programs may tend to be used routinely and uncritically and that the primary need to examine one's data in the first instance in terms of simple descriptive statistics, and with a copious use of graphs and plots, will be omitted.

REFERENCES

ACKNER, B., HARRIS, A., and OLDHAM, A. T. (1957) Insulin treatment of schizophrenia, *Lancet*, i, 607–11.

ARMITAGE, P. (1960) The construction of comparable groups, in *Controlled Clinical Trials*, ed. Hill, A. Bradford, Oxford.

COCHRAN, W. G., and COX, G. M. (1958) *Experimental Design*, 2nd ed., New York.

COX, D. R. (1955) A design in which certain treatment arrangements are inadmissible, *Biometrika*, **41**, 287–95.

FISHER, R. A. (1935) *The Design of Experiments*, London.

FISHER, R. A., and YATES, F. (1957) *Statistical Tables for Biological, Agricultural and Medical Research*, London.

HINTON, J. M. (1961) The actions of amylobarbitone sodium, butobarbitone and quinalbarbitone sodium upon insomnia and nocturnal restlessness compared in psychiatric patients, *Brit. J. Pharmacol.*, **16**, No. 1, 82.

MAXWELL, A. E. (1958) *Experimental Design in Psychology and the Medical Sciences*, Chapter 9, London.

FURTHER READING

ARMITAGE, P. (1971) *Statistical Methods in Medical Research*, Oxford.

COX, D. R. (1958) *Planning of Experiments*, New York.

HILL, A. BRADFORD (1960) *Controlled Clinical Trials*, Oxford.

MAXWELL, A. E. (1961) *Analysing Qualitative Data*, London.

MAXWELL, A. E. (1970) *Basic Statistics in Behavioural Research*, London.

6

DATA HANDLING

A. B. LEVEY

The 'handling' of data, like the handling of horses, babies, aubergines, sports cars or the opposite sex, serves a multiplicity of ends and is likely to be a matter of experience. The term has quietly entered the vocabulary of research jargon, with all its connotations intact, largely because it summarizes a number of aspects of research activity which cannot otherwise be neatly categorized. Thus we 'handle' a set of data in a number of different senses: to bring it under control; to make the most efficient use of it; to learn its inward structure; or simply to get the feel of it. In this chapter the beginning researcher is introduced to those aspects of data processing which have more to do with management than with analysis. The treatment is intended to be elementary and practical, and no reader should feel patronized if it is too much so. On the other hand it is hoped that those aspiring to do good research may find here a useful preview of the type of information which is usually acquired by trial and error, on the job, rather than in the standard textbooks.

To begin, it is worth considering where data come from. Data are simply observations; the given information in experiences or situations. Research data are observations collected systematically, and with a minimum of interference or bias from the observer. Clinical histories, case records and hospital files are collections of observations about individual patients, gathered by the various people responsible for their assessment and treatment. Similarly every physical examination or mental status, every domiciliary or admission interview is a series of observations—a data collection. Research begins with the *organization* of data. A formal theory, a hunch, a clinical conviction leads to the *selection* of certain sets of data, items of information, which form recurrent patterns or relationships. Such patterns have meaning or interest because they summarize information in a way which makes it understandable, often in a sense which appears to be causal. The object of research activity is to establish the generality of such patterns, or more accurately the limits of their generality. In more technical terms, the aim is to establish invariant relations between and among sets of observations. Knowing the content of one set of observations, we wish to use this information to predict new information in other sets.

In the classical period of the physical sciences this process led to the formulation of general laws. In psychiatric research we are unlikely to be concerned with general laws, and likely to be concerned with trends and tendencies which are repeated often enough to be useful in understanding the behaviour of psychiatric patients. To assess the generality of a pattern of observations, research methods have evolved which control the quality of information in two very important ways which are shared by all the sciences. Two or more independent observers must be able to agree, on the basis of separate observation, that the pattern exists, that it is publicly verifiable. The information must be repeatable, that is the pattern must be seen to occur in more than one situation as well as by more than one observer. These two criteria, verifiability and replicability carry the implication that the data are relatively free of error. In order to fulfil them, the research process ensures that the pattern of interest is confirmed by observations collected systematically and objectively. In psychiatric research we usually include the use of statistical techniques to ensure independence and to minimize error. The overall strategy of research methods, then, is intended to ensure objectivity in the data, and this is particularly important in psychiatric research.

This brief, highly selective résumé of the philosophy of science contains by implication most of the concerns which arise in data handling. In summary, we are concerned to clarify the patterns and relationships within the data, to identify the situations in which these patterns occur, and to ensure that the data are as free from error as possible. Needless to say, the first place to ensure these aims is during the phase of data collection. Data should be collected as carefully as possible, and with a clear notion of the kinds of statistical analysis for which they will be suitable. It is usually good practice, in fact, to lay out first a dummy set of numbers, representing the data to be collected, and to analyse it, at least in fantasy, to make sure that the analysis will really answer the questions being asked. However, for the present purpose it will be assumed that the data have been collected. Thus the remainder of this chapter will be concerned chiefly with methods of data preparation and data storage, and the problems to which they give rise. The problems chosen for discussion are those which, in the writer's experience, are most frequently embodied in the questions asked by research novitiates and students engaged in research.

Some of these problems are related to the role of the computer in research. Any discussion of data handling is necessarily overshadowed by the towering presence of the computer—the friendly giant of modern research. It should be said at the outset that all or most of the problem of data handling, as well as the actual statistical analysis, can be dealt with by the computer. At the same time, the point of view advocated here is that the investigator, particularly the novice, should undertake a good deal of data preparation by hand. One of the disadvantages of the large computer, hidden among its many advantages, is that the investigator can easily lose sight of his data. Thorough inspection and exploration of the data is an intrinsic part of research activity. In the discussion to follow, it will be assumed that computer facilities are available, and that the student intends to learn to use them effectively. It will also be assumed that the more he knows about his data, before submitting them to the computer, the better he will understand the results it returns to him.

DATA PREPARATION

Most sets of data require some preparation before they are ready for analysis. The two main aims of this preparation are to render the data as 'clean' as possible, and to organize it into the forms required by the analysis. To these should be added the important aim of exploring and understanding the structure of the data and its interrelationships. A great deal is learned by getting a preview of the formal analysis, and by inspecting alternative forms of analysis. Indeed, it can be stated almost dogmatically, that the results of the final analysis can only be fully understood in terms of this preliminary exploration.

The standard statistical texts usually contain introductory chapters on the preparation of graphs, tables, and other diagramatic ways of representing data (e.g. Dubois, 1965; Guilford, 1965). Often they omit to mention how exceedingly useful these methods can be. No attempt will be made here to outline these techniques, but the student is urged to review them, remembering that they involve a certain expertise which needs to be learned and practised. In applying them to a set of data it is useful to identify clearly the situation or situations represented in the data.

In general, psychiatric research is usually concerned with three situations. One common situation involves counts which have been made of the presence or absence of a characteristic, or a set of characteristics, in each of two or more groups of individuals. These individuals, or units, are likely to be individual patients or subjects, but they may also be drawn from other categories. The characteristics counted may be graded or they may be all-or-none. The distinguishing feature of this situation is that each unit is counted only once for each characteristic and the groups are compared on the basis of these counts.

Examples: (a) A group of patients diagnosed as depressive and a group diagnosed as non-depressive, counted separately for presence or absence of early wakening, constipation, and tremor. (b) Three groups of communities, small, medium and large in which counts are made separately of the presence or absence of several voluntary mental health organizations. (c) Two wards, an active care unit and a custodial ward, in which records are made of the number of aggressive incidents occurring in two hour periods throughout the day, categorized as 'none', 'one only', 'more than one'.

A second situation involves two or more groups in which measurements have been made of each individual on one or more characteristics. The characteristics are measured with some appropriate degree of precision ranging from a ranking across both groups, through scaling of subjective or objective ratings, questionnaire responses or precise physiological measurements. The distinguishing feature of this situation is that each individual in each group is measured separately on each of the characteristics and the groups are then compared on the basis of these measures.

Examples: (a) A group of patients classified as anxious, and a group classified as non-anxious are compared by measuring for each individual: blood pressure on rising, rate of habituation of eye-blink responses to a light puff of air, and scores on a personality test. (b) All the group practices in a given area are divided into two groups: those in which one or more of the G.P.'s specialize in caring for psychiatric conditions, and those in which psychiatric patients are seen on a rota basis; for each practice the rate of psychiatric referrals, the average dosage of tranquillizers and sedatives and the number of prescriptions for these drugs is obtained. (c) Medical students in their final year, divided into those who take a psychiatric elective and those who do not, are given an attitude questionnaire on mental illness before and after the elective, their grades in basic science subjects are recorded, and the students are ranked within the class as a whole by three of the clinical staff in terms of all round proficiency.

The third common situation involves two or more measures taken for each of a set of heterogeneous individuals, who are not further divided into groups. Again the individuals may be drawn from several categories, but the distinguishing feature of this situation is that the comparison is not between groups of these individuals, but between the measures themselves.

Examples: (a) Patients in an admission ward are each rated for hostility to nursing staff, estimated duration of illness is recorded, and a personality test administered to each patient. (b) For each of the county boroughs of a given area the rates for accidental deaths and suicides are separately recorded. (c) All the candidates for admission to a school of psychiatric nursing are given a battery of selection tests, followed by periodic ratings of progress.

The content of the above examples is trivial, though in each case it should be possible to see a number of uses to which the data might be put. The points to note are that for each of these common situations, the units measured or counted are not necessarily individual persons, though they are likely to be; the measures may take several forms, including varying levels of precision; and measures of the same characteristic may be repeated in the same units, or several characteristics measured or counted. The three situations have much in common and in practice will be found to overlap. The essential feature shared by all of them is that the same characteristics are measured in the same way for each of the units in the samples. Bearing this in mind it can be seen that, though the arrangements of the data differ, as do the statistics appropriate to their analysis, each of the situations represents a set of relationships between measures which enable the investigator to use the information in one set, to predict the information in another.

An important aspect is that the classification of individuals or units into groups is itself a form of measurement. If, for example, we divide patients into an anxious and a non-anxious group we are using a scale containing two measurement steps. In this type of classification we may also be implying that there is an underlying scale of a great many more steps—on a continuum of 'anxiety'—from which the two categories have been condensed. Conversely, for many of the individual measures the subjects can be re-grouped into discrete categories which represent levels of the characteristic measured. To put this fairly important point in another way: the observations with which a research project is concerned may usually be thought of in terms of the precision with which they separate the individuals in the study. At the highest level of precision each individual occupies a unique position on the scale. At the lowest level the scale simply divides the individuals into two sets. In between these extremes, are varying degrees of precision within which a greater or lesser number of individual units fall at the same place. When a set of data are considered in this way it becomes possible to make useful sets of comparisons, in which precision of measurement is sacrificed to gain a clearer picture of the relationships. Two extreme cases are of interest because they illustrate the concept of scaling. In the situation in which a heterogeneous sample of individuals is measured on two or more characteristics, each individual may be regarded as a group of one, from the standpoint of any one of the characteristics on which there are no tied measures. Conversely, where subjects are divided into groups, they may be lumped together into a single group which then represents a measuring scale of one step. In the next section the relevance of these considerations to data handling will be underlined in more practical terms. First, however it will be useful to consider a general strategy based on this essentially practical way of looking at data.

It will be recalled that the three aims of data preparation are to 'clean' the data, i.e. to reduce the amount of error; to arrange the data into the form suitable for statistical analysis; and to arrive at an understanding of the relationships within the data. An essential step in any data preparation can be used to fulfil all these aims, namely the plotting of frequency distributions of each of the measures. The frequency distribution shows the number of units or cases falling within equal steps of the measuring scale. A clear step-by-step description of procedures is given by Guilford (1965, pp. 27–40). It is a useful strategem to do this chore first, since it offers an opportunity for a preliminary scan of the data, and the information gained from the frequency distributions is usually essential to the interpretation of subsequent plots or comparisons. In plotting distributions the data situation should be identified clearly. If the data are drawn from separate groups or categories it is useful to plot the distributions separately (using the same intervals) for each of the categories or subcategories included in the samples. These sub-plots can then be combined to yield a picture of the whole of the sample.

The process of plotting frequency distributions requires the investigator to examine each observation separately. He may thus be alert to detect any observation which is unexpected or surprising. These may be values which appear too large or too small, or simply inconsistent with the remainder of the data. The basis on which an individual score is 'unexpected' will depend on the observer's knowledge of his data, the expected range of measures and so on. Every unexpected value should be checked in the original source data, and corrected if an error is discovered. Depending on the quality of the data, the rigours of the research design and the size of the sample, individuals whose scores are suspect may legitimately be discarded.

Extreme scores, or 'outliers', represent a special case, in which, if no error of measurement is found, the possibility must be considered that the observation is drawn from a different population than the rest of the sample. The problem is in defining what is meant by extreme, and statistical techniques are available (e.g. Chauvenet's criterion, Parrat, 1961, p. 175) which make this decision objective. The point to be firmly made, is that if data are to be discarded the decision to do so must be made before the results of any analysis. Alternatively, extreme scores may be adjusted by arbitrarily assigning an adjacent value to them. This procedure, sometimes called 'Winsorising', must be used with some caution. Some of the pros and cons of the method are discussed by Dixon and May (1968, p. 111) in an interesting account of the choice of strategies in this and related matters adopted in an actual research project.

In the course of plotting the distributions the number of missing observations, if any, can also be considered. The problem of missing data has no solution, and the ideal answer is to collect more data if possible. Advanced statistical textbooks usually describe optimum techniques for replacing missing observations with estimates (e.g.

Scheffe, 1959) and modern computer programs often make these estimates. The point to remember, however, is that no technique for replacing data, however sophisticated, can possibly add information, and the more elaborate procedures simply ensure that the disruptions caused by missing data are reduced to some minimum. If the data are thoroughly familiar, there is sometimes a case for substituting a best guess. This is likely to be group or subgroup mean—illustrating the fact that no information is added. If a number of measures has been collected it may be preferable to estimate an approximate value on the basis of the remaining measures, and a practical illustration of this method is discussed by Dixon and May (1968) in the chapter referenced earlier. The problem of missing data is most likely to be troublesome in research based on large scale surveys. In this case many investigators adopt a per cent criterion for excluding both subjects and measures for which there is insufficient data.

Another useful piece of information which can emerge in the course of plotting frequency distribution is the detection of small numbers in one or more subgroups. It is frequently a source of concern to embryo researchers, and of astonishment to their advisors to find at the completion of an analysis that the numbers are too small to afford meaningful comparisons. During the phase of data preparation it may, therefore, be useful to judge whether the samples are large enough. This can be guessed, with a little experience, from the amount of overlap among distributions, but formal methods are better (e.g. Cohen, 1969), and are easy to apply. The techniques enable a fairly precise estimate of the number of subjects needed, based on the variance of the measures in a preliminary sample, in relation to the particular statistic to be used in the analysis. If the numbers are small, it is useful to find this out during the phase of data preparation, and to collect further observations while the machinery and techniques for doing so are still intact. Investigators are sometimes worried, however, that conclusions based on small samples are inherently less significant, in the statistical sense, than those based on large numbers of individuals. This is a misunderstanding based on the fact that small samples are less *likely* to exhibit statistical significance. If the result of interest is shown by the statistical test to be significant, this information tells us of itself that the sample is large enough. If, however, the comparison of interest is shown to be non-significant, but in the expected direction, the possibility is open that the numbers in the sample are too small.

Having met and resolved the problems of missing data, small numbers and so on, at an early stage, the way is clear to examine the information conveyed by the frequency distributions themselves. If the data are in the form of counts the frequency distributions may convey directly an impression of the results of the study. Most of the information is contained in the shape of the distribution, and the chief concern is usually whether the shape conforms to the normal distribution. While a certain mystique surrounds the concept of normality for data in the life sciences, our interest at this stage is more practical. Most of the more powerful statistical analyses assume, among other things, that the measures represent an underlying normal distribution. While the statistical techniques are able to tolerate fairly wide departures from normality they do so at the expense of their discriminating power. At the same time those procedures which do not require the assumption of normality, the non-parametric statistics, are invariably less powerful than those which do.

Most statistical textbooks offer chapters on sampling and sampling distributions, and describe techniques for estimating the goodness of fit of an observed distribution to the normal curve. They should be consulted if they are not already familiar, bearing in mind that the techniques are not formidable (e.g. Dubois, 1965, p. 295; Guilford, 1965, p. 242). In small samples, the frequency distribution may not look much like a normal distribution, depending partly on how the intervals have been chosen. The simplest way of deciding is to apply the appropriate test. If the test shows that the data are not normally distributed there is usually no cause for alarm. In many cases the data can be transformed, i.e. adjusted mathematically so that they conform more nearly to the normal distribution. It is usually preferable to attempt such a transformation before turning to the less powerful non-parametric statistics.

Many investigators feel intuitively that transformation of the raw data violates the original observations. It may be useful to reflect that at some point the observations, together with the tender care which has been lavished on them, and the subtle operational processes which underlie them, have got to be reduced to mere numbers. As such they represent the points on a measuring scale, of which the simplest example is the common yardstick. When we use a yardstick, however, we have reasonable assurance that six inches at one end are the same as six inches at the other, or in the middle. With many of the measurements undertaken in psychiatric research this assurance is not possible. An increase in physiological activity, for example, above a high initial level, is not the same as an increase above a low level. Again, there is no way of knowing whether the distance from, say, 'quite tense' to 'very tense' in a self-rating scale, is the same as the distance from 'slightly tense' to 'quite tense'. If the units of measurement are unequal their variations will also be unequal and this will be reflected in the shape of the distribution. All that a data transformation does is to adjust, mathematically, the units of the underlying scale towards more nearly equal intervals. The choice of an appropriate transformation may be made on mathematical grounds, on the basis of some knowledge of the characteristics of the measuring instruments, or on purely empirical grounds. A practical outline is given in Maxwell's indispensable book (1958, p. 71), and the matter is treated in detail in many of the larger texts. An important step in the procedure is to re-plot the distributions after applying a transformation, to find out whether it has had the desired effect.

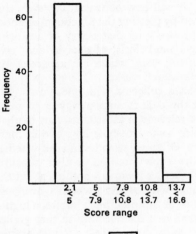

FIG. 6.1. Frequency distribution of raw data for alpha abundance in EEG recordings. (Reproduced by kind permission of Dr. J. C. Shaw.)

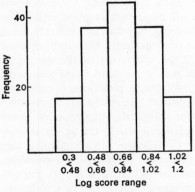

FIG. 6.2. Frequency distribution of the data in FIG. 6.1 after logarithmic transformation. (Reproduced by kind permission of Dr. J. C. Shaw.)

FIGURE 6.1 shows the frequency distribution of data from an experiment in which alpha abundance was averaged for five-second epochs of subjects' EEG records. They give the misleading impression that most of the subjects produced low amounts, with fewer and fewer subjects falling at each higher interval. In FIGURE 6.2 the same data are plotted after having been converted to natural logarithms. They now show that most of the subjects fell in the middle range while a few subjects had scores at either extreme, and this is what we might expect of a normal population.

The foregoing paragraphs can be summarized by saying that there is much to be learned about any set of data, simply by looking carefully at every observation; and that this can be conveniently done while plotting its frequency distributions. This probably represents the absolute minimum of data preparation which it is desirable to undertake before the data are analysed. It will now be urged, however, that there are rich dividends to be gained by plotting the functional relationships within the data. There is probably no better way of acquiring familiarity with the various 'shapes' and 'feels' of data in ones own field, and of developing the heuristic skills which are a part of the armamentarium of the experienced research worker.

The data will hopefully have been collected with specific aims in view and the first step is to plot the data in such a way as to make explicit the comparisons which are relevant to those aims. Any method of representation can be used which serves to show how two or more variables are related to one another. Often we wish to find out whether a low score on one measure implies a low score on another measure, whether it implies a high score, or whether it implies nothing about the other measure. Alternatively, we may wish to know whether membership in a certain group (e.g. 'anxious' or 'hospitalized') implies a higher or lower score on some variable than non-membership in that group. For counts, these comparisons will mean cross-tallies, e.g. two-by-two tables, while for measures the data will be plotted on graph paper. Each unit or individual will furnish two scores, one for each variable, which are represented as a single tally or data point in the table or graph. Means and variances, estimated at this stage, enrich the description of the data, but the chief objective is to get a good visual representation of the relationships between and among measures. If more than one set of measures has been collected, the plots of relationships between separate pairs of measures within the categories or groups of the sample are likely to prove interesting. If the study involves correlation, the data plots of pairs of measures are an essential step. In examining the plots the investigator will be alert to the possibility of non-linear relationships, remembering that a zero or near-zero linear correlation may conceal a non-linear relationship of significance. The object of these plots and tables is to form a clear and familiar picture of the data. Brief but useful illustrations of these principles are provided by Dubois (1965, pp. 125 ff.), by Guilford (1965, pp. 106 ff.) and by Jolley (1968, pp. 83 ff.) for simple data sets.

A practical example is illustrated in FIGURES 6.3 and 6.4, in which data from a study of orienting responses and conditioned responses are

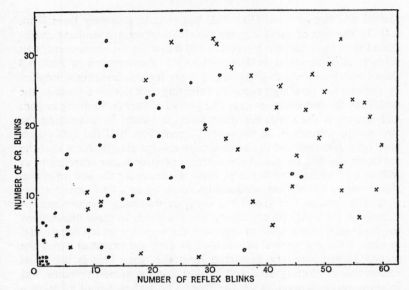

FIG. 6.3. Plot of raw data comparing the frequency of conditioned responses for each individual as a function of number of orienting responses given by the same individual.

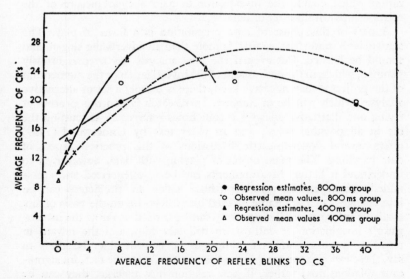

FIG. 6.4. Summary of the data in FIG. 6.3, showing the averaged data points and the curves fitted to them by regression formulae in the final data analysis.

plotted first in raw form [FIG. 6.3] and then in summary form [FIG. 6.4]. In the first of these Figures the circles represent subjects conditioned at an interstimulus interval of 400 ms, while the crosses represent subjects conditioned at an 800 ms interval. Examination of FIG. 6.3 shows that for each sub-group a low score for conditioning is implied by either a low or a high score for orienting, but not by a score in the middle of the respective ranges. The overall picture (combining crosses and circles) is the same, but information is gained by examining the two groups separately. In the second figure [FIG. 6.4] the data points have been averaged and the relationships emerge clearly. Note that the curve for the 400 ms group represents a positive linear correlation, as well as a curvilinear relationship, while the curve for the 800 ms group shows only a curvilinear relationship, resulting in a near zero correlation. The broken line shows the curve representing the two groups combined, for which no correlation was observed. In these illustrations the horizontal axis is used to represent the response which occurs first in time, while the vertical axis is used to show the extent to which the second response can be predicted from the first. This is the usual convention in plotting data, and implies that the second response was in some sense dependent on the first. The techniques of plotting a dependent variable can be extended by using distinctive colours as well as shapes to represent data subsets of interest. A little experience with data plots of this sort will quickly establish skills of pattern recognition which enable the investigator to gain a clear picture of the relationships within a set of data.

A part of this phase of data preparation is a form of play. The statistician's motto 'see me first' is more than an advertising slogan, and should be heeded. But even if the final analysis has been rigorously planned, which, in the enthusiasm of the investigation or the momentum of the project it may not have been, there is usually a set of alternative analyses which will be of interest. In research jargon this process of trying out alternative analyses is sometimes referred to as 'cutting the pie in all possible ways', and an older text by Underwood (1959) offers several down-to-earth discussions of this practical aspect of data handling. The main object of playing with data, however, is to understand it better. Measurements can be re-categorized and cross-tallied; the dependent variables (those which are predicted) can be interchanged; or the sample divided into categories on the basis of any available information. This process can be carried as far as the investigator's imagination or enthusiasm will take him, and the reward in terms of increased understanding can be considerable. Needless to say, these exercise are not designed as a search, after the fact, for significant relationships; rather, if new relationships emerge, they can be used as the guide lines for new hypotheses.

An interesting example of this kind of data manipulation concerns a problem which is often raised in psychiatric research. One of the criteria of scientific observation, mentioned earlier, is agreement between or among observers. When two physicians examine, say, an oral thermometer they are likely to agree fairly closely on the patient's temperature. When two psychiatrists attempt to assess a patient's degree of depression, or a more subtle interpersonal reaction, they are less likely to agree. Suppose that an investigation is planned in which outcome of psychiatric treatment is the dependent variable. Wisely, the investigator asks three of his colleagues to rate improvement, intending to pool the ratings and use the common judgement as a final criterion. However, he may also ask himself what it means when the raters disagree. Either two are wrong and one is right, or all of them are wrong, or two or more of them are right but in different ways.

By playing with the data, that is by plotting and tallying the results for each rater separately, he may notice that one rater marks a patient improved if and only if he is free of symptoms. Another may score improvement for those patients who are working effectively, whether symptoms are present or not. The investigator concludes that more than one kind of improvement is being measured, and in his next study he provides separate scales for symptom remission, and work effectiveness. This naïve example can be extended in principle to sophisticated levels of observation, for example of complex interpersonal processes, which are likely to be of interest in psychiatric research. The point it illustrates is that the understanding of a set of data can be increased, either intuitively or empirically by searching among its relationships.

A final comment on this kind of exploration concerns publication of the results. *Ad hoc* findings should never be reported as research results, though they can be mentioned as speculations of interest. At the same time, an editor and his readers are entitled to expect that the author of a research report knows considerably more about his subject than he reports. Thorough exploration of the data, and familiarity with its workings enhance the authority with which conclusions can be drawn and results reported.

DATA STORAGE

The storage of data may be considered as a separate phase of data handling. The desirability of clear and consistent records, bearing unambiguous labels is probably self evident. It is useful to prepare data sheets, typed and duplicated in advance of the data collection, on which all of the data for a single individual are recorded in the same format. Alternatively, the various forms of ruled paper available commercially can be used to summarize the data in an orderly fashion.

At some point, however, the original data should be stored in a more convenient and permanent form than that provided by separate sheets of paper. A variety of methods have evolved which enable large amounts of data to be stored in a form which reduces their bulk, allows for quick location and sorting of specific data items, and provides physically durable materials which can be handled frequently with reduced risk of loss or damage. These devices, described below, are sometimes called 'data vehicles' since they convey the data through the various phases of manipulation and analysis in an efficient manner. This is particularly desirable if analysis is planned using a computer, and the permanent store is likely to be in a form which is usable directly by the computer. In any case, the concept of a data 'bank', i.e. a cumulative store of information to which data can easily be added, has been popularized by computer techniques and is useful even if the computer is not involved in the analysis.

The common forms of data storage include feature cards, edge-clipped cards, column punch cards, paper tape and magnetic tape. The first three of these are illustrated in FIGURES 6.5 to 6.7. Each type of card has acquired a bewildering variety of names, though their functions are entirely distinct. The feature card is used to record the code numbers of each of the individuals who display a specific characteristic. In the example shown in FIGURE 6.5, the numbered fields allow for representation of 1,000 individuals. The card may be used to record, for example, all those patients using Stelazine, and a hole punched through a particular patient number would show that that patient is using the drug. Cross comparisons are possible by aligning the cards representing two or more features and noting the correspondence of holes.

Edge-clipped cards are used to store the data items for a single individual or unit. In the example illustrated in FIGURE 6.6 each of the holes is assigned to a particular item; if that hole is clipped the individual whose data is represented on the card is shown to fall in the category, e.g. depression, which the item represents. Cross-comparisons are made by inserting probes through one or more holes, allowing the cards which have been clipped in those holes to fall free of the remainder. Both types of cards represent methods of data storage developed before the advent of the computer. They both remain popular, particularly for large-scale surveys on long-term projects for which data accumulate in small amounts.

It is probably fair to say that the choice between the two types of card is largely a matter of familiarity and individual expertise, though advantages are claimed for each by their users. Variants of the two types are in use, and extended techniques of information coding provide highly sophisticated applications of these simple devices. A

GMP

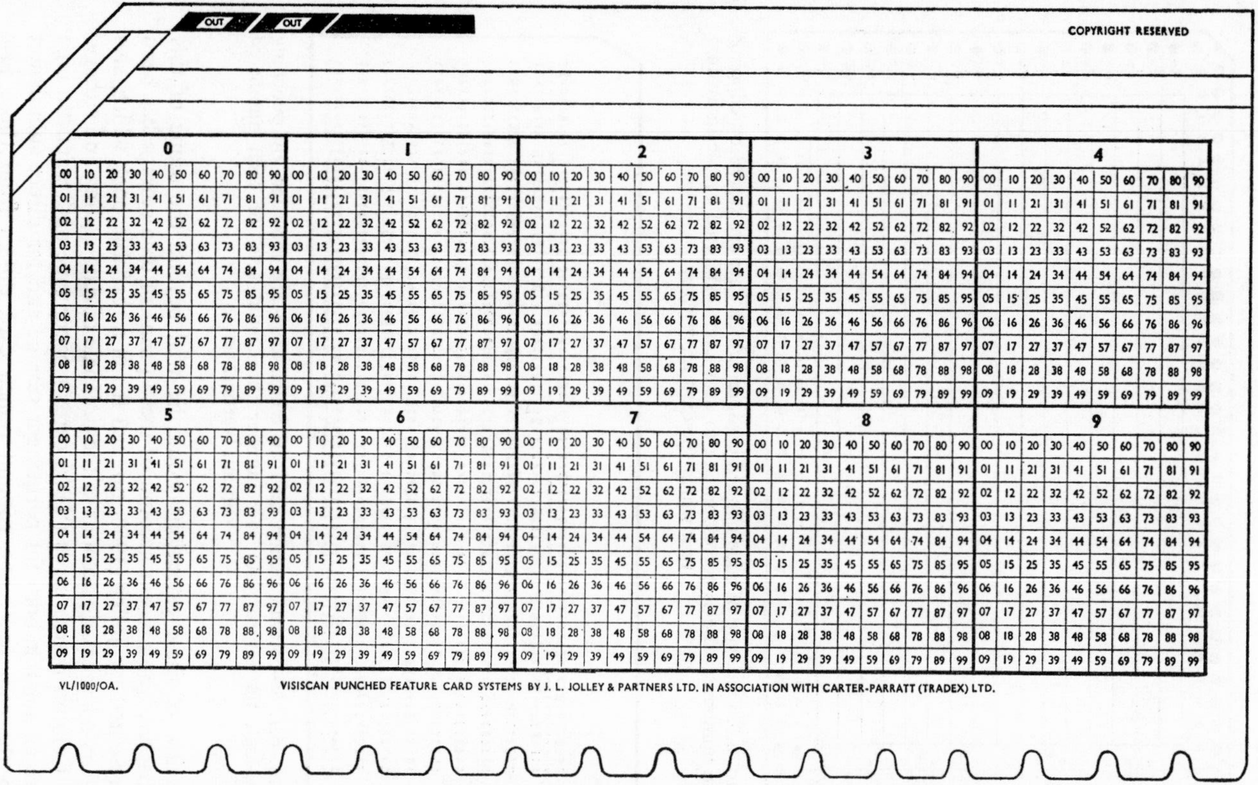
OUT
OUT
COPYRIGHT RESERVED
0
1
2
3
4
5
6
7
8
9
VL/1000/OA.
VISISCAN PUNCHED FEATURE CARD SYSTEMS BY J. L. JOLLEY & PARTNERS LTD. IN ASSOCIATION WITH CARTER-PARRATT (TRADEX) LTD.

FIG. 6.5. One type of feature card, on which data are recorded by punching out the number corresponding to each of the individuals who possess the characteristic represented by the card.

FIG. 6.6. One type of edge-clipped card, on which data are stored by clipping the numbered wholes corresponding to data items exhibited by the individual unit which the card represents.

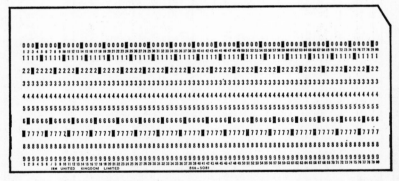

FIG. 6.7. 80-column punch card on which data are recorded by punching through the appropriate row number (horizontal sets) of each numbered column (vertical sets).

review of these extensions would lie well beyond the scope of this chapter, but a recent account of these forms of data storage has been presented by Jolley (1968, pp. 168 ff.) in a readable book which also offers a systematic account of the rationale of data coding and storage.

Column punch cards ('IBM cards') paper tape and magnetic tape are all suitable both for permanent storage and for direct submission to the computer. The column punch card differs from those just described, in that numbers of any size are directly represented. In the illustration in Figure 6.7, for example, columns 1 to 3 may be reserved for the subject number, which may be any value between 000 and 999 depending on the row number which is punched. Column 4 may be reserved for, say, sex, a punch in row one indicating 'male', a punch in row 2 'female'. It can easily be seen that this type of card is extremely versatile, and combines the functions of both the cards described above; though it is unsuitable for hand sorting.

Both punch cards and paper tape are prepared on machines designed for the purpose, on which data is typed in from a standard keyboard. The typing is error prone, even in skilled hands, and data are usually punched twice and checked automatically. Data are punched from coded forms which the trained punch operator learns to use very efficiently. For this reason the data should be prepared on the standard forms, since punching from non-standard layouts is likely to be slow, costly, and subject to a high rate of error. Figures should be clearly legible, and it is good practice to print the numbers from 0 to 9 at the top of one form so that the operator knows the convention of printing used by the coder. The data are laid out so that all the observations for each individual occur in the same order, and in the case of punch cards in the same numbered card column. It is good practice to number each individual, and to code all identifying information first, followed by the observations.

Individual workers have individual preferences for either punch cards or tape, but in practice this decision is usually determined by the available punching facilities and the type of input accepted by the computer. Paper tape is somewhat easier to store, being less bulky, and there is no danger of the data becoming shuffled by accident, since they are recorded on a continuous strip. By the same token it is cumbersome to add new data and to make alterations since the tape must be unwound, rather like a papyrus scroll, to find the location of a specific item. Punch cards offer two distinctive features which paper tapes do not: they can be shuffled and sorted very rapidly by machine, and they can accept new data by inserting new cards into the stack. Cards should always contain the subject number, and a card number for each card used for an individual subject, in order to facilitate identification, and to enable the stack to be reassembled if it is accidentally shuffled. Both cards and tape require reasonably careful handling, and very careful storage (usually at between 60° to 70° Centigrade and 40 to 60 relative humidity) if they are to be kept safe for long periods.

Magnetic tape storage of data has become more popular in recent years, and facilities for recording directly on to magnetic tape are becoming available. The advantages of magnetic tape stem from the fact that it is the form in which data is used by the computer. A reel of tape can be kept at the computer installation under ideal conditions of preservation, and mounted on the machine when it is required, without the intermediate step of reading from cards or paper tape. It is seldom damaged in use, whereas both cards and paper tape are fairly easily damaged by the machines which read them. The investigator who is engaged in a large-scale project or in serial projects may be well advised to rent or purchase a magnetic tape for storage of all his data. Subsets of the data for individual analyses may then be read from the tape by a simple program which puts the required data directly into the store used by the computer, where it can be used by the program which performs the actual analysis.

As a final comment, it might be noted that one of the influences of computer technology has been to draw attention to the concept of data storage. The data 'bank' mentioned earlier, is a research tool in its own right, and the role of information storage and retrieval, as part of the research process, is being increasingly appreciated. It might be predicted that further developments in the use made of data storage, and the stratagems of data collection and analysis which derive from storage methods, may influence the nature and style of scientific research profoundly.

THE COMPUTER

The foregoing pages have attempted to provide the aspiring research worker with a kind of orientation to the use he will make of his data collection. They are intended for the novice, and some of the points which may seem self-evident to him should not on that account be dismissed. In the same spirit the final section will discuss very briefly a practical orientation to the use of computer facilities, intended for those who wish to use the computer in their research.

The modern-high-speed-giant-electronic-digital-computer, like transatlantic commuting and the Pill, is probably here to stay. Most discussions of research topics, including this one, refer rather solemnly to its 'Advent' in the tones once reserved for an earlier advent and nativity. This can be seen as a propitiating gesture which reflects our alarm at the changes it has wrought, and the awe those changes inspire. The first step, then, in using the computer, is to remind oneself sternly that it is only a machine—a servant of its user. It is not even a 'thinking machine', and the concept of the electronic brain invoked by popular journalists is misleading. The computer does exactly what it is told to do—rather like the regiment of mindless servants conjured up by the Sorcerer's Apprentice. It behoves the reseacher, therefore, to know exactly what he is telling it to do.

Fortunately, this knowledge need be neither detailed or esoteric provided it is precise. The chief responsibilities of the research worker who wishes to make use of the computer in his research are to find out what facilities it offers, to learn to use those facilities effectively and to be clear about what he wants to do. This usually means learning less about the computer itself, than about the installation in which it is run. A certain general administrative format has been evolved to ensure the best use of the computer, and it may be useful to outline its essential components. These components are departments or administrative units of the computer installation. Terminology varies, but the usual computing centre includes an intake group ('Reception', 'User Services') responsible for the acceptance processing and discharge of work submitted; a 'Systems' group responsible for planning and renewing the detailed strategies which control the computer's activities; an operating group responsible for the actual running of the machine; and a maintenance group responsible for keeping it running. These groups are listed roughly in the order in which they are likely to be contacted in the process of using the computer and the last three will not be considered further.

The services offered to the user by the intake group are likely to include, in addition to actual job processing, an advisory service, library of programs and reference materials, facilities for data preparation (i.e. preparation of punched cards, paper tapes, and magnetic tapes) and provision of training courses, among others. If it is planned to use the computer in a research project, these facilities should be explored with reasonable thoroughness. Rather often, an investigator preoccupied with completing a particular data analysis, uses only a fraction of the facilities available to him. It might be suggested that the decision to use the computer at all, implies a certain obligation to use it meaningfully. Apart from becoming familiar with the available services, however, it is essential to learn the routine of job submission and retrieval, the program facilities available and the cost of the computer services to the user.

The cost of using the computer should be inquired into carefully, since computer time can be very expensive. If the work setting of the investigator includes computer facilities, he should inquire whether he will be charged for their use. If computer facilities are not a part of the setting, the first decision may be which computer to use, and cost should figure largely in the decision. For various historic and administrative reasons the cost of computer services, as it is charged to the user doing non-profit research, can vary from centre to centre with almost psychotic abandon. Indeed it may be cheaper to submit jobs by post to a computer at the other end of the country, than to use your friendly neighbourhood centre. In general, the university-based computing centres are able to provide research services at reduced rates, though the size of the reduction varies considerably. Some commercial data processing firms offer substantial academic discounts for bona-fide research, and while, in general, the commercial centres are prohibitively costly in terms of data preparation, they may provide standard statistical analysis fairly cheaply. Private firms, local government offices, and so on having their own computer can be approached, particularly for help with data preparation since it is in their interest to keep the machinery going, but are unlikely to be able to undertake data analyses of the type required. Ideally, then, an academically orientated, preferably university-based computer installation can be found by inquiring among colleagues or by writing to one of the larger universities.

Having located a computer, having determined that it can be afforded within the research budget (which should have allowed for computing costs, see CHAPTER 2), the next steps are to find out how to use it and what it will do. At this point it is advisable to visit the installation and talk to one of the advisers. One aim of this meeting is to learn well in advance the routine required in submitting work, the form in which work may be submitted, and the extent to which help is available with data preparation as well as analysis. Every computer unit has a set of rules and procedures which should be accepted as given, no matter how arbitary they may appear at first. It is a matter of professional philosophy to assume that the procedures required of the user are those which operate for the most efficient overall use of the computer.

With regard to the types of the analysis available, the second aim of the meeting is to find out what programs are available. This will usually mean reading, with some care, the catalogue of available programs. However, in this area the opposite philosophy prevails, and one does not merely accept what is first offered. The computer staff are willing and able to provide new programs, to borrow programs from elsewhere, to provide lists of programs which may be borrowed or to run programs brought by the user. Computer technology is still in a formative stage, and the *esprit de corps* of a new profession is still very much alive. The staff of any large computer unit are in general eager to facilitate any reasonable request, and to extend their services in order to show what they can do. It is at this point that the research worker should know precisely what he wants the computer to do.

Lists of programs are prepared by various agencies (e.g. Mitchell, *et al.*, 1972) from time to time which give an over-view of the types of programs and analyses currently available. (The one just referenced also provides a list of University computers and a glossary of computing terms). The potential user should be willing to study these lists carefully and to ask the advice of a statistician if necessary. The range of data analyses which the computer makes available enables the research worker to apply techniques of analyses without understanding either their computational procedures or the logic of the analysis. This is not in itself undesirable, provided the investigator is willing to study the rationale of the analysis, and to understand its requirements in terms of the assumptions it makes about the data. Put another way, research is improved if new techniques are explored, and the computer makes available a wide range of techniques. The use of these techniques demands of the investigator a non-technical understanding at least of what the analysis accomplishes, and places on him the responsibility of using the techniques correctly.

A final word concerns the degree of involvement in data processing which the investigator is willing to undertake, about which every investigator must make his own decision. Research workers are not required to be either statisticians or computer programmers; they should expect to know, however, the requirements of both fields. It has been suggested here that a great deal is to be learned, particularly in the early stages of a research career, by preparing data by hand. Beyond this there is no simple division of labour. Temperament and training will partly determine how deeply an individual becomes involved in data handling as opposed to theorizing, observing or simply collecting data. Probably the simplest formulation of this problem is that time spent in any one of these areas is time taken away from the others.

REFERENCES

COHEN, J. (1969) *Statistical Power Analysis for the Behavioural Sciences*, London.

DIXON, W. J., and MAY, P. R. (1968) Methods of statistical analysis, in *Treatment of Schizophrenia*, ed. May, P. R., New York.

DUBOIS, P. M. (1965) *An Introduction to Psychological Statistics*, London.

GUILFORD, J. P. (1965) *Fundamental Statistics in Psychology and Education*, 4th ed., London.

JOLLEY, J. L. (1968) *Data Study*, London.

MARCHANT, J. P., and PEGG, D. (1967) *Digital Computing: a Practical Approach*, London.

MAXWELL, A. E. (1958) *Experimental Design in Psychology and the Medical Sciences*, London.

MITCHELL, J. C., THOMPSON, J., THORN, G., and WEIR, D. (1972) *Computerguide 3: Programs for Social Scientists*, Manchester.

PARRAT, L. G. (1961) *Probability and Experimental Errors in Science*, New York.

SCHEFFE, H. (1959) *The Analysis of Variance*, New York.

UNDERWOOD, B. J. (1957) *Psychological Research*, New York.

7

THE EVALUATION OF TREATMENT IN PSYCHIATRY

MICHAEL SHEPHERD

The relatively short history of modern psychiatry has witnessed the rise and fall of many different forms of treatment. At the present time few branches of medicine stand more in need of reliable methods for the assessment of therapeutic claims. If this unsatisfactory state of affairs springs in some measure from an uncertainity about the causes and nature of most psychiatric illness it also reflects a failure on the part of many workers to have applied well-recognized principles of clinical investigation. Since the establishment of the Therapeutic Trials Committee of the Medical Research Council in 1931 a number of studies in other medical fields have demonstrated the value of collaboration between the clinician, the statistician, the laboratory scientist and, more recently, the clinical pharmacologist. Their combined skills have shaped and developed the modern controlled clinical trial, a procedure which has been defined as 'an experiment carried out with the object of seeing whether a treatment has any effect on the course of a disease' (Doll, 1965).

It should be emphasized at the outset that in its fully developed form the clinical trial takes its place as the cornerstone of the late confirmatory stage of evaluation. The stage of early evaluation calls for more empirical procedures which may have to be uncontrolled and in some measure intuitive. In the case of the drug treatment of mental disease, for example, a report from the World Health Organization suggests that the stage of early evaluation be sub-divided into two phases, the first concerned with dose-range, side-effects and toxic reactions and the second with therapeutic range and effectiveness (WHO, 1967). Only in the third phase are strictly controlled techniques employed, ideally in an attempt to validate the observations already made in the two earlier stages. In the field of psychiatry, there have been very few attempts to explore the early stages of evaluation, and formal clinical trials have suffered in consequence (Blackwell and Shepherd, 1967).

In principle, the clinical trial consists in a comparison between the outcome of two identical groups differing only by virtue of the remedy which one of them receives [see FIG 7.1]. The logic of the controlled, or comparative, trial is therefore clearest when its aim is prophylatic as, for example, when attack rates are estimated after the vaccination of

ESSENTIALS OF A COMPARATIVE TRIAL

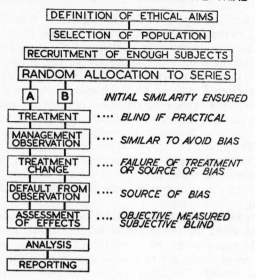

FIG. 7.1.

populations which are initially free of disease and so theoretically homogeneous. When the population is already diseased the comparative trial may not always be necessary: an untreated illness may, for example, carry a 100 per cent mortality rate, or the effectiveness of a new treatment may be so dramatic as to be self-evident. To most instances of physical disease and to virtually all psychiatric disorders, however, such conditions do not apply; the primary question is not so much whether a particular treatment is effective as how it compares in efficacy with some alternative. In general, the controlled trial is likely to be most valuable when rational treatment is administered to a clearly defined disorder of known aetiology whose outcome can be established by unequivocal criteria. Excellent models have been provided by the treatment of several acute bacterial infections and of some chronic physical illnesses, e.g. pulmonary tuberculosis, whose nature and course are well understood. With chronic physical disease of obscure aetiology and uncertain outcome, however, the comparative trial encounters difficulties which are essentially similar to those which arise in the treatment of most psychiatric disorders. These issues may be considered conveniently by a brief discussion of some of the principal problems posed by the investigation.

ETHICS

Although the ethical aspects of the clinical trial in psychiatry differ in no respect from those which apply to other forms of illness, the burden is lightened to some extent by the small number of established remedies. While the patient should not suffer by having effective treatment withheld for more than a limited period of time, in this branch of medicine experience suggests that the moral imperative is as likely to be exercised against the over-treatment of mental disease, especially when the symptoms impair the patient's capacity for rational communication and affect his ability to participate freely in the therapeutic procedure. The physical treatment of psychiatric disorders has provided some unfortunate examples of therapeutic zeal in the past, and the newer fashions in pharmacotherapy have already illustrated the dangers of administering compounds with uncertain properties in large quantities over long periods of time.

Ethical arguments have been advanced by some clinicians when they are trying to avoid the use of controlled therapeutic experiments. A characteristic example may be taken from the current vogue for the supposedly prophylactic use of lithium carbonate in the management of depressive illnesses. Thus two of the advocates of this practice write as follows: 'Since a striking prophylactic action of lithium became apparent with the first patients studied, it would have been difficult as well as painful to distribute the patients into two groups, one to receive lithium and one to be given placebo or the traditional, and in most cases rather ineffective, therapy. Since prophylactic rather than therapeutic effects were studied the patients—many of them severely handicapped by frequent relapses—would have had to remain in their group for a number of years' (Baastrup and Schou, 1967).

The response to this mode of reasoning has been clearly stated by Pickering: '. . . all therapy is experimentation. Because what in fact we are doing is to alter one of the conditions, or perhaps more than one, under which our patient lives. This is the very nature of an experiment, because an experiment is a controlled observation in which one alters one or more variables at a time to try and see what happens. The difference between haphazard therapy and a controlled clinical trial is that in haphazard therapy we carry out experiments without design on our patients, and therefore our experiments are bad experiments from which it is impossible to learn. The controlled clinical trial means merely introducing the ordinary accepted criteria of a good scientific experiment' (Pickering, 1960).

In practice, while each case must be treated on its merits every investigator concerned with the problems of therapeutic evaluation can profitably address himself to the six questions posed by Bradford

Hill who has played a major role in the development of the modern clinical trial (Hill, 1963):

1. Is the proposed treatment safe or, in other words, is it likely to do harm to the patient?
2. Can a new treatment be ethically withheld from a new patient in the doctor's care?
3. What patients may be brought into a controlled trial and allocated randomly to different treatments?
4. Is it necessary to obtain the patient's consent to his inclusion in a controlled trial?
5. Is it ethical to use a placebo or dummy treatment?
6. Is it proper for the doctor not to know the treatment being administered to his patient?

CONSTRUCTION OF PATIENT-POPULATIONS

The guiding principles of this phase of the investigation have been expounded clearly by Bradford Hill (1960): 'In a simple experiment in the laboratory the scientific worker wishes to see what happens to A if he manipulates B. He tries to keep constant all other factors that may upset or influence the relationship. Similarly in the controlled trial we endeavour to keep constant the characteristics of those on treatment A and those on treatment B. Some of those characteristics we can keep constant by stratification—by keeping equal in the two groups such obvious features as age and sex. Other characteristics we cannot deliberately equalize and our aim is to achieve it by the random allocation which, in the long run, offers no favour to one or other group.' The securing of homogeneity in groups of diseased subjects is greatly facilitated by knowledge of the aetiology and course of the illness concerned. In an MRC trial of the treatment of tuberculosis by streptomycin, for example, it was possible to define succinctly the patients entering the trial as suffering from 'acute progressive bilateral pulmonary tuberculosis, believed to be of recent origin, bacteriologically proved, unsuitable for collapse therapy, age group 15–30'. By contrast, the clinical criteria for inclusion in the first MRC trial of therapy in depressive illness could not be defined more objectively than in the following terms: 'The clinical features of the illness must reveal as its primary manifestations a persistent alteration of mood exceeding customary sadness and constituting a major symptom of the illness. This should be supported by one or more of the following symptoms: self depreciation with a morbid sense (or delusional ideas) of guilt; sleep disturbance; hypochondriasis; retardation of thought and action; agitated behaviour' (MRC, 1965).

Diagnostic categories which depend on such uncertain criteria are open to large 'observer variation'. Further, psychiatric populations defined in these terms are inevitably heterogeneous: in consequence, it is imperative to recruit sufficient subjects in each group for random allocation to equalize bias. For this reason it may prove necessary to organize a multi-centred trial, a complex undertaking which demands considerable time and resources.

BIAS

When treatment has been instituted bias may arise from several sources. After the random allocation of patients there can be changes of treatment and drop-outs in the course of therapy which might distort the composition of the groups significantly. Such factors can be minimized by careful attention to practical management. In addition, however, a major bias may be introduced by the expectations of the medical attendant and the patient, a matter of particular importance in the management of many psychiatric conditions where subjective factors enter so intimately into the nature of the illnesses and their outcome In these circumstances the double-blind technique, designed to keep the observer and the patient in ignorance of the treatment prescribed, can be valuable in conjunction with a placebo or standard therapy for the control group. It is important to stress, however, that it may be inapplicable when a drug has side-effects which can be detected, when a placebo must not be administered for ethical reasons or when the nature of the therapeutic procedure cannot be disguised (Rickels *et al.*, 1970).

THE CRITERIA OF RESPONSE

Inasmuch as the objectives of any treatment must be defined before its success can be estimated, psychiatric illnesses have suffered by comparison with physical illnesses in the past. The reason has been underlined by Zubin (1953) as follows: 'In the case of physical disorders the goal of therapy is usually self-evident. The corresponding goal in mental disorder is more difficult to define since we do not know the level to which the patient is to be returned. Should it be to his premorbid level; should it be to the level which he is capable of attaining when one takes into consideration the disease process and its after-effects; or should it be to the average level of the general population who never had the illness? The following criteria have been proposed by various workers for gauging the goals of therapy: (a) ability to withstand pressure of external events; (b) capacity to tolerate uncertainty, deprivation and frustration; (c) absence of blindly compulsive activity; (d) freedom from symptoms; (e) increased productivity; (f) adjustment and pleasure in social and sexual life; (g) good interpersonal relationship and sufficient insight. It is clear that such criteria cannot constitute the objective framework required for scientific evaluation.'

But even when agreement can be reached on the aims of treatment, it remains necessary to set up measurable indices of response. These indices should be both valid, in that they are closely associated with the severity of the disease in question, and discriminating, in that they reflect responses to treatment; they should also be repeatable, preferably simple and as objective as possible. As a rule the physical correlates of illness conform to such requirements more readily than social or psychological criteria but in the present state of knowledge there are relatively few such physical indices of psychiatric disorder. With depression, for example, Eugen Bleuler's statement that 'the affect is the index of the whole picture' still remains substantially true and enforces the use of necessarily subjective criteria in evaluating treatment.

The difficulty of standardizing subjective responses resulted in their virtual neglect for many years, but their patent importance for clinical research in psychiatry has recently led to a quickening of interest in their measurement and assessment. Much work in this sphere has been focused on the construction of rating-scales (Wittenborn, 1964; see also CHAPTER 12). It is necessary for these scales to contain items of behaviour which are appropriate to the investigation. The items should be pre-tested to ensure that they are clearly comprehensible, that they apply to the relevant sample of patients and that they form a progressive continuum. If possible, the scale should be empirically validated before it is adopted for use in clinical trials. Elaborate but essentially meaningless statistical procedures cannot be justified for their own sake.

THE ANALYSIS OF RESULTS

Since the therapeutic trial is designed to refine clinical experience in quantifiable terms the statistician must be involved in every stage of the experiment if he is to make his maximal contribution. He should be able to help decide on whether the standard comparison of groups is to be preferred to some other design, such as the self-controlled, self-recorded trial (Hogben and Sim, 1953) or to the newer sequential techniques (Sainsbury and Lucas, 1959): he should be consulted on dosage-schedules as well as on the more specialized problems of the recording of data and the analysis of results. Only when the statistician is familiar with the material from the outset can full benefit be obtained from his advice, which will be directed towards obtaining clear-cut results whenever possible: in the context of the clinical trial Bradford Hill has pointed out that the term 'not statistically significant' should be equated with the verdict of 'non proven' rather than that of 'not guilty'.

'SPECIFIC' AND 'NON-SPECIFIC' EFFECTS OF TREATMENT

It is evident that in theory the modern clinical trial can be modified to evaluate any form of remedy for any form of illness. If in practice it has proved to be most effective when the physical components of the treatment and of the illness have been salient this is principally because these dimensions can be measured most accurately. At present the majority of physical treatments in psychiatry are empirical and precise indications for their use are lacking; clinical trials often yield no more than a broad area of information whose relevance to individual patients may be remote. When somatic treatment rests on a rational basis, however, the clinical trial can be employed to tackle questions of a different order. Speculations about the mode of action of the psychotropic drugs, for example, has led to a number of hypotheses, of which the role of monoamine oxidase inhibition in the treatment of depression is among the most prominent. Thus the substance iproniazid (isopropylisonicotinic acid hydrazide), which has been used in the treatment of depressive states following the observation of its euphoriant action in the treatment of tuberculosis, is known to exercise an inhibiting effect on monoamine oxidase, the enzyme largely responsible for inactivating 5-hydroxytryptamine, and also on a proportion of naturally occurring catecholamines. One clinical trial carried out with this drug was designed to learn not merely whether iproniazid benefited depressed patients but also whether those patients who responded could be distinguished clinically and biochemically (by estimations of urinary 5-hydroxyndoleactic acid) and, still more precisely, whether the positive responders exhibited any evidence to suggest that their responses were related to changes in the brain concentration of 5-HT or of catecholamines (Pare and Sandler, 1959). Another example of a biologically-orientated experiment carried out within the framework of a clinical trial was designed to test the hypothesis that depressed patients who respond to desmethylimipramine metabolize the drug more slowly than those who do not, thereby giving the drug more time to exert its pharmaco-dynamic action (Watt et al., 1970).

　 Such investigations are being rendered more feasible by the development of newer methods of estimating plasma-levels of drug in man (Curry, 1971; Walter, 1971). Their potential importance is enhanced by the possibility that information obtained in a therapeutic setting may be used to shed light on the physiopathological mechanisms of the disease under treatment. This type of biological 'specificity' is often contrasted with the 'non-specific' social and psychological factors which can assume an important role in the outcome of many physical illnesses, especially those which run a chronic course. A number of studies have shown how powerful are the effects of these 'non-drug' or 'non-specific' factors in the treatment of psychiatric illness, where the interplay between physical and psychosocial factors is more complex and always demands consideration (Shepherd, 1961).

A great deal of evidence has now accumulated about the influence of *social factors* on the outcome of mental disease. Controlled experiments have indicated the degree of improvement which can be related to environmental change even with chronic schizophrenics (Pasaminck *et al.*, 1967), and it has been demonstrated that the attitudes of such patients are important for the course of their rehabilitation. Only when it is possible to evaluate these supposedly 'non-specific' therapeutic forces can most current physical methods of treating the major psychoses in institutions be properly assessed, a point which has been well illustrated schematically by Rashkis and Smarr (1958) [FIG. 7.2].

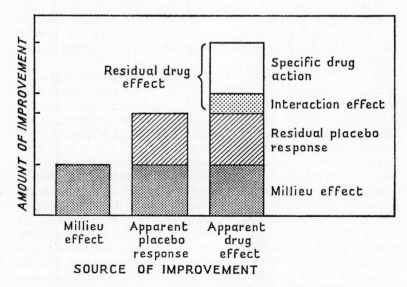

FIG. 7.2. Specific and non-specific factors affecting pharmacotherapy in psychiatric institutions.

In one form or another *psychological treatments* are widely used in the treatment of mental disorders. Not many workers, however, have been prepared to apply the principles governing therapeutic evaluation and, indeed, it has been shown that such an exercise may not be feasible for some forms of psychotherapy (Candy *et al.*, 1972). On the other hand, the introduction of psychological treatments based on learning theory, so called 'behaviour therapy', has shown clearly that such measures can be subjected to formal evaluation and have stimulated comparison with psychotherapy (Gelder *et al.*, 1967).

While the claims on behalf of formal psychotherapy have been pressed chiefly by enthusiastic but uncritical practitioners and rebutted by equally dogmatic sceptics, very few investigators have so far preferred to study the central problem to which Rosenthal and Frank have drawn attention, namely that: 'improvement under a special form of psychotherapy cannot be taken as evidence for: (a) correctness of the theory on which it is based; or (b) efficacy of the specific technique used, unless improvement can be shown to be greater than or qualitatively different from that produced by the patient's faith in the efficacy of the therapist and his technique—"the placebo effect". This effect may be thought of as a non-specific form of psychotherapy and it may by quite powerful in that it may produce endogenous changes and relief from stress of considerable duration.' One of the few investigators who has faced this issue squarely is Leder who has furnished some evidence suggesting that the psychotherapeutic process be divided into two phases: an initial phase of passive learning when the 'placebo effect' occurs, followed by a phase of specific active re-learning (Leder, 1968).

In view of the complexities of this field it is not surprising that much of the most clear-sighted work has come from experimentally-minded psychologists who are more sophisticated than most clinicians in the complexities of experimental design (Edwards and Cronbach, 1952). One of the more convincing of these investigations has been the treatment of delinquent behaviour in the U.S. Navy by a form of psychotherapy carried out in small closed communities called 'living groups' where twenty offenders were placed under the care of three supervisors for 6 or 9 weeks. A consultant psychologist conducted five 90-minute group-therapy sessions weekly which the men and their supervisors attended. Among the many variables manipulated by the design were the predicted effectiveness of individual supervisory teams, the level of maturity of group members, the duration of supervisor-group relationships and a variety of interpersonal rating-scales. It emerged that the simpler breakdowns of the data failed to do justice to the results; therapeutic success and failure in terms of subsequent behaviour could be explained only when account was taken of the interaction between predicted supervisory effectiveness and the estimated levels of the subjects' interpersonal maturity.

THE EVALUATION OF MENTAL HEALTH SERVICES

Over the past few years the growing appreciation of the burden of mental disorder on the community has been accompanied by an awareness of the need to introduce and modify the mental health services, both intra- and extra-mural. Unfortunately, although a large variety of measures have been adopted in different societies for different purposes, only a minority of these have been subjected to adequate evaluation. The reasons for this situation are manifold, arising partly out of the complexity of the task of evaluation, and partly out of the understandable proclivity of health administrators to impose their own values on whatever system of care they adopt. Nonetheless, the need for an objective assessment of such systems is now widely acknowledged, and in this country it has been recognized that there is a need to show that 'the technique of the controlled trial can be adapted and developed, using sociological and economic as well as clinical measures, so as to play at least a part in the evaluation of complex services' (Matthew, 1971).

A number of studies in several areas of the National Health Service are currently under way with this objective. Among the investigations of psychiatric interest there may be mentioned a Scottish case-register study (Baldwin, 1971), the Wessex study of mental subnormality (Kushlik, 1967), and the community-based programme at Chichester (Grad and Sainsbury, 1966). The interest of the Department of Health and Social Security in such work should ensure its occupying an important place in the future plans which are now being formulated.

CONCLUSION

The evaluation of psychiatric treatment should be regarded as no more than a complex variant of a general procedure. Kety (1961) has pointed out that: 'Every therapist, be he surgeon, internist, or psychotherapist, accepts a patient for treatment without knowing all of the individual factors which will determine the final outcome, but on the basis of hypotheses that he can help such patients.' While there is still much to learn about the individual determinants of outcome in psychiatric illness the psychiatrist's therapeutic hypotheses must be put to the test as rigorously as those of other clinicians. Though the task may be a formidable one the scientific future of treatment in psychiatry depends on the integrity and imagination with which it is tackled.

REFERENCES

BAASTRUP, P. C., and SCHOU, M. (1967) Lithium as a prophylactic agent, *Arch. Gen. Psychiat.*, **16**, 162.

BALDWIN, J. A. (1971) *The Mental Hospital in the Psychiatric Service*, London.

BLACKWELL, B., and SHEPHERD, M. (1967) Early Evaluation of psychotropic drugs in man, *Lancet*, ii, 819.

CANDY, J., BALGOUR, F. H. G., CAWLEY, R. H., HILDEBRAND, H. P., MALAN, D. H., MARKS, I. M., and WILSON, J. (1972) A feasibility study for a controlled trial of formal psychotherapy, *Psychol. Med.*, **2** (4), 345–62.

CURRY, S. H. (1971) Chlorpromazine: concentrations in plasma, excretion in urine and duration of effect, *Proc. roy. Soc. Med.*, **64**, 285.

DOLL, W. R. S. (1965) Clinical Trials, in *Evaluation of New Drugs in Man*, ed. Zaimis, E., p. 159, Oxford.

EDWARDS, A. L., and CRONBACH, L. J. (1952) Experimental design for research in psychotherapy, *J. clin, Psychol.*, **8**, 51.

GELDER, M. G., MARKS, I. M., and WOLFF, H. H. (1967) Desensitisation and psychotherapy in the treatment of phobic states: a controlled enquiry, *Brit. J. Psychiat.*, **113**, 53.

GRANT, J. D., and GRANT, M. Q. (1959) Group dynamics approach to nonconformists in the navy, *Ann. Amer. Acad. polit. soc. Sci.*, Mar., 127.

GRAD, J. C., and SAINSBURY, P. (1966) Evaluating the community psychiatric service in Chichester: Results, *Milbank Mem. Fd Quart.*, **44**, 246.

HILL, A. B. (1960) In *Controlled Clinical Trials*, ed. Hill, A. B., p. 169, Oxford.

HILL, A. B. (1963) Medical ethics and controlled trials, *Brit. med. J.*, **1**, 1045.

HOGBEN, L., and SIM, M. (1953) The self-controlled and self-recorded clinical trial for low-grade morbidity, *Brit. J. prev. soc. Med.*, **7**, 163.

KETY, S. S. (1961) The heuristic aspects of psychiatry, *Amer. J. Psychiat.*, **118**, 385.

KUSHLIK, A. (1967) A method of evaluating the effectiveness of a community health service, *Soc. Econ. Admin.*, **1** (4), 29.

LEDER, S. (1968) Psychotherapy: placebo effect and/or learning? in *The Role of Learning in Psychotherapy*, ed. Porter, R., p. 114, London.

MATTHEW, G. K. (1971) Measuring need and evaluating services, in *Portfolio for Health*, ed. McLachlan, G., p. 27, London.

MEDICAL RESEARCH COUNCIL (1965) Report by its Clinical Committee, Clinical trial of the treatment of depressive illness, *Brit. Med., J.*, 1, 881.

PARE, C. M. B., and SANDLER, M. (1959) A clinical and biochemical study of a trial of iproniazid in the treatment of depression, *J. Neurol. Neurosurg. Psychiat.*, 22, 247.

PASAMINCK, B., SCARPITTI, F. R., and DINITZ, S. (1967) *Schizophrenics in the Community*, New York.

PICKERING, G. W. (1960) In *Controlled Clinical Trials*, ed. Hill, A. B., p. 165, London.

RASHKIS, H. A., and SMARR, E. R. (1958). A method for the control and evaluation of sociopsychological factors in pharmacological research, *Psychiat. Res. Rep. Amer. psychiat. Ass.*, 2, 121.

ROSENTHAL, D., and FRANK, J. D. (1956) Psychotherapy and the placebo effect, *Psychol. Bull.*, 53, 294.

RICKELS, K., LIPMAN, R. S., FISHER, S., and PARK, L. C., (1970). Is a double-blind clinical trial really double-blind? *Psychopharmacologia*, 16, 329.

SAINSBURY, P., and LUCAS, C. J. (1959) Sequential methods applied to the study of prochlorperazine, *Brit. med. J.*, 2, 737.

SHEPHERD, M. (1961) The influence of specific and non-specific factors on the clinical effects of psychotropic drugs, in *Neuropsychopharmacology*, ed. Rothlin, E., p. 183, Amsterdam.

WALTER, C. J. S. (1971) Clinical significance of plasma imipramine levels, *Proc. roy. Soc. Med.*, 64, 282.

WATT, D. C., CRAMMER, J. L., and ELKES. A. (1970) *V Conferentia Hungarica pro Therapia et Investigatione in Pharmacologia*, Societas Pharmacologica Hungarica, p. 125.

WITTENBORN, J. R. (1964) Comments on the selection and use of symptom rating scales for research into pharmacotherapy, Vol. 7, in *International Review of Neurobiology*, ed. Smythies, J. R., and Pfeiffer, D.C., New York.

WORLD HEALTH ORGANIZATION (1967) Research in psychopharmacology, *Tech. Rep. Ser.*, No. 371.

ZUBIN, J. (1953) Evaluation of therapeutic outcome in mental disorders, *J. nerv. ment. Dis.*, 117, 95.

FURTHER READING

HARRIS, E. L., and FITZGERALD, J. D., eds (1970) *The Principles and Practice of Clinical Trials*, Edinburgh.

LEVINE, J., SCHIELE, B. C., and BOUTHILET, L., eds (1971) Principles
and problems in establishing the efficacy of psychotropic agents,
U.S. Public Health Service Publication, No. 2138.

SHEPHERD, M., LADER, M. H., and RODNIGHT, R. (1968) *Clinical Psychopharmacology*, London.

TRUELOVE, S. C., ed (1975) *Medical Surveys and Clinical Trials*, 3rd
ed., London. [In the press.]

8

DEFINING DIAGNOSTIC CRITERIA
FOR RESEARCH PURPOSES

R. E. KENDELL

Diagnosis is an imperfect business, particularly where mental illness is concerned. Several studies have shown that if two psychiatrists interview and diagnose non-organic patients independently of one another under ordinary working conditions, they are likely to make the same diagnosis only 30–40 per cent of the time (Ash, 1949; Hunt, *et al.*, 1953; Schmidt and Fonda, 1956) and even when both are experienced and share the same orientation agreement is rarely better than 60 per cent (Kreitman *et al.*, 1961; Beck *et al.*, 1962). In addition to this widespread evidence of low reliability it is becoming increasingly clear that there are major differences in the usage of key diagnostic terms like schizophrenia between one country and another, and even between different centres in a single country (Rawnsley, 1967; Kendell *et al.*, 1971). Faced with this situation, and also for other reasons, some American psychiatrists have advocated abandoning diagnoses completely and substituting comprehensive formulations of the predicament of each individual patient (e.g. Menninger, 1963). Unfortunately, however useful such formulations undoubtedly are for some purposes, they are in no sense a substitute for a diagnosis. In order to communicate at all with others, even to learn from our own previous experience, we have to classify our patients somehow; we have to have a means of recognizing features that are common to some but not to all of them, and of distinguishing between similarities which are important and those, like eye colour, which are not. We may decide to represent these relationships by a set of dimensions rather than by the discrete mutually exclusive categories of a typology, or to replace our existing classification by an entirely different one, perhaps based on psychodynamic defence mechanisms or cognitive variables, but we cannot avoid the necessity of classifying patients in some way or other.

Whether we like it or not, now and for the foreseeable future we are very dependent on diagnostic distinctions, not only in everyday clinical practice but perhaps even more so in our research. The subject matter of over 60 per cent of the papers published in the *British Journal of Psychiatry* in 1971, for instance, was defined wholly or in part by reference to diagnostic categories; and most of the studies that did not involve diagnostic distinctions either did not involve patients at all, or else were concerned purely with administrative groupings—all patients admitted to a given hospital during a specified time period, for instance. Although there are many other criteria[1] which could in theory be used, in practice when distinctions need to be drawn between one type of patient and another diagnostic criteria are used, either alone or in combination, in the bulk of contemporary clinical research.

A fundamental requirement of all scientific work is that it should be carried out and described with sufficient precision for others to be able to repeat it, and this principle applies to the definition of the subject matter just as much as it does to the experimental procedures involved and the results obtained. The evidence we have of the unreliability of psychiatric diagnosis, and of systematic differences in the diagnostic criteria used in different places, make it clear that at present this requirement is met very imperfectly. The information that the subjects of a particular study had all been diagnosed as schizophrenic may tell us remarkably little about them, certainly not enough for us to be able to assemble another group of patients with any confidence that they would be comparable. Indeed, it is probably true to say that this failure, or inability, to define adequately the essential common characteristics of the patients who constitute its subject matter (and those of the population from which they were drawn) is the most serious defect of contemporary psychiatric research. The literature is full of studies, highly sophisticated in other respects, with elegant monitoring techniques and complex statistical handling, which are rendered almost valueless by their neglect of this crucial issue. The purpose of this chapter is to describe various ways in which diagnostic criteria may either be made more precise or replaced by other more reliable criteria.

Because the potential unreliability of psychiatric diagnosis is widely recognized, attempts are often made to deal with the problem by ensuring that diagnostic assignments for research purposes are made only by experienced diagnosticians, or that they are agreed by two diagnosticians working independently, or simply by excluding all atypical cases. The literature is full of such phrases as 'diagnosed by Board-certified psychiatrists', 'diagnosed independently by two experienced clinicians', 'all with typical symptoms', 'in no case was there any doubt about the diagnosis', and so on. Unfortunately, although there

---

[1] Possible alternative criteria are legion but obviously include (a) individual symptoms, like depersonalization or phobic anxiety; (b) psychodynamic defence mechanisms, like denial or projection; (c) physiological anomalies, like a spike focus in the EEG; (d) biochemical anomalies like phenylketonuria; (e) forensic status, such as having been convicted of shoplifting; (f) therapeutic status, like having failed to respond to phenothiazines; (g) performance on cognitive or projective tests; and so on.

is probably some value in each of these strategies, they are all inadequate. Experienced psychiatrists are perfectly capable of disagreeing with one another, as anyone who has ever attended a case conference will know; even when two have agreed a third may still fail to do so; and what is regarded as typical schizophrenia in New York may be nothing of the sort in London or Manchester.

For the most part psychiatric diagnoses are based on symptomatology. Indeed, as Scadding's (1967) lucid analysis of our concept of disease implies, at present the defining characteristic of every non-organic psychiatric diagnosis is simply its syndrome, the constellation of symptoms and signs typically associated with that diagnosis. It is convenient to distinguish two main contributors to the low reliability of this type of diagnosis: disagreements about which symptoms are present; and disagreements about which symptoms, or combinations of symptoms, are necessary to establish the diagnosis under consideration. It may be simplest to consider the second of these, the question of diagnostic criteria, first and defer that of symptom detection until later.

DEFINING THE RELATIONSHIP BETWEEN SYMPTOMS AND DIAGNOSIS

The basic problem is that in ordinary clinical practice the relationship between symptoms and diagnosis is inadequately specified. Usually all the characteristic features of any given condition do not have to be present in order to establish that diagnosis. To be diagnosed as a schizophrenic, for instance, a patient does not have to possess all the typical symptoms of schizophrenia, only some of them. But which are essential and which are not, which may be regarded as alternatives to one another, how many must be present altogether, and which other symptoms must be absent, are rarely specified.

Authors sometimes attempt to clarify the diagnostic criteria they were using by stating that they were 'in accordance with the description in Mayer Gross and Slater's (or someone else's) textbook'. Such statements are unfortunately of little value. Textbooks almost invariably provide descriptions of the typical features of syndromes, rather than criteria for establishing their presence, and there is good evidence that psychiatrists may use diagnostic categories in quite different ways in practice, in spite of agreeing on the characteristics possessed by typical members of that category (Hordern et al., 1968).

It is often suggested that this problem of defining diagnostic criteria could largely be solved by the provision of glossaries containing definitions of all the diagnostic categories recognized in a given nomenclature. It was largely with this intention that, twenty years ago, the

American Psychiatric Association introduced its Diagnostic and Statistical Manual (American Psychiatric Association, 1952) and, sixteen years later, that the Registrar General's advisory committee in this country provided a glossary to the Eighth Revision of the International Classification (General Register Office, 1968) when that nomenclature was first introduced. In practice, however, both these glossaries have achieved only limited success. This is partly because of the inherent defects of the present International Classification, particularly the way in which it chops and changes between symptomatology and aetiology as a basis for classification, but to a large extent it is due to the type of definition provided in these two glossaries. Neither really provides adequate working definitions of its various diagnostic categories, much less the true operational definitions advocated by Hempel (1961). For the most part their definitions consist of brief descriptions of the characteristic features of each condition, which provide a useful summary of the essential elements of the clinical concept in question, as ordinary textbook descriptions do, but are of little help in indicating how patients with mixed or atypical symptoms should be classified. For this purpose a set of clearly defined criteria which *must* be fulfilled, rather than a description of the typical features of the condition, is what is needed. Glossaries composed of operational definitions of this type do exist and Feighner *et al.* (1972) have recently published the criteria used in St. Louis for the fifteen major diagnostic categories which they recognize. Others may disagree with some of their criteria, or even question some of their categories, but the need for unambiguous criteria of this type can hardly be questioned.

The difference between these two types of definition—the descriptive and the operational—is best illustrated by example. In the Registrar General's glossary anxiety neurosis is defined as:

'A disorder in which the principal manifestation is excessive anxiety, often amounting to panic, presenting in the psychic and/or somatic field, diffuse in quality, in which other psychoneurotic components such as obsessional or hysterical phenomena, though possibly present, do not dominate the clinical picture.'

By contrast, Feighner and his colleagues give these criteria:

A. The following manifestations must be present: (1) Age of onset prior to 40. (2) Chronic nervousness with recurrent anxiety attacks manifested by apprehension, fearfulness, or sense of impending doom, with at least four of the following symptoms present during the majority of attacks:

(a) dyspnoea, (b) palpitations, (c) chest pain or discomfort, (d) choking or smothering sensation, (e) dizziness and (f) paraesthesiae.

B. The anxiety attacks are essential to the diagnosis and must occur at times other than marked physical exertion or life-threatening situations, and in the absence of medical illness that *could* account for symptoms of anxiety. There must have been at least six anxiety attacks, each separated by at least a week from the others.

C. In the presence of other psychiatric illness(es) this diagnosis is made *only* if the criteria described in A and B antedate the onset of the other psychiatric illness by at least two years.'

To know that a group of patients were diagnosed using the Registrar General's criteria is in practice not much more informative than knowing that they were diagnosed 'by experienced psychiatrists', or 'in accordance with the description in so and so's textbook', but to know that the St. Louis criteria were used gives a fairly precise indication of which patients would and would not have been included. This latter approach does, however, have one important disadvantage: a number of patients will fail to fulfil the criteria of any category and as a result will have to be assigned to a 'rag bag' category, or else labelled simply as 'undiagnosed psychiatric disorder'. In fact this is the fate of about a quarter of all patients, both inpatients and outpatients, in St. Louis. In theory there is no reason why this should not be avoided, but in practice it is difficult to do so without either making the classification so simple that it fails to represent the clinical concepts it is concerned with, or alternatively making the diagnostic criteria for each condition so complex and interdependent that they can barely be understood. Part of the problem is that ordinary language is not an appropriate medium for expressing the complex rules needed to cope with innumerable combinations of symptoms. The notation of symbolic logic (Ledley and Lusted, 1959) is really required in this situation, but any glossary couched in these terms would be quite unsuitable for ordinary clinical use.

In some kinds of research, particularly biological studies, it is vital to ensure that all those who are included are correctly diagnosed but immaterial how many others are excluded or left undiagnosed in the process. In a situation like this there are a number of acceptable ways in which the diagnostic composition of the subject matter could be defined. A publicly available set of operational criteria, of the type described by Feighner and his colleagues, could be used for each diagnostic category involved. In many ways this is the ideal solution as there are obvious advantages in a single set of criteria becoming widely accepted and used in many different centres. But often no suitable criteria are available and the research worker has to produce a working definition of his own which corresponds reasonably well to the clinical concept in question and at the same time stipulates exactly which patients should and should not be included. For instance, manic depressive depression could be defined as severe depression of mood in the presence of any two of the following—severe weight loss, early morning wakening, guilt feelings, diurnal variation of mood, retardation and a 'distinct quality' to the depression. Or schizophrenia could be defined as an illness characterized by the presence of any one of Schneider's 'symptoms of the first rank' (Mellor, 1970) in the absence of evidence of brain disease. If suitable rating scales exist it is usually preferable to frame the definition in terms of scores on these, because in this way relatively complex criteria, involving numerous alternative combinations of symptoms, can be expressed quite simply without any loss of clarity. Manic depressive depression, for instance, might be defined by a score of 8 or more on the Newcastle Scale (Carney *et al.*, 1965), and if it were important to ensure that every patient was fairly severely depressed it might also be stipulated that each should have a score of 14 or more on the Hamilton Scale (Hamilton, 1960).

If only a small number of patients are needed, but it is important for them to be classical cases, criteria of this sort can easily be made more stringent. For a diagnosis of schizophrenia two first rank symptoms could be required instead of one, for manic depressive illness a score of 10 on the Newcastle Scale might be required instead of 8, and so on. In practice where the line is drawn will depend on how many patients are needed and how much time is available. In a drug trial, for instance, criteria that were too restrictive might jeopardize the chances of the trial ever being completed. What matter is that there should be clear and uniform criteria for each diagnostic category; what those criteria are and how restrictive they are are subsidiary issues.

Situations in which it is necessary for every subject in a population to be allocated to a diagnostic category, as is the case in epidemiological studies, are much harder to deal with. As no one can be rejected or left undiagnosed, rules of class membership must be laid down within a unitary framework and as a result they usually become very complex. If the number of symptoms recognized and the number of diagnostic categories involved are both fairly small these rules can be instituted by hand, as in Silbermann's CHAM system (1971), but it is generally necessary, for reasons of both speed and accuracy, to utilize a computer and most existing systems do so.

It is convenient to distinguish three different types of computer program used for this purpose: those based on a logical decision tree, those based on probability theory, and those based on discriminant function procedures. A logical decision tree consists of a series of questions, the answer to each of which eliminates one or more diagnoses or groups of diagnoses and also determines the next question asked, until eventually every diagnosis but one has been eliminated. For example, the first question, based on a group of items concerned with cognitive function, might be used to determine whether the illness was organic or not. If the answer was 'no' the second question, based perhaps on a series of items about delusions and hallucinations, might determine whether the illness was psychotic or neurotic, and so on. The formal structure is, in fact, the same as that of the familiar flora used to identify flowers from the shape and number of their leaves and petals and stamens, and can be likened to a branching tree, or to a railway marshalling yard with every question serving the function of a set of points. Spitzer's Diagno (Spitzer and Endicott, 1968), based on the scale scores of a structured mental state interview known as the Psychiatric Status Schedule [see p. 112] was the first such program to be developed and allocates every patient to one of 27 diagnostic categories, including 'not ill' and 'non specific illness with mild symptomatology'. It was followed by Diagno II (Spitzer and Endicott, 1969), a more complex program using history data as well as current mental state items and generating a wider range of diagnoses, including personality disorders. The authors were able to show that agreement between the diagnoses generated by this program and those made by clinicians was as good as that between two groups of clinicians provided independently with the same data, thus demonstrating that the computer's diagnoses possessed adequate face validity as well as being reliable. More recently Wing has developed a similar program, Catego (Wing et al., 1972), based on his structured Present State Examination (see p. 113). The second approach is a probabilistic or statistical one based on Bayes' theorem. The basic algebraic statement of this theorem is given in the appendix. The essential principle is to determine the probability of a patient with a particular group of symptoms belonging to one or other diagnostic category.

Most of the early programs for deriving diagnoses by computer were of this type (Overall and Gorham, 1963; Overall and Hollister, 1964; Smith, 1966) but, in spite of the obvious relevance of probability theory to diagnosis, the Bayesian model has several disadvantages. It assumes that each of the diseases is equally probable, that each is independent of the others, and that symptoms are also independent of one another, and as Zubin (1967) has pointed out none of these assumptions is justified. It also requires a reasonable estimate of the incidence of the various symptoms in each of the diseases encountered in the population under consideration. In practice these data are rarely available and in fact both Overall and Smith were forced to resort to the questionable procedure of using ratings of hypothetical typical cases instead.

The third group of techniques is based on discriminant function procedures. In its simplest form discriminant analysis involves two populations, one whose members have been assigned a clinical diagnosis A and the other a diagnosis B, and all of whom have been rated for the presence or absence of N items relevant to the distinction between A and B. Starting with these data the analysis produces a linear variable (the discriminant function) consisting of a set of weights for the N items calculated so as to maximize the ratio of between-group to within-group variance. As a result, when a score is derived for each patient by adding together his weighted scores on the N items, the separation between those with diagnosis A and those with diagnosis B is maximal. Subsequently, this discriminant function can be used to allocate any patient who has been rated on the N items to the appropriate diagnosis, A or B. In practical several diagnoses are usually involved, not just two, which means using a multiple stepwise discriminant procedure, but the basic principle remains unchanged. Techniques of this sort have been used by Melrose et al., (1970) and Sletten et al. (1970) and the latter at least were able to obtain a level of agreement between clinical and computer diagnoses comparable to that achieved by Spitzer with Diagno II.

All these ways of generating diagnoses by computer have the great advantage over ordinary clinical methods that they guarantee consistency; any given combination of symptoms will always be assigned the same diagnosis by any given program. It is arguable which of the three approaches described here is most useful, or which corresponds most closely to the reasoning processes employed by clinicians. The decision tree method is the simplest, and also the easiest to construct, but it is rather unadaptable as each program is useable only with the particular rating scale or structured interview for which it was designed, and individual diagnostic distinctions are necessarily based on rather crude criteria. The probabilistic and discriminant function procedures share the important advantage that, although each patient is assigned to a single category, the probability of his belonging to other categories can also be given, thereby identifying doubtful or borderline cases. Of the three methods discriminant function procedures probably hold the greatest promise. Although their main use in medicine is in the assessment of differential therapeutic response—helping forecast whether a patient with symptoms or laboratory findings A, B and C is more likely to respond to treatment X or treatment Y—viewed simply as a diagnostic tool they have many advantages. They are more flexible and have greater discriminating power than decision trees, and involve fewer unfulfilled assumptions than Bayesian models. In addition, the diagnostic criteria they impose are determined by, and reflect, the actual usage of clinicians rather than being arbitrarily imposed by the program designer. The outline description given above is illustrated in FIGURE 8.1.

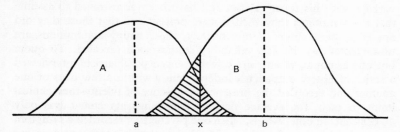

FIG. 8.1. Hypothetical discriminant function.

The two curves represent the distribution of scores obtained by the population A and B on the discriminant function. Their respective means are a and b, and x is the midpoint between a and b. In practice there is likely, as here, to be some overlap between the two populations with some A patients obtaining scores on the function greater than x and some B patients scores less than x. What the program does in this situation is rediagnose all patients with scores less that x as A and those with scores greater than x as B [the hatched areas in FIGURE 8.1]. As the weights given to the N items constituting the discriminant function are ultimately determined by the clinical criteria originally employed to identify the two populations A and B, what this procedure does, in effect, is impose on every patient the pooled or averaged diagnostic criteria employed by the clinicians responsible for the original diagnoses. In a study involving several diagnosticians, inspection of those patients whose clinical and computer diagnoses are different may reveal that individual clinicians have idiosyncratic diagnostic criteria. For instance, if an individual rater had several patients he had diagnosed as A rediagnosed by the computer as B, but none he had diagnosed as B rediagnosed as A, this would strongly suggest that his criteria for diagnosis A were wider than those of his colleagues.

SYMPTOM DETECTION

Up to this point we have been concerned entirely with various ways of ensuring that any given combination of symptoms always leads to the same diagnosis, without considering how the presence of those symptoms is established in the first place. Unfortunately disagreements about symptomatology are just as common as those about diagnosis, and even harder to eliminate.

Traditionally psychiatrists, like other physicians, have detected symptoms by holding a free-ranging interview with the patient, and perhaps with his relatives also, and have been accustomed to assume that the symptoms they elicited were present and that those they did not elicit were absent. Unfortunately, these happy assumptions are unwarranted, as the first reliability studies soon revealed. To quote but one example, when pairs of experienced psychiatrists interviewed a series of ninety outpatients independently within a few days of one another and recorded the presence or absence of twenty-four clinical items in each, the average positive percentage agreement was only 46 per cent; in other words, when one psychiatrist recorded a symptom as present there was less than a 50–50 chance of his colleague agreeing with him (Kreitman *et al.*, 1961).

Many factors contribute to this low reliability. There are differences in behaviour between one psychiatrist and another; they ask different questions, show interest and probe further in different places, establish different sorts of relationship with the patient, and so on. Then there are differences in expectation, which tend in a variety of ways to facilitate the detection of what is expected and militate against the detection or recognition of the unexpected to a quite surprising extent (Kendell, 1968). Finally important conceptual differences are often involved. Common technical terms like anxiety, delusion, thought disorder and so on may be used in quite different ways by different psychiatrists without their being aware that this is so (see, for instance, Rosenweig *et al.*, 1961); and even where there is no disagreement over the meaning of a term there is often disagreement over the extent to which graded characteristics like worry or tension have to be present to justify a positive rating.

A growing awareness of these problems has led to the development of three fairly distinct groups of instruments—self-assessment questionnaires, rating scales and structured interviews. They avoid or minimize the shortcomings of the traditional clinical interview in different ways and to differing extents [see TABLE 8.1] and each has important advantages and disadvantages.

Self-assessment questionnaires eliminate the interview completely. In this way they remove at one stroke all the problems produced by the vagaries of the clinician, but in doing so create several others instead. Patients who are agitated, retarded, unable to concentrate, or badly disturbed in any way, may give very misleading answers and it is comparatively easy for symptoms to be denied; patients' actual behaviour, as opposed to their views about it, cannot be examined at all; and there is no more guarantee that different patients all mean the same by words like anxious, depressed and hostile than there is that different interviews do so. For these reasons questionnaires are usually

TABLE 8.1

THE MAIN SOURCES OF UNRELIABILITY IN THE CLINICAL INTERVIEW
and the effect of these on questionnaires, rating scales and structured interviews

SOURCE OF UNRELIABILITY	SELF-ASSESSMENT QUESTIONNAIRE	RATING SCALE	STRUCTURED INTERVIEW
The Interviewer's behaviour	Eliminated	May be limited to some extent	Severely limited by procedural rules
The Interviewer's expectations	Eliminated	Largely unaffected	Limited by procedural rules
The Interviewer's interpretation of the technical terms involved	Problem transferred to the patient	Can be reduced by providing definitions	Reduced by the provision of definitions

inappropriate in situations where it is necessary to establish accurately the presence or absence of particular symptoms in individual patients. In general they are most useful for measuring overall levels of pathology in populations which do not contain a high proportion of disturbed or psychotic people, for measuring change in particular aspects of psychopathology like depression or anxiety, and as screening devices for the detection of psychiatric disturbance. In fact the majority of widely used questionnaires were specially designed for one of these three purposes. The Beck Inventory (Beck *et al.*, 1961) and the Zung Self Rating Depressive Scale (Zung, 1965), for instance, were designed specifically to measure change in depressive symptomatology over time and the Taylor Manifest Anxiety Scale (Taylor, 1953) was designed to fulfil an analogous function for symptoms of anxiety. Goldberg's General Health Questionnaire (Goldberg, 1972) was developed specifically to detect patients with significant psychiatric problems in general medical populations and Hathaway and McKinley's Minnesota Multiphasic Personality Inventory (MMPI), though originally introduced as a screening instrument for military recruits, has since been used most successfully for comparing overall levels or patterns of symptomatology in different populations.

Rating scales provide a convenient means of ensuring that a predetermined range of topics will be covered in a clinical interview and that the information elicited in these areas will be recorded in a uniform way. They hold strong attractions for statistically minded researchers because they ensure that the data arrive in a form suitable for whatever statistical manipulations are envisaged and, because they are so easy to construct, they are often designed on an ad hoc basis for individual pieces of research. If adequate working definitions are provided for the various items of psychopathology contributing to the scale reliability may be quite high, in spite of the fact that the interviewer is left to elicit the necessary information however he likes. If this is not done, however, a rating scale is simply an unstructured clinical interview covering a particular range of topics and retains all the shortcomings of an ordinary interview beneath its veneer of respectability. Lorr's In-Patient Multidimensional Psychiatric Scale (Lorr and Klett, 1967) and Overall's Brief Psychiatric Rating Scale (Overall and Gorham, 1962) have both been widely used and cover the whole range of psycho-pathology likely to be elicited in a clinical interview. Lorr's IMPS contains 89 items, mostly rated on 9-point scales, and the need for definitions is circumvented fairly successfully by a careful avoidance of all technical terms. The first question, for instance, asks not whether the patient is verbally retarded but whether 'compared to the normal person' his speech is 'slowed, deliberate or laboured'. Overall's BPRS consists of 16 7-point scales embracing different areas of symptoma-tology and reasonably adequate working definitions are provided for each of them. The main use of both these instruments is for com-paring levels and patterns of symptomatology in different populations—English and West Indian schizophrenics for example—or for measuring change in a single population, as in drug trials. Like self-rating question-naires they are not usually suitable in situations in which it is necessary, for diagnostic or other reasons, to establish the presence of individual items of psychopathology.

Structured interviews are of more recent origin than questionnaires or rating scales and to some extent their development is the result of an increasing recognition of the inadequacies of these other instruments. In a structured interview the manner in which symptoms are elicited is prescribed as well as the way in which they are recorded. The questions the patient is asked, and their order, are both laid down in advance, ratings are made serially as the interview progresses rather than at the end, and definitions, implicit or explicit, are provided for each item. Actually the degree of standardization involved varies considerably from one 'structured interview' to another. In some, as in Burdock's Structured Clinical Interview (Burdock and Hardesty, 1969) what the interviewer can say and do is so tightly controlled that the instrument is very close to being a verbally administered questionnaire; in others the interviewer still retains some control over the exact wording of the questions he asks and even over his interpretation of the patient's replies.

The differences between these two approaches are exemplified by the two most well known and widely used structured interviews—Spitzer's

Psychiatric Status Schedule (Spitzer *et al.*, 1970) and Wing's Present State Examination (Wing *et al.*, 1972). The Psychiatric Status Schedule (PSS) is designed to elicit and record the symptoms experienced by the patient and his role functioning during the preceding seven days and consists of a booklet containing an interview schedule and a matching inventory of 321 dichotomous items. The schedule stipulates the exact form of words to be used for each question and the corresponding ratings are closely tied to the wording of the patient's reply. Further probing is allowed if his reply is incomplete or ambiguous, but only to a limited extent, by means of general queries like 'Can you tell me more about that?' or 'What do you mean by that?'. The Present State Examination (PSE) is less highly structured and also differs in other ways. It is concerned more exclusively with symptoms, particularly psychotic phenomena, and covers a longer period of time—the previous four weeks rather than the previous seven days. Suggested probes are provided for each item but with this instrument the interviewer is free to ask additional questions if he feels this is necessary, and the rating he finally makes represents *his* judgement whether or not the symptom in question is present, rather than the patient's initial reply to his original probe.

In theory the PSS, as the more highly structured of the two, should have higher reliability. In practice it is possible to obtain equally good reliability with the PSE, though only after prolonged training. Both interviews can be used comfortably with a wide range of patients and are equipped with decision tree computer programs (Diagno and Catego) to convert symptom profiles into diagnoses. The PSS requires less training, can be used by non-psychiatrists and is perhaps most suitable for population comparisons. The PSE can only really be used by trained psychiatrists but its flexibility makes it particularly suitable for use with psychotic patients or in situations where the patient's symptoms need to be elicited in detail. Several other structured interviews have been developed, including history interviews; indeed Spitzer and his colleagues (Spitzer *et al.*, 1967) have produced a veritable arsenal of instruments for use in different situations.

Their relative lack of flexibility, and the training needed to use them fluently and reliably, makes structured interviews inappropriate for ordinary clinical purposes. They are essentially research instruments. Whether they should be regarded as essential in any given piece of clinical research depends on the situation. In cross-cultural comparisons where it is vital for geographically separated groups of patients to be interviewed in identical ways, or in any multicentre study involving more than one team of interviewers, clearly they are essential. In a situation where only a small group of interviewers and one patient population are involved the need is less obvious, particularly as in situations of this sort it is often possible to demonstrate adequate reliability using a rating scale. Even here though the general requirement of all scientific work—that what is done should be stipulated and described with sufficient precision for others to be able to do the same—makes it difficult to defend unstructured interviewing, especially if operational definitions are not provided for all the technical terms involved.

The crucial role of adequate definitions is a constant theme running through this discussion. They are as important for symptoms or individual items of psychopathology as they are for diagnoses and it is much easier to provide them for some symptoms than for others. Weight loss can easily be defined as 'loss of at least 3 kg in 6 months in the absence of relevant organic disease or deliberate dieting' and early morning wakening as 'waking, and failing to get any more satisfying sleep, at least 2 hours before normal at least 3 nights a week'. Items like 'good previous personality' and 'immaturity' pose a much harder problem. It is relatively easy to provide terms such as these with 'syntactical' definitions which provide rules of substitution, but much harder to provide 'semantic' definitions providing rules of application (Reid and Finesinger, 1952). For example, it is relatively easy to define immaturity as 'failure to develop the attitudes and behaviour patterns generally accepted as appropriate to the individual's chronological age', but syntactical definitions like this do not make it any clearer which people the term is applicable to. All they really do is provide an alternative form of words allowing us, if we wish, to avoid using the word immaturity. A sematic definition, on the other hand, would have to specify precisely which attitudes and behaviours were evidence of immaturity and which were not, and in practice this is very difficult to do. For this reason terms like immaturity and good previous personality are best avoided. In general all definitions which remain heavily dependent on inference, as purely syntactical definitions inevitably do, are likely to prove inadequate, as there is abundant evidence that inferential judgements are consistently less reliable than those based on directly observable criteria (Heyns and Lipitt, 1954; Lehmann et al., 1965). In principle there is no reason why patients should not be classified on the basis of the defence mechanisms they utilize rather than their overt symptoms, particularly as many psychiatrists believe that such a classification would be more useful and valuable than what we have at present. The problem is that the majority of the psychoanalytic concepts involved cannot be provided with semantic or operational definitions, or at least their advocates are not prepared to reformulate them in such a way as to make this possible. As a result the reliability of these terms remains so low that any attempt use them as a basis for classification is hamstrung from the start.

Sometimes it is possible to use physiological or psychological test results as defining criteria, though usually only as an adjunct to clinical criteria. For instance, a minimum level of 'basal' forearm blood flow of 4ml/100ml/min (Kelly 1966) might be used as a qualifying condition in a study of anxiety states, or a stipulated range of intensity and consistency scores on the Bannister Fransella Grid Test as a qualifying condition in a study of thought-disordered schizophrenics (Bannister and Fransella, 1966). In general opportunities of this sort should always be taken as physiological or psychological tests are likely to be more reliable than purely clinical criteria, if only because they do not depend on subjective or inferential judgements. However it is important to establish the reliability of any test in the circumstances in which it is to be used before deciding to use it. A test that has been shown to be reliable when administered by its originator to student volunteers will not necessarily be reliable when administered by others to chronic schizophrenics. Validity must also be considered. In some circumstances a clinical rating of anxiety may be preferable to physiological measures like palmar skin conductance or forearm electromyography in spite of its comparatively low reliability because it is a direct measure of the variable in question, the subjective experience of anxiety, whereas the others are only indirectly related to it.

Finally, even after adequate means have been found for defining the essential common characteristics of the subjects, attention must be given to two other almost equally important matters: the extent and composition of the population from which subjects with these characteristics will be drawn, and the manner in which they will be drawn—as consecutive cases presenting at a particular facility, or by sampling methods. Both these issues are dealt with in some detail in other chapters. Here it is appropriate only to draw attention to a general problem encountered in all clinical research described so clearly by Feinstein (1964). The members of any given diagnostic category encountered in any given setting will never be an unbiased sample from the universe of all members of that category: they will always tend to be restricted in some way by the characteristics of the limited population from which they were drawn. The range of schizophrenics encountered in any given hospital, for instance, will inevitably be limited by the demographic characteristics of that hospital's catchment population, by the innumerable factors influencing the conditions under which members of that population come to medical attention, by the criteria used by other physicians for referring patients to the hospital, by the criteria for admission of the hospital staff, and so on. This problem can never be overcome completely, even in community studies. The best that can be done is to choose a population, bearing in mind the objects of the study, whose inbuilt biases will not restrict the range of patients to an unacceptable extent, and then describe the composition and define the boundaries of that population clearly and comprehensively.

APPENDIX

The basic statement of Bayes' theorem is:

$$P(d_i/s_j) = \frac{P(d_i) \cdot P(s_j/d_i)}{\sum P(d_k) \cdot P(s_j/d_k)}$$

where

$P(d_i/s_j)$ is the probability that a patient with the constellation of symptoms s_j has the disease d_i

$P(d_i)$ is the probability (or incidence) of the disease d_i in the population under consideration.

$P(s_j/d_i)$ is the incidence of the symptoms s_j in the disease d_i

$P(d_k)$ is the incidence of each disease $1 \to k$ in the population.

and

$P(s_j/d_k)$ is the incidence of the symptoms s_j in each of the diseases $1 \to k$.

REFERENCES

AMERICAN PSYCHIATRIC ASSOCIATION (1952) *Diagnostic and Statistical Manual of Mental Disorders (DSM I)*, Ist. ed., Washington, D.C.

ASH, P. (1949) The reliability of psychiatric diagnoses, *J. abnorm. Soc. Psycho.*, **44**, 272–6.

AUBIN, J. (1967) Classification of the behaviour disorders, *Ann. Rev. Psychol.*, **18**, 373–406.

BANNISTER, D., and FRANSELLA, F. (1966) A grid test of schizophrenic thought disorder, *Brit. J. Soc. Clin. Psychol.*, **5**, 95–102.

BECK, A., WARD C., MENDELSON, M., MOCK, J., and ERBAUGH J. (1961) An inventory for measuring depression, *Arch. gen. Psychiat.*, **4**, 561–71.

BECK, A., WARD, C., MENDELSON, M., MOCK, J., and ERBAUGH, J. (1962) Reliability of psychiatric diagnoses: 2. A Study of Consistency of Clinical Judgements and Ratings, *Amer. J. Psychiat.*, **119**, 351–7.

BURDOCK, E. I., and HARDESTY, A. S. (1969) *Structured Clinical Interview Manual*, New York.

CARNEY, M. W. P., ROTH M., and GARSIDE F. R. (1965) The diagnosis of depressive syndromes and the prediction of E.C.T. response, *Brit. J. Psychiat.*, **111**, 569–674.

FEIGHNER, J. P., ROBINS, E., GUZE, S. B., WOODRUFF, R. A., WINOKUR, G., and MUNOZ, R. (1972) Diagnostic criteria for use in psychiatric research, *Arch. gen. Psychiat.*, **26**, 57–63.

FEINSTEIN, A. R. (1964) Scientific methodology in clinical medicine. 2. Classification of human disease by clinical behaviour, *Ann. Inter. Med.*, **61**, 757–81.

GENERAL REGISTER OFFICE (1965) *International Statistical Classification of Diseases, Injuries and Causes of Death*, Eighth Revision, London, H.M.S.O.

GOLDBERG, D. P. (1972) *The Detection of Psychiatric Illness by Questionnaire*, Maudsley Monograph No. 21, London.

HAMILTON, M. (1960) A rating scale for depression, *J. Neurol. Neurosurg. Psychiat.*, **23**, 56–62.

HEMPEL, C. G. Introduction to problems of taxonomy, in *Field Studies in the Mental Disorders*, ed. Zubin, J., New York, pp. 3–22.

HEYNS, R. W., and LIPPITT, R. (1954) Systematic observational techniques, in *Handbook of Social Psychology*, ed. Lindzey, G., Vol. I, pp. 370–404, Cambridge, Mass.

HORDERN, A., SANDIFER, M. G., GREEN, L. M., and TIMBURY, G. C. (1968) Psychiatric diagnosis: British and North American concordance on stereotypes of mental illness, *Brit. J. Psychiat.*, **114**, 935–44.

HUNT, W. A., WITTSON, C. L., and HUNT, E. B. (1953) A theoretical and practical analysis of the diagnostic process, in *Current Problems in Psychiatric Diagnosis*, ed. Hoch, P. H., and Zubin, J., pp. 53–65, New York.

KELLY, D. H. W. (1966) Measurement of anxiety by forearm blood flow, *Brit. J. Psychiat.*, **112**, 789–98.

KENDELL, R. E. (1968) An important source of bias affecting ratings made by psychiatrists, *J. Psychiat. Res.*, **6**, 135–41.

KENDELL, R. E., COOPER, J. E., GOURLAY, A. J., COPELAND, J. R. M., SHARPE, L., and GURLAND, B. J. (1971) Diagnostic criteria of American and British psychiatrists, *Arch. gen. Psychiat.*, **25**, 123–30.

KREITMAN, N., SAINSBURY, P., MORRISEY, J., TOWERS, J., and SCRIVENER, J. (1961) The reliability of psychiatric assessment: an analysis, *J. men. Sci.*, **107**, 887–908.

LEDLEY, R. S., and LUSTED L. B. (1959) Reasoning foundations of medical diagnosis, *Science*, **130**, 9–21.

LEHMANN, H. E., BAN, T. A., and DONALD, M. (1965) Rating the rater, *Arch. gen. Psychiat.*, **13**, 67–75.

LORR, M., and KLETT, C. J. (1967) *Inpatient Multidimensional Psychiatric Scale*, Palo Alto, California.

MELLOR, C. S. (1970) First rank symptoms of schizophrenia, *Brit. J. Psychiat.*, **117**, 15–23.

MELROSE, J. P., STROEBEL, C. F., and GLUECK, B. S. (1970) Diagnosis of psychopathology using stepwise multiple discriminant analysis, *Comprehens. Psychiat.*, **11**, 43–50.

MENNINGER, K. (1963) *The Vital Balance*, New York.

OVERALL, J. E., and GORHAM, D. R. (1962) The brief psychiatric rating scale, *Psychol. Rept.*, **10**, 799–812.

OVERALL, J. E., and GORHAM, D. R. (1963) A pattern probability model for the classification of psychiatric patients, *Behav. Sci.*, **8**, 108–16.

OVERALL, J. E., and HOLLISTER, L. E. (1964) Computer procedures for psychiatric classification, *J. Amer. med. Ass.*, **187**, 583–8.

RAWNSLEY, K. (1967) An international diagnostic exercise, in *Proceedings of the Fourth World Congress of Psychiatry, Amsterdam*, Excerpta Medica Foundation, Vol. 4, pp. 2683–6.

REID, J. R., and FINESINGER, J. E. (1952) The role of definitions in psychiatry, *Amer. J. Psychiat.*, **109**, 413–20.

ROSENZWEIG, N., WANDENBERG, S. G., MOORE, K., and DUKAY, A., (1961) A study of the reliability of the mental state examination, *Amer. J. Psychiat.*, **117**, 1102–8.

SCADDING, J. G. (1967) Diagnosis: the clinician and the computer, *Lancet*, **ii**, 877–82.

SCHMIDT, H. O., and FONDA, C. P. (1956) The reliability of psychiatric diagnosis: a new look, *J. abnor. soc. Psychol.*, **52**, 262–7.

SILBERMANN, R. M. (1971) *CHAM: A Classification of Psychiatric States*, Amsterdam.

SLETTEN, I. W., ULETT, G., ALTMAN, H., and SUNDERLAND, D. (1970) The Missouri Standard System of Psychiatry, *Arch. gen. Psychiat.*, **23**, 73–79.

SMITH, W. G. (1966) A model for psychiatric diagnosis, *Arch. gen. Psychiat.*, **14**, 521–9.

SPITZER, R. L., and ENDICOTT, J. (1968) Diagno: a computer program for psychiatric diagnosis utilising the differential diagnostic procedure, *Arch. gen. Psychiat.*, **18**, 746–56.

SPITZER, R. L., and ENDICOTT, J. (1969) Diagno II: further developments in a computer program for psychiatric diagnosis, *Amer. J. Psychiat.*, **125**, Jan. Suppl., pp. 12–20.

SPITZER, R. L., ENDICOTT, J., and FLEISS, J. L. (1967) Instruments and recording forms for evaluating psychiatric status and history: rationale, method of development and description, *Comprehens. Psychiat.*, **8**, 321–43.

SPITZER, R. L., ENDICOTT, J., FLEISS, J. L., and COHEN, J. (1970) The psychiatric status schedule: a technique for evaluating psychopathology and impairment in role functioning, *Arch. gen. Psychiat.*, **23**, 41–55.

TAYLOR, J. A. (1953) A personality scale of manifest anxiety, *J. abnorm. soc. Psychol.*, **48**, 285–95.

WING, J. K., COOPER, J. E., and SARTORIUS, N. *Instruction Manual for the Present State Examination and Catego*, in press.

ZUNG, W. K. A self-rating depression scale, *Arch. gen. Psychiat.*, **12**, 63–70.

9

THE USE OF CLINICAL RECORDS IN
RETROSPECTIVE RESEARCH

NORMAN KREITMAN

The terms 'retrospective' and 'prospective' research may be defined in more than one way. Perhaps the most accurate use is to designate as 'retrospective' those inquiries in which we start by observing B and then seek information about a preceding event A; conversely, a prospective study is one which comprises observing A and then following the patient to see if B ensues. In psychiatric research, however, the distinction between the two methods usually devolves upon whether we start our investigation with observations already recorded or collect wholly new data, and it is in this rather looser sense that the term will be used here. It is important to note that the operative word is 'start': it is *not* implied that a retrospective study can always be completed without seeking further information about our patients, and in fact this will often be required.

The retrospective method has come in for a good deal of criticism from experimentally minded statisticians, and many of their strictures have considerable weight. At the same time it is worth noting that a very substantial proportion of research in psychiatry is of the retrospective kind and has led to valuable results. There are also situations in which the retrospective method is the *only* one applicable, and many more in which it is certainly the most practical. We may well start by considering some of these circumstances; practical aspects will be discussed subsequently.

INDICATIONS
PAST EVENTS AND SITUATIONS

Perhaps the most obvious use of retrospective research is when dealing specifically with events now past, or in other words, with history. The period of time covered may range from a few months to a century or more; indeed, it is only limited by the duration for which adequate records have been kept. Studies of this kind are usually concerned with a relationship between some changing clinical feature on the one hand, and, on the other, with a variety of social or administrative factors which might be judged responsible. For example, using the old

Bethlem Hospital records of patients admitted during the nineteenth century and who would now be diagnosed as schizophrenic, Klaf and Hamilton (1961) have shown interesting changes in the content of schizophrenic delusions over that time and have put forward explanations for this. There is still a great deal to be done in determining the effect of booms, slumps, unemployment and war on the incidence and nature of mental illness. 'Historical' studies of this kind verge upon cross-cultural psychiatry, using differences in time rather than of geography to secure specimen cultures. Others relate more to the effects of changing legislation and hospital practice.

In the latter context we may note that this kind of question is nowadays of particular importance. Although most hospitals passed through a major administrative and therapeutic evolution in the mid-1960s, important changes are still going forwards—or perhaps backwards! There have been similar revolutions before, but the ground they gained has often been lost, largely through lack of adequate documentation. Second generations are frequently sceptical of the doctrines of their forbears, and only hard facts can convince them. This is but one of the indications for careful studies of these developments. To illustrate the retrospective method in this connexion we might ask what effect a therapeutic community regime has upon the need for restraint of patients. Indices of the latter are not hard to come by: there is by statute a record kept of all patients forcibly secluded; there are records of the quantities of sedatives ordered by ward sisters; there are often the details given in the nurses' notes—often much more valuable than the doctors' records for obtaining a clear idea of what a patient actually did; there may even be a log book by the hospital maintenance staff of the number of broken windows in the ward. Some of these measures have been used in published studies, and ingenuity may suggest others, but whatever the criteria a demonstration that any such index has systematically reflected changes in ward management would be a most valuable contribution.

A similar approach might well serve in questions such as the effects of community-care methods of treatment on prognosis. More will be said later concerning the actual use of recorded data and about prognostic criteria, but here we may simply note that a comparison of readmission or re-referral figures before and after the introduction of such a scheme could prove a preliminary attack on the problem, though a number of other considerations such as the comparability of the patients would also require attention. Or again, one might be interested to determine whether the apparent enlightenment of psychiatric services has resulted in patients coming earlier for treatment than was formerly the case. The interval between the onset of an illness and the point at which the patient was referred would afford a suitable index. The comparison of such intervals in similar groups of patients seen before and after the introduction of a new policy would again be one method of tackling a most worthwhile project.

Many questions relating to the effects of changing psychiatric practice can also be approached by using hospital statistics. Sometimes these are used alone but usually the value of such data is much enhanced by complementary study of the clinical notes. As an illustration we may note the study by Shepherd (1957) who compared the prognosis of two cohorts of admissions to a county mental hospital for 1931 and 1945; he concluded that changes in hospital policy and the impact of administrative measures contributed more to the better outcome of the later group than did the introduction of specific therapies. There are many studies of a similar kind which will provide further models: those interested should consult the review by Brown (1960) which, though limited to studies of schizophrenia, provides an admirable introduction.

RARITIES

The second situation in which the use of existing data is well-nigh obligatory is that in which we wish to study some unusual phenomenon, such as an uncommon symptom or a rare disease. For straightforward descriptive studies it is usually wise to confine oneself to cases personally observed, but such descriptive accounts with the very limited numbers of patients that the individual worker can collect are becoming less common.

This trend is unfortunate; there is still an important place in research for careful clinical description, especially of uncommon disorders. But establishing any general statement about the phases of a catatonic schizophrenia, the sex ratio in Gerstmann's syndrome or the characteristics of anorexia nervosa in men would almost certainly necessitate looking back into the records of one or more hospitals.

Uncommon variations on otherwise common conditions, such as depressive stupor or the rarer types of specific mental defect form an analogous group. These may be especially valuable by displaying clearly characteristics which are less easy to perceive in more typical cases. 'To study nature we must go to her extremes.'

With only a few cases in the series it is in general misguided to attempt formal statistical tests of hypotheses. It is more profitable to use the data to provide a descriptive account and perhaps as a basis for informed speculation, but occasions may also arise when numerical comparisons are appropriate, especially if some form of reference group can be used. There is no reason against using a larger number of 'controls' than there are 'rare' patients, preferably with each patient matched against several of the control or comparison subjects. A statistician will have valuable guidance to offer on the use of these small-sample techniques.

LONG PERIODS OF TIME

There is another important circumstance in which the retrospective method is invaluable, namely, when we are concerned with the effects of relatively long periods of time. The cardinal example here is in studies of the natural history of illness, and in particular, prognostic follow-up studies. To determine by prospective means the prognostic significance over ten years of, let us say, acute schizophrenic thought disorder would require the resources of a large and securely based institute, a guarantee that no radically different method of treatment would be introduced in the next few decades, a similar guarantee that sufficient new cases will be forthcoming in the future, and the devotion of a saint prepared to wait perhaps twenty or thirty years to amass enough data. This is a formidable list. Most of what has been established about the natural history of psychiatric illness is in fact based on methods which are retrospective in the sense here employed.

Much of what we shall shortly be considering concerning the practical conduct of inquiries which begin with existing data will be applicable to follow-up studies. The subject is a large one, however, and here we can only note the main points. All start with the identification of the patients it is desired to study, and securing their case records. Once this is achieved, one may then proceed to seek additional *documentary* data elsewhere. For example, one way to determine the life expectation in various geriatric disorders would be to consult the death registers in the appropriate districts to determine precisely when the patients died. Such information may be extremely valuable, and enable one to categorize an otherwise mixed group of senile illnesses. In such studies it is important, of course, to choose a group of patients sufficiently far back in time to ensure that a reasonable number will have died in the interim. Parallel uses of the technique might be to determine the number of children seen at a child guidance clinic who subsequently are charged before the courts, or who fail in educational examinations.

If patients discharged from hospital subsequently attended a follow-up clinic or if they maintained contact with their GP's, their progress since departure from hospital can be determined retrospectively from existing medical records. Documentary inquiries of this kind based either on hospital records exclusively or on additional sources of information have certain advantages, especially if applied to clear-cut questions, but are often handicapped by incomplete coverage of the sample or defects in the available records. Commonly, then, it is necessary to establish contact with the patients and to re-examine them; additional documentary information can of course also be used. To those whose interests are chiefly clinical, new contact with a patient is usually the superior approach. From the patient and his family it will be possible to amplify (cautiously) the original account of the illness, to learn how he has fared in the interim, and to examine in detail his clinical state at the time of the interview. This procedure represents a combination of retrospective and prospective techniques and all the advantages of the latter—in particular the systematic collection of specified information based on current examination—are then added to the practical convenience of the former. Most follow-up studies are in fact of this kind. The major difficulty encountered is the fall-out rate due to patients having been lost sight of, or having died, or being otherwise unavailable. There are, however, techniques for dealing with such losses, provided they are not too great (Reid, 1959).

OTHER CONSIDERATIONS

Before concluding this account of the indications for retrospective methods, a few miscellaneous points may be considered. In general the decision about whether to undertake any piece of research is determined by the seriousness of the question asked, the methods available for its solution, and the availability of suitable data and facilities. Any one of these three may act as the generative point, though for some reason it is often thought rather improper to begin with the last one, i.e., with considerations of what lies to hand. But if it is known that the records of a hospital happen to contain interesting data, it may well be rewarding to start from there, so to speak. It could be that a particular hospital is fortunate in enjoying the services of a good non-psychiatric specialist consultant to whom patients are frequently referred and whose observations are systematically recorded in the notes. Or the laboratory or X-ray department may for years have carried out some routine procedure on all new cases (see, for example, the study by Parker et al., 1961). Perhaps the hospital tends to admit a particular type of patient; I am referring not only to units for special disorders, but also to characteristics of the patient population such as an uncommon proportion of coalminers or stockbrokers, or of some particular age group. It may be that the catchment area contains some interesting feature such as a new housing estate or a monastery. If so, provided one is reasonably sure that these points are duly recorded in the records, all sorts of possibilities for research may emerge, and it will often be found that for the reasons already discussed such programmes will usefully and perhaps uniquely be served by the retrospective method.

Lastly, we may note there are many studies in which forward-planned research is hampered by the fact that an investigator in the very act of inquiry alters what he seeks to study. This is particularly true in social investigations, or when assessing the outcome of psychotherapy. In such circumstances a retrospective approach may be a way of overcoming the difficulty.

PRACTICAL ASPECTS

Let us assume that one is about to undertake research based on hospital records. Before one so much as sets foot in the records department of the hospital, one will have carefully considered all the patients one is *not* going to find there, because their absence may have an important effect on the nature of the sample. These 'missing' patients will at least comprise all those people suffering from the disorder but who have failed to consult their general practitioners, or if they have, did not progress to the out-patient department, or if they did, were successfully treated there or died or moved away while under therapy. The remaining patients, then, represent a heavily biased group skewed in the direction of greater severity. This may or may not be a disadvantage. If one wishes to elaborate some aspect of the clinical features of an illness, it will usually be helpful to deal with fully developed cases rather than with mild forms. If, on the other hand, one is interested in determining the frequency with which a particular symptom occurs in a certain disorder, there is a risk of being misled by considering only severe cases, unless it is clear that the study relates only to this category.

In all probability there will be other biases too, such as a preponderance of females and of lower social-class patients, characteristics which seem to apply to most of the diagnostic categories of in-patient admissions. If the hospital has an active community-care programme it will also be true that those admitted differ in still further respects from all those referred (Sainsbury and Grad, 1962).

If these various selective factors are irrelevant to the purpose (or, more likely, are to be regretted but stoically borne in the absence of any other sample) one may proceed to the records department. What is found there will vary enormously according to the quality of the record-keeping traditions of the hospital: the difference between various centres is quite astonishing. At the better hospitals there will no doubt be an index or register of the records, to which one will now apply oneself. Here the next difficulty arises, in that doubts about the completeness of such index lists are only too often justified. It is well worth spending a good deal of time speaking to *all* the personnel involved to enquire *in detail* how the index is compiled: one is often surprisingly ignorant of the administrative machinery operating in one's own area. It is always well to check, for example, that emergency admissions are eventually included, as they may by-pass the usual recording system on arrival. If by any chance it is necessary to use out-patient records, it is particularly important to ensure that all the avenues by which the patient may come to hospital are adequately covered, as are patients seen on domiciliary visits and in general hospitals.

Assuming that the index is reasonably accurate, one will next consider the details recorded therein. Age, sex, date of admission and discharge, and perhaps marital status, will usually be the minimum given. Diagnosis may or may not be recorded, but in either event one would want to examine the records of all patients who *might* fall within the sample in order to confirm the recorded diagnosis, and to correct any misclassified according to the criteria being used in the study. It is evident, then, that one is in a relatively strong position if the sample can be defined, at least initially, in terms of age and sex. Suppose one is interested in involutional melancholia in women. In order to exclude possible misdiagnosis of schizophrenic and senile disorders, it would be desirable on clinical grounds alone to limit the group to first admissions between forty and fifty-five or sixty years of age. By doing so one reaps the additional advantage of being able to use the age and sex data from the index or register as the starting point of the quest for material.

Once one has obtained a list of names or case numbers one may proceed at last to lay hands on the records. It is probable that a number of these are missing. This may seem a trite observation, unless it is borne in mind that such omissions may represent a serious source of bias. It is important to discover just why the notes are not where they should be. Some may have been sent temporarily to another hospital where the patients concerned are currently being treated. If so, the remainder will under-represent those with a poor prognosis or a relapsing course. Sometimes notes are missing for the elementary reason that someone else is using them for his own research. If this is the case, one must discover from the colleague exactly how your interests overlap: at a large hospital this situation can occur not infrequently.

Paradoxically, it is also possible to have more case folders than there should be. In almost all hospitals the records of each admission for any given patient are contained in the same folder. Nevertheless, studies on computer-based record linkage systems have revealed how often a patient is regarded as a new case when in fact he has been admitted previously. This can easily happen if his name permits of variant spellings; for McLauchlan, for example, there are seventeen different versions. Women who change their surnames on marriage may also be unrecognized by the records staff. The final case material must be scrutinized with these dangers in mind, using ancillary data such as date of birth, address and of course the previous clinical history as recorded at each admission.

Occasionally it may be found that although all the different patients are correctly identified the number of separate admissions ascribed to them is based more on administrative than clinical reality. For example, a young patient transferred to the local general hospital for appendicitis or an elderly patient briefly admitted there for treatment of fracture will be usually considered to have been discharged and subsequently readmitted. If questions of the number of admissions per patient over a given interval, or duration of hospital stay, are germane to the enquiry these details will require close attention.

Sometimes one wishes to use only a proportion of the available cases. To do so in an unbiased way means a proper randomizing technique. Of these the simplest is to give the list of names serial numbers and then consult a table of random numbers. Equally simple is to write the name of each patient on a card, shuffle thoroughly and then deal out as many as are required—honestly and from the top of the deck. A third way is to stack the notes along a rack and then to pull out every second or third, repeating if necessary till the numbers are made up. It is not good technique to select by initial letters of surnames, as this may lead to bias by various ethnic groups, nor to use particular months during which the patients were admitted, since many areas are subject to seasonal migration and the migrants may well be atypical.

Extracting the relevant information from the final sample is the next stage. I do not wish to say too much about the reliability of the data recorded since the reader will know how trustworthy are his own hospital procedures better than any outsider, but a few general points are important.

The identifying data will probably be correct. Points to watch are, that foreign names are especially likely to be spelt incorrectly and hence lead to difficulties in genetic studies if other family members are to be traced; that addresses based on the patient's statement will sometimes prove to be inaccurate; that age is subject to the same error, while in older records the date of birth is rarely given, so that accurate determination of age on discharge etc. will not be possible; and that data regarding divorce and cohabitation are often suppressed. Occupational data are usually very sparse and their use presents many difficulties. To use the Registrar General's classification of social class requires considerable detail regarding occupation, and this is rarely available in the notes. The Hall-Jones system (see Glass, 1954) provides an alternative which has the advantage of requiring less precise data, but against this must be set the difficulty of comparing the findings with other studies or with the national statistics published by the Registrar General's Office. Perhaps for these reasons the method has not become popular. Married women in both systems are classified according to their husband's occupation, and since this is often not mentioned in mental hospital records, it is generally wiser not to attempt any formal classification on female samples.

The clinical data which comprise the bulk of the record are more likely to be the focus of attention. The problems that arise here are crucial, and can be grouped into three main categories.

First, there are errors of omission. To read other doctor's clinical notes in quest of some specific item of information is apt to be a heartbreaking experience. One may firmly believe, for example, that retardation is a cardinal feature of depressive states. Try to confirm this by reading through a collection of records of such patients, and it will probably be found that its presence or absence is noted in only a minority of cases. Clearly this can mean (1) that the examiner did not think about the matter at all, or (2) that retardation was present in some degree but that the examiner did not note this for a variety of reasons, or (3) that it was not present. Usually there is no way of deciding between these three possibilities: to be safe one may only take it that a symptom was present or absent where there is a precise statement to that effect.

This difficulty is so prevalent with record data that a number of devices have been worked out to circumvent it. The only one worth mentioning here is to assume that all the doubtful or incomplete cases go against the hypothesis. The applicability of this method to a specific piece of research is best discussed with a statistician.

Secondly, there are what may be termed errors of commission. Here I have in mind those situations in which special attention is paid to certain features of the patient if he happens to fall into some particular category. An example is the question of the role of homosexuality in the paranoid delusions of schizophrenics. The notion that a homosexual basis may exist for persecutory delusions has been current for many years and is familiar to most psychiatrists. One may therefore expect that with a paranoid patient inquiry will be made concerning sexual predisposition, while with non-paranoid schizophrenics the question may not be raised at all. If one is collecting only positive statements, therefore, it may well be possible to report that, say, 60 per cent of a large group of paranoid schizophrenics gave a history of homosexual experience as compared with 10 per cent of a matched group of non-paranoid schizophrenics. The statement would be both strictly accurate and totally misleading. Other examples could be multiplied. Selective reporting is particularly apt to occur in the less formal sections of the examination, such as in descriptions of personality or of parental attitudes in child guidance work.

Bias of this kind is due to the psychiatric education we have received, or the hospital we work in, and may operate in the most subtle ways; remember too that the biases of previous decades were often different from ours. The important point is to be aware at every stage of the possibility of distortion creeping in, and to question almost reflexly each step taken in the investigation. Once the principle has been grasped it should not be difficult to spot whether any such distortions are affecting the argument.

Lastly we must mention, though we cannot solve, the question of the criteria used in the classification of data. Mention has already been made of the need for preliminary diagnostic criteria in terms of age and perhaps sex. A major problem to be faced is whether to accept the diagnosis given in the notes, or to attempt to use the details given in the records to derive a diagnosis based on one's own nosological scheme. One must consider that the doctor who saw the patient at the time was in a much better position to reach a diagnosis, and that at best one can only see the patient through his eyes. Against this must be set the fact that the research criteria may be different, if only because they are designed for some specific purpose, and further, that the records were probably written by many different people, possibly from different hospitals, so that a single diagnostic label may have been applied to a heterogeneous group of patients. Usually the desirability of uniformity will tip the balance in favour of adopting specified criteria, but the question always deserves careful consideration.

It is sometimes difficult to devise a simple yet satisfactory list of diagnostic features, despite the considerable freedom of choice. On the one hand, a detailed list will result in both a small number of cases and in a group so closely defined that the findings are of limited application. A less stringent set of requirements will yield a group of larger size and one from which it is easier to extrapolate to other groups. For example, let us suppose the effects of ECT on depressive illness are being investigated. One might stipulate that the patient should have a positive family history of depression, be of pyknic build, have an extraverted personality which is subject to mood swings, be not less than thirty-five nor over fifty-five, show sadness of mood and depressive affect, with retardation, anorexia and lack of energy, be free of any suspicion of paranoid delusions and have no evidence of physical illness. This will ensure a small—perhaps vanishingly small—homogeneous group of patients, but it would not be possible, logically, to apply the findings regarding treatment to any patient who does not have *all* the features listed. On the other hand the omission of most of

KMP

these characteristics will lead to a larger group, and one can be more confident that the findings will be applicable to the majority of patients usually regarded as having an affective disorder. The decision must always be taken in the context of a particular inquiry, but I would add that progress, in my opinion, is more likely to come from the study of small and carefully described groups. (See CHAPTER 8 for other aspects of diagnostic definition.)

THE USE OF 'MINISTRY CARDS'

Hospitals in the United Kingdom are required by the Government to make returns on standardized forms (MHE in England and Wales, SMR(MH) in Scotland) for all admission, discharges, deaths and transfers. The data which has to be supplied concern identification characteristics, including age and address, the date on which the event occurred, the diagnosis and a number of other items, the details of which vary from year to year (and also between England and Wales, and Scotland), but include matters such as the type of treatment the patient received prior to admission, after-care arrangements and legal status. Data concerning discharge, death and transfers are appended to the information about admission on the same card. Hospital record officers invariably retain a duplicate set of cards.

There thus exists a comprehensive body of data on a number of major variables, systematically collected and available over a number of years. The layout and coding of the data are designed for transfer to machine punch-cards, and it may even be possible, by diligent enquiry, to extract from the authorities (The Department of Health and Social Security or the Scottish Home and Health Department) copies of the punch-cards they have prepared from the information supplied by the hospital. Failing that, the precise coding instructions used by these official bodies can be readily obtained, and the data coded by the investigator. (If others are to assist important questions of confidentiality must be considered.)

This national system of data collection, which is often envied by other countries, has many strengths but some weaknesses (reviewed by Ashley, 1972). From the viewpoint of the individual researcher it is particularly tempting if he has in mind operational research on the way his own hospital functions. Two major defects must however be pointed out. There is firstly the problem of adequate linkage of data relating to events befalling the same individual. Since a reasonable amount of identifying data is available on admission, there are probably only few instances where the discharge data are ascribed to the wrong person. But each new admission leads to the preparation of a new document, and it is sometimes difficult to link together all the epsiodes of care for given individuals. Ambiguities and errors can lead to individuals being recorded as having more or fewer episodes of care than they actually experienced. There is also the problem already noted of purely 'administrative' discharges and readmissions. Secondly, diagnosis is often poorly recorded. Sometimes quite junior clerical staff are entrusted to make this entry, and they may use anything they can find in the case notes or correspondence when no diagnosis is clearly written on the front sheet of the record.

In practice, therefore, studies initially designed to be carried out on the 'cards' will end up with consulting case-note folders. These are laborious to use and unwieldly, and operational studies covering more than a brief period of time which use such a method represent a formidable undertaking. The ultimate answer lies in the establishment of area case registers, or on a more modest scale, in computerized record systems with record-linkage facilities for individual hospitals. Simpler resources may suffice if a particular study is planned in advance, but this takes us out of the present review of retrospective methods.

SPECIAL RECORD SHEETS

It is difficult to conclude without a passing reference to the apparent paradox of considering retrospective studies to be carried out at some time in the future. Quite frequently one becomes interested in a certain type of clinical problem without having any testable hypothesis in mind. In these circumstances we look more closely at our patients. Since we cannot systematically record *everything*, it is important to ensure that for every case certain minimum data are collected; a special sheet in the notes is the best way to do this. If the research is to be carried out in the midst of everyday practice, the number of items noted must be kept small particularly if one has recruited the assistance of colleagues, but there is no reason why some of these items should not be changed from time to time if a new idea should arise. Once a suitable number of cases have been seen, the information can be marshalled with the assurance that on a number of cardinal points the data are precise, relevant, and systematic.

CONCLUSION

It is evident that a retrospective research requires as much care and detailed planning as any other kind of enquiry, and indeed exactly similar principles must be observed. Nevertheless, in execution it is relatively economical in money and time (though no royal road to quick results) and provided due care is paid to the snags awaiting the over-optimistic, can make a useful—and sometimes unique—contribution to psychiatric research.

REFERENCES

ASHLEY, J. S. (1972) Present state of statistics from hospital in-patient data and their use, *Brit. J. prev. soc. Med.*, **26**, 135–47.

BROWN, G. (1960) Length of hospital study and schizophrenia, *Acta psychiat. scand.*, **35**, 414.

GLASS, D. (1954) *Social Mobility in Great Britain*, London.

KLAF, S., and HAMILTON, J. (1961) Schizophrenia—a hundred years ago and today, *J. ment. sci.*, **107**, 819.

PARKER, J., THEILE, A., and APIELBERGER, C. (1961) Frequency of blood types in a homogeneous group of manic-depressive patients. *J. ment. Sci.*, **107**, 936.

REID, D. (1959) Epidemiological Methods in the Study of Mental Disorder. Wld Hlth Org. Publ. Hlth Pap., No. 2, Geneva.

SAINSBURY, P., and GRAD, J. (1962) *The Burden on the Community*, Chapter VI, London.

SHEPHERD, M. (1957) *A Study of the Major Psychoses in an English County*, Maudsley Monographs, No. 3, London.

FURTHER READING

DOLL, R. (1959) Retrospective and prospective studies, in *Medical Surveys and Clinical Trials*, ed. Witts, L. J., London.

10

PSYCHOPHYSIOLOGICAL METHODS IN CLINICAL PSYCHIATRY

M. H. LADER

Psychophysiology uses the techniques of physiology in a psychological context, a typical experiment consisting of the measurement of one or more physiological variables while behavioural factors such as direction of attention or degree of motivation are controlled. Thus, the physiological variable is being studied for its psychological connotations yet that variable is primarily carrying out a physiological function. For example, forearm blood flow increases under conditions of anxiety, either occurring clinically or induced by a stressful situation. Blood flow also increases during and after exercise of that limb but it is naive to conclude from this that exercise is a psychological stress. Consequently, in order to use physiological measures in a psychological framework, the subject must be in conditions of physiological 'neutrality'; in other words, no extra physiological demands must be made on the system under study.

Ethical considerations are important in psychophysiology. It is justifiable to measure arterial blood pressure with an intra-arterial catheter in a patient with heart disease, unjustifiable in psychiatric patients because there is no benefit to the patient and the small risk involved outweighs any possible scientific gain. Many psychophysiological techniques utilize surface electrodes and transducers, and radioactive isotopes are rarely used.

Some techniques are used differently in physiology and psychophysiology. For example, the neurophysiologist concerned with the electrical activity of individual muscle fibres inserts a needle electrode; the psychophysiologist is more interested in the overall activity of a muscle or group of muscles (reflecting 'tension') and uses disc electrodes attached to the skin. Some physiological measures are neglected by physiologists, the prime example being the palmar skin conductance which hardly merits a mention in most textbooks of physiology and yet is the most widely used psychophysiological measure. Furthermore, physiologists usually examine fairly clear phenomena and elicit obvious changes in these measures, e.g. the firing rate of neurones. Psychophysiologists commonly deal with less clear-cut effects which may require statistical evaluation.

In this chapter, the commoner psychophysiological techniques are outlined with the emphasis being on their range of application and usefulness rather than on technical coruscations. Two large source-books exist to which the reader should refer for full technical details: Brown (1967), and Venables and Martin (1967). It is also assumed that the reader will have perused CHAPTER 11, in order to provide himself with some elementary technical background.

AUTONOMIC MEASURES

SWEAT-GLAND ACTIVITY, SKIN CONDUCTANCE AND SKIN POTENTIAL

One direct method of estimating sweat-gland activity is to measure the moisture content of gas passed over an area of skin. Another consists of counting active sweat-glands by using moisture-sensitive papers (such as starch-iodide) on which each active gland is represented by a spot. Although these methods are relatively simple, they are tedious and can provide only intermittent readings.

Electrical methods rely on the fact that the skin is a better conductor of electricity when the sweat-glands are active than when the skin is dry. The measurement technique, though simple in principle, is very liable to artefact (Montagu and Coles, 1966). There are two main methods: in the 'exosomatic' method, a voltage is impressed on the skin and the current which flows is proportional to the conductance; in the 'endosomatic' method the naturally occurring potential differences between two skin sites are amplified and recorded. Skin conductance responses to stimuli are always increases, representing more sweat-gland activity; skin potential responses are usually biphasic. The skin potential measure is also more demanding technically and should only be used under expert guidance.

An additional complication is that until quite recently it was easier to record skin resistance by passing a constant current through the skin, the voltage produced being proportional to the resistance rather than the skin conductance. One is, of course, the reciprocal of the other. However, there is evidence that conductance bears the more direct relationship to sweat-gland activity and even if resistance is measured the reciprocal transformation to conductance is essential before any further analysis (Lykken and Venables, 1972). Abrupt responses to stimuli are generally termed 'galvanic skin responses' (GSR's) and are superimposed on the background skin conductance level [FIGURE 10.1] The GSR reflects an increase in pre-secretory activity of sweat-gland cell membranes.

There are certain essential precautions in recording skin conductance (or resistance):

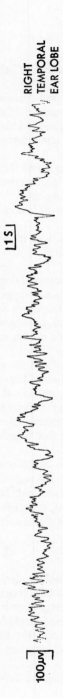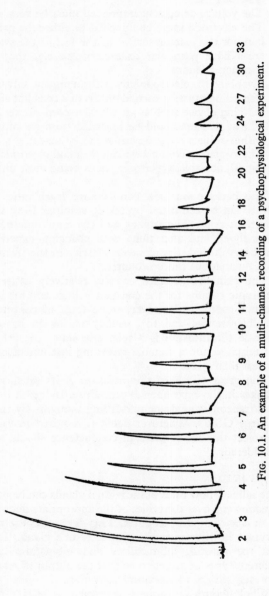

RIGHT
TEMPORAL
EAR LOBE

|1 S|

100μV

Fig. 10.1. An example of a multi-channel recording of a psychophysiological experiment.

1. The electrodes must be non-polarizable, silver–silver chloride being generally used.
2. The voltage or current impressed must be very small and constant.
3. The electrode must be attached to either the palmar surface of the hand or the plantar surface of the feet as the sweat-glands in these areas have particular characteristics, e.g. they are not normally thermoregulatory.
4. Swabbing the electrode sites with an organic solvent is inadvisable.
5. Recording must be carried out from a constant area of skin so that a masking device such as an adhesive corn-plaster must be used.
6. The same site should be recorded from on successive occasions if within-subject comparisons are to be made.
7. The contact medium between skin and electrode should be physiological, abrasive hypertonic jellies being most unsuitable.

The background skin conductance level varies continuously and trends can be estimated by taking readings from the trace at appropriate intervals. The latency and the amplitude of the responses can be analysed and alterations with changing experimental parameters can be evaluated. Spontaneous activity in the tracing also occurs and such fluctuations can be counted.

The skin conductance can be relatively easily measured as the electronic circuits for the constant voltage and the initial amplification are not complex. However, some form of continuous 'write-out' is usually essential and this usually means an ink-writing polygraph. Because the measure is a relatively slow one, a fat pen-response is not required and a suitable recording instrument can be put together for less than £100.

The great virtue of this measure is its sensitivity to quite small changes in the experimental procedure. Indeed it is often too sensitive as extraneous sounds or perturbing thoughts by the subject can lead to large GSR's. Wherever detail is required in following changes in a subject the use of the skin conductance should always be carefully considered.

SALIVATION

The salivary flow rates of individual glands can be measured by placing a suction cup over the orifice of the appropriate duct with a tube leading to an electronic drop-counter. This device has the advantage that it is accurate in measuring the output of one gland. The disadvantage is that the parotid, submaxillary and submandibular glands produce different types of secretion so that the output of one gland may not be representative of whole-mouth salivation.

Whole-mouth salivation is estimated by placing pre-weighed dental rolls in the mouth for a standard time and calculating the saliva secreted by re-weighing the rolls. Three rolls are usually used, being placed in the mouth for 2 minutes. At least three repetitions should be carried out. Care must be taken that the subject has not eaten, drunk or smoked for at least an hour and has been lying quietly with his mouth closed for at least 15 minutes. This method, despite its simplicity, is very useful in practice, especially in studying depressed patients.

HEART RATE

Heart rate is a commonly used measure because it is sensitive to a wide variety of influences. It is easy to monitor because it consists of a series of discrete, identifiable events. Electrocardiography is the most widely available technique and adequate for background levels. Other pulse detectors include a microphone to pick up heart sounds, photoelectric detectors over the finger-tip and pressure transducers attached to the skin over an artery. If finger or forearm blood flow is being recorded, pulse rate can be obtained from the record.

To obtain greater detail, beat-to-beat intervals must be recorded to the nearest 5 or 10 ms. To do this, the pulse signal is converted into an electrical pulse. The time between pulses is displayed in some convenient way and written on a channel of a polygraph from which tracing the beat-to-beat interval can be measured [FIG. 10.1]. This type of display allows the measurement of responses to discrete stimuli. If this amount of detail is unnecessary the pulses can be integrated to give a running average pulse rate.

BLOOD PRESSURE

The only accurate method of measuring blood pressure is to place a catheter containing a pressure transducer into an artery. This is not usually feasible in psychiatric patients for both technical and ethical reasons. The classic method, the sphygmomanometer and arm cuff, can be automated to take readings every thirty seconds or so, the Korotkoff sounds being detected with a microphone over the brachial artery. The obvious drawbacks are the intermittent nature of the readings and the disturbance to the subject.

Systolic pressure alone can be recorded automatically by a small inflated cuff on the finger with a pulse detector sited distally. The cuff is inflated until the pulse disappears, the pressure is then lowered until the pulse reappears and this cycle is repeated giving an estimate of systolic pressure. The technique is suitable for ambulant patients but the cuff must be deflated frequently to restore the circulation.

Because of all these technical problems blood pressure has been relatively unpopular as a psychophysiological measure.

BLOOD FLOW

During the systolic phase of the pulse cycle, inflow into the limb or digit excedes outflow and the part enlarges. During diastole the reverse occurs. The transient increase in digit volume is termed the pulse volume or blood volume pulse. There is a close correspondence between the rate of blood inflow and the pulse volume. Over the long term the blood flow into a limb must equal the outflow but short term variations in limb volume (blood volume) can occur. Thus, by recording the volume of a limb or digit, alterations in volume can be seen upon which are superimposed blood volume changes corresponding to each pulse beat [FIG. 10.1].

There are several ways of measuring the volume changes in a limb or digit. Direct measurement of fluid displacement can be carried out by encasing the part in a rigid container (oncometer) and measuring the volume of the system with a volumetric transducer. Air is usually used as the fluid and, for a digit, the pulse volume changes are so small that high-gain stable amplification is necessary. Alternatively, the girth can be measured with a mercury-in-rubber or other strain-gauge wrapped around the part as changes in circumference usually correlate highly with volume changes. Electrical impedance or photo-electric devices are also commerically available and are convenient although calibration is a problem.

To obtain an absolute measure of blood inflow, venous occlusion plethysmography must be used. A cuff is inflated to a pressure just above venous pressure so that venous return is prevented without imparing arterial inflow. The increase in volume of the limb is then equal to the rate of inflow. This method can be automated but readings cannot be taken more frequently than once every thirty seconds.

There is such a variety of techniques available for measuring different aspects of blood flow that expert advice should always be sought before embarking on the establishment of any blood-flow techniques.

A special form of girth plethysmography is penile plethysmography where a strain-gauge is wrapped around the shaft of the penis and is a sensitive index of sexual arousal.

PUPILLOGRAPHY

Techniques for the measurement of pupil size range from the very expensive with infrared detectors and on-line computer analysis to the simple disc comparison found on many ophthalmoscopes. One simple technique comprises a perspex strip out of one side of which a series of semi-circles of varying sizes is cut. The strip is mounted in a metal tube about 30 cm long in which is housed a small light. The observer places one end of the tube against the subject's face and presses his own face to the other end. He moves the perspex strip up and down in front of the subject's eyes until a semi-circle matches the pupil. This advice yields intermittent readings only but is useful for detecting drug effects.

GASTRO-INTESTINAL FUNCTION

The contents of the stomach can be aspirated via a gastric tube and analysed. Gastric movements can be detected by an inflated balloon on the end of a tube but such a bulky object may itself initiate contractions. The stomach's electrical activity can be recorded using surface electrodes in the left hypochondrium but this technique is relatively untried. The radiosonde pill can detect both pressure and pH and relay the data by telemetry.

SOMATIC MEASURES

RESPIRATION

The most relevant variable for the psychophysiologist is usually minute volume which is the depth of respiration (tidal volume) times the respiratory rate. The former is monitored using a spirometer but this is cumbersome and the subject needs practice in order not to over-breathe. Respiration rate can most conveniently be assessed using a girth plethysmograph around the chest. This technique gives only a semi-quantitative estimate of tidal volume as the pattern of respiration may not be constant. However, using one strain-gauge around the chest and one around the abdomen gives good estimates of both rate and depth of respiration. A simpler way of measuring respiratory rate is to fix a temperature-sensitive device such as a thermistor in the nostril.

Respiration is not only studied in its own right as a useful psychophysiological measure but is often added as an important monitoring variable when cardiovascular measures are being taken.

ELECTROMYOGRAPHY

The most convenient measure of muscle activity is to amplify and integrate the electrical activity of the contracting fibres. There is a linear relationship between the voltage-time integral of the electrical activity and the isometric voluntary tension, *i.e.*, when no movement actually occurs. Any superficial muscle in the body can be recorded from, the most commonly used being the frontalis, neck and forearm muscles.

For each muscle mass, standard electrode placements have been devised. At these sites, the skin is abraded, hypertonic electrode jelly rubbed in and EEG-type electrodes affixed. The muscle-action potentials are amplified using a high-gain AC amplifier, an EEG machine being most suitable. Some form of integration is desirable converting a series of spikes into a relatively smooth tracing [FIGURE 10.1].

The distinction between 'relevant' and 'irrelevant' muscle activity is important, the psychophysiologist usually confining his attention to the latter. Relevant activity refers to EMG activity during necessary movement; irrelevant activity occurs in muscles not directly involved in a task or in maintaining posture, and reflects emotional arousal.

GROSS MOVEMENTS

Limb movements can be assessed by attaching an accelerometer which transduces acceleratory forces into electrical signals which can be amplified and recorded. Finger tremor is a particular application of this technique which has been used in the study of anxiety states and drug effects. Whole body movements may be quantified using ultrasonic waves which are reflected from the subject.

EYE MOVEMENTS

The most commonly used technique relies on the presence of a standing voltage between the front and back of the eye, the corneo-retinal potential. If the eye moves, the potential field also moves and changes in it can be determined by suitably placed electrodes around the orbits. The number of movements, e.g. during REM sleep periods, can be roughly estimated using AC recordings but for accurate quantitative work the technically more difficult DC techniques must be used.

ELECTROENCEPHALOGRAPHY

This technique is more readily available to the psychiatrist than most and has the added advantage that there is usually a highly skilled technician available to help with the recordings. Several textbooks exist which deal with this technique (e.g. Cooper *et al.*, 1969) and the techniques used on psychophysiology are identical in principle with those used clinically. If anything, the recording techniques used in the research context are simpler and many psychophysiologists make one or two channels suffice and do not bother with a full montage of electrodes.

It is in the analysis of the recordings that the clinical and the research applications of the EEG diverge. The clinical electroencephalographer is concerned with abnormal waves and spikes, with phase reversals, etc., all essentially the recognition of abnormal patterns for which visual analysis is sensitive and convenient; the psychophysiologist is searching for empirical correlates with psychological states. As visual analysis, e.g. measuring the percentage time of the record occupied by alpha waves, has proved very limited, sophisticated mathematical analyses using computers have been developed.

The most easily available quantitative technique is the Walter wave analyser which is a device that splits up a ten-second epoch of EEG into its constituent sine-waves, displaying the voltage at each frequency as a vertical deflection on a special pen overwriting the EEG trace [FIG. 10.2]. Many EEG departments have such an instrument and it should certainly be utilized in psychophysiological experiments. Similar analyses can be carried out using digital computers but this is a complex proceeding for experts only.

A simpler method of analysing the EEG is to process it through broad-wave band-pass filters. For example, a filter can be built to pass EEG waves between 7·5 and 13·5 Hz (cycles per second), roughly corresponding to waves of alpha frequency. The output of the filter can be integrated to give a measure of energy in that frequency band.

EVOKED RESPONSES

It has been possible to assess background EEG activity since the 1930s, but only in the last decade or so have techniques become available to measure EEG responses to such discrete stimuli as tones, clicks, light flashes and electric shocks (Regan, 1972). The responses are very small and usually obscured by the background activity. To bring out the response (signal) from the background (noise), the stimulus is repeated and the EEG epochs of, say, 500 ms following each stimulus are added together and finally averaged. Any electrical activity at the scalp which is time-locked to the stimuli builds up, any random background noise cancels out. The averaging is carried out using computer techniques, either a special-purpose small instrument ('computer of average transients', CAT), a small general-purpose laboratory computer, or, less conveniently, a big computer. The EEG technique is essentially the same as for clinical recordings except a non-standard electrode placement such as vertex to ear-lobe is generally used. The wave-form of the averaged evoked response is complex but some components are related to attentional factors, some to level of activation and others to information content of the signal.

A related technique is the 'contingent negative variation' (CNV) or expectancy wave'. A warning stimulus is given followed by a stimulus to which the subject makes a response such as a key-press. After a few trials a steady negative potential can be seen between the two stimuli, terminated by the key-press. To record the CNV, a long time-constant amplifier is essential and averaging techniques must be used to delineate the signal.

Sleep studies have burgeoned recently following the advances in our

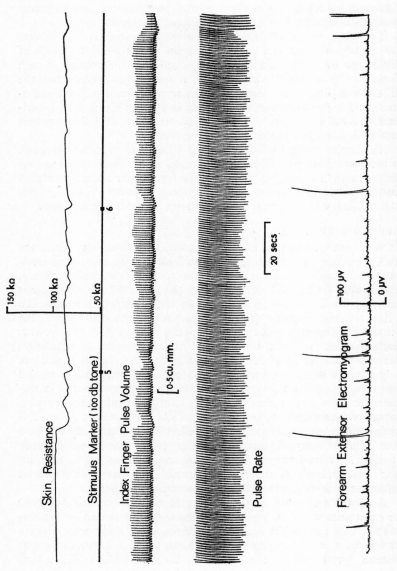

FIG. 10.2. Wave analysis of the EEG. The deflections of the lower pen represent the proportions of energy at each of the frequencies shown. (By courtesy of Dr. M. Driver, EEG Dept., The Maudsley Hospital.)

understanding of this phenomenon and its relevance to psychiatric conditions such as severe depression. A special laboratory is necessary but the EEG techniques are fairly standard. Eye movements and EMG are often recorded as well.

THE RECORDING INSTRUMENT

In the past the 'end-product' of a psychophysiological experiment has almost invariably been a paper tracing on a polygraph. After amplification of the electrical signals picked up by the electrodes or provided by the transducer, the output voltage is fed into a pen oscillograph, the deflection of the pen being proportional to the voltage. Ink-writing pens on ordinary chart paper or heated pens on special heat-sensitive paper are both available, the former being much cheaper but more fiddly to maintain.

The drawback of the polygraph is that its output is 'static' as manual intervention is necessary to extract information from the tracing. This can be unbelievably tedious especially if several measures have been recorded simultaneously. Consequently, in many laboratories, the polygraph has been demoted to being a monitoring instrument while the data is recorded on an instrumentation tape-recorder. This resembles an ordinary audio tape-recorder except it is machined to a higher standard and provision is made for recording low frequencies right down to steady potentials by the use of frequency-modulation. Like an audio tape-recorder, the recordings can be played back and the data retrieved as an electrical signal, *i.e.* in 'dynamic' form. Furthermore, because the recorder has several speeds, recording can take place at a slow speed and playback at a fast one, thus saving a great deal of analysis time. Several channels can be recorded, a running commentary of the experiment placed on a voice-track, and some recorders use $\frac{1}{4}$-inch tape which keeps costs very low.

Most experiments are carried out with leads trailing from the subject who sits or lies in the experimental room. In some cases, especially real-life situations such as in desensitization procedures or when recording from restless subjects, there are advantages in transmitting the recorded variables from the patient to the recording equipment using telemetry. Commercial devices are now available. An alternative technique which has advantages for recording slowly changing variables is for the patient to carry a miniaturized tape-recorder in his pocket.

COMPUTERS IN PSYCHOPHYSIOLOGY

This is a rapidly developing and naturally complex topic. Nevertheless, psychophysiological experiments are particularly appropriate for computer applications because large amounts of data are generated, complicated stimulus parameters required, and complex statistic analyses often essential.

There are several ways in which computer methods can be harnessed to the psychophysiologist's needs. The most obvious method is for the researcher to score his polygraph records, transfer the data onto punched cards and use a central computer as with any data. More direct computer applications require the conversion of the electrical signal, a varying voltage, into digital form, a number. The device which does this is called an analog-to-digital converter which can be programmed to sample the signal at pre-determined intervals, to compute the digital equivalent to that sample voltage and then to leave this value accessible to the rest of the computer for further processing and storage. The simplest digital method is the data logger which consists of an A/D converter and some form of output such as punched paper tape. The paper tape can then be taken to a central computer for analysis. A more direct method, recently available, is the instrumentation coupler which links the central computer directly to the recording equipment via a teletype terminal. The computer is programmed to present stimuli and to take samples via an A/D converter, the data being transferred and stored centrally. However, as it would be uneconomic to use a large computer for one such experiment only, time-sharing is necessary, with several users often with different requirements operating simultaneously. This is a complex procedure and it is not yet clear how practical such a device will be.

Special purpose computers such as the CAT have been used for averaging evoked responses and for several other applications. They are very fast, e.g. they have been used in biophysics, relatively inflexible and the output of data is often clumsy.

General purpose laboratory computers are being increasingly used and provide complete flexibility, rapid and versatile data acquisition and useful computational facilities for statistics, all at a price within the resources of most University Departments. They have the additional advantage of feed-back experiments where the patient's responses are immediately analysed and information relayed back to him. The user has to familiarize himself with the general working of the machine and with the elements of programming but the time and money is amply repaid in both volume and complexity of studies carried out.

CHOICE OF EQUIPMENT

The choice of equipment is so dependent on factors such as funds available, type of research envisaged, previous experience, and local expertise that only general guidelines can be given. One is to explore all possible computer facilities first. Most clinicians and research workers should have access to a computer in the region and to use it one need only learn a simple programming language like Fortran. Usually there will be someone at the computer installation deputed to help the tyro. If computer facilities are available, the obvious choice for the main item of equipment is a data logger which provides a paper tape (or even magnetic tape) output. Monitoring of the measures is still necessary but it is usually sufficient to have a cheap, single channel pen-recorder which can be switched from channel to channel as necessary. If the computer facilities include A/D converters, a transportable instrumentation recorder should be bought which can be carried to the computer and tapes played back. If adequate funding is available, a small general-purpose computer should be sought: it can do almost all a large computer can, much more cheaply and conveniently, and it is always available for the unscheduled experiment, e.g. a patient coming for testing on the wrong day. If no computer facilities are available, manual analysis of polygraph records must be resorted to, but the time necessary for such analyses should not be underestimated.

If little money is available, the budding researcher should scour his hospital, university or laboratory for discarded pieces of equipment. An obsolete EEG machine or old pen recorder can often be pressed back into service after overhaul. Wherever possible equipment should be borrowed from a colleague to ensure its suitability before it is ordered from the manufacturer. It is worth remembering that delivery dates of equpiment may be optimistic.

The local electronic experts should be cultivated as their help is often essential both to advise and to build instruments. Nevertheless, some components such as integrated circuits are now so cheap that it is a mistaken economy to try and build the equivalent out of components.

NEUROENDOCRINOLOGICAL MEASURES

Few psychiatrists would wish to get involved in setting up the complex techniques required for the analysis of hormones in the body fluids. Indeed, some of the techniques are sufficiently onerous and capricious for one laboratory only in a group to undertake them. The biochemistry of the adrenal cortex in particular is very complicated with a wide range of steriods. In this area, the help of the specialized area laboratory should be solicited and work in the psychiatric context carried out in collaboration with them. The following brief account lists the measures which are available.

LMP

ADRENAL CORTEX (JENKINS, 1968).

Cortisol is the main glucocorticoid, corticosterone being secreted in much smaller quantities in man. There is appreciable diurnal variation in plasma cortisol levels so the time of venepuncture must be standardized. The plasma level can be estimated fluorimetrically and, by the administration of a small quantity of radioactively labelled cortisol, the rate of secretion can be estimated. In the urine, techniques are available to measure the 17-oxosteroids, which are derived from androgens as well as cortisol, and the 17-oxogenic steroids which are metabolites of cortisol.

The assessment of pituitary-adrenal function can be carried out: (a) by injecting ACTH to stimulate the adrenal cortex; (b) by administering metyrapone which inhibits the synthesis of cortisol, thus stimulating ACTH production and in turn the cortisol precursor, 11-deoxycortisol; and (c) by giving large doses of a synthetic glucocorticoid such as dexamethasone which suppresses ACTH secretion and hence plasma cortisol levels.

Aldosterone plasma levels and rate of production can be measured but the techniques are highly specialized.

ADRENOMEDULLARY FUNCTION

Both biological and chemical methods exist for the estimation of adrenaline and noradrenaline in the plasma, the latter methods being more convenient but a little less specific. Small quantities of catecholamines are excreted unchanged in the urine where they can be estimated giving a semi-quantitative time-integral of catecholamine production (Levi, 1972).

THYROID FUNCTION

The level of circulating thyroid hormones is estimated by analysing the protein-bound iodine in the plasma. The functioning of the thyroid gland is assessed using the radioactive iodine uptake test.

STIMULATION PROCEDURES

Firstly, it must be decided whether any stimulation procedures will be used or whether 'resting', background measures are sufficient. It must be remembered that the experimental situation, such as the attachment of electrodes, itself acts as a stimulus. Repeated sessions may be necessary for the patients, especially anxious ones, to acclimatize to the procedures.

An alternative approach is to attempt to relax the individuals either spontaneously or by administering a sedative. The changes with the onset of sedation are then quantified.

Most stimuli used in psychophysiological studies fall into one of the following categories: (a) physical, e.g. electric shocks; (b) physiological, e.g. injection of ACTH; (c) pharmacological, such as the injection of methacholine; (d) behavioural, as in carrying out mental arithmetic; and (e) psychiatric, e.g. a psychotherapeutic interview.

EXPERIMENTAL STRATEGY

This is the nub of a research project and follows from the 'natural history' of the problem under study. Often a chance clinical observation will seem sufficiently important for it to be formulated as a testable hypothesis or for more systematic observations to be worthwhile gathering in a standardized laboratory situation. The physiological measure may require estimation as a direct index, e.g. how altered is the cardiovascular system in anorexia nervosa ? This use of the measures is unexceptionable and straightforward.

The problems arise when the physiological measures are used as concomitants of psychological functioning, e.g. plasma cortisol levels as an index of 'stress' or skin conductance as a measure of 'arousal'. The relevance of such indices to psychiatric problems has to be established empirically. Even so, it is always worth searching for psychiatric phenomena which promise to have some relationship to physiological measures, for example, psychomotor retardation in depression.

The adequate provision of controls is a major problem. In one approach, a group of patients, putatively homogeneous for some feature such as acute paranoid schizophrenia, is compared with a group of normal control subjects, matched for a series of factors such as age and sex. Or non-psychiatric patients in hospital for, say, orthopaedic conditions, can be used as controls. Thirdly, psychiatric patients lacking the feature of interest may be used. The more control groups, the more likely the research worker is to detect genuine physiological concomitants to the psychiatric feature of interest.

An alternative approach is to use patients as their own control, for example, before and after recovery. However, the treatment itself may affect the measure so that one cannot tell whether changes in that measure are due to the treatment or to the recovery.

Normal subjects can be used if the feature of interest, e.g. anger, is believed to be elicitable in normals and to be only quantitatively and not qualitatively different from that feature in patients.

A particular current problem is that most patients are receiving some form of treatment. As many psychotropic drugs have physiological effects, e.g. on the autonomic system, drug-free patients should be used wherever possible despite this prolonging the study.

Admission to hospital acts as a stress in most patients and produces alterations in many measures, e.g. a rise in plasma cortisol levels. Patients should be left for a few days before testing providing treatment is not being deliberately withheld.

CONCLUSIONS

As with any research in which expensive equipment is involved, problems of cost colour all the scientific solutions to the experimental questions which are asked. Access to a fully equipped laboratory changes the question 'What can I do ? 'to 'What shall I do ?'. Nevertheless, if a problem is worth tackling, it is worth tackling thoroughly because otherwise the germ of orginality in the idea for the experiment will be wasted by inadequate methods. Advice should be sought, firstly, regarding whom one should ask for advice: as techniques become more and more complex and expensive, few people will have had the opportunity to assess these techniques in detail. Secondly, when approaching the appropriate expert, it always helps to have some smattering of the subject so that a dialogue results. The purpose of this chapter is to provide that background for clinical psychophysiology. Nevertheless, the worth of the project really depends on the soundness of the basic ideas and these should be based on unbiassed clinical observation.

REFERENCES

BROWN, C. C. (1967) *Methods in Psychophysiology*, Baltimore.

COOPER, R., OSSELTON, J. W., and SHAW, J. C. (1969) *EEG Technology*, London.

JENKINS, J. S. (1968) *An Introduction to Biochemical Aspects of the Adrenal Cortex*, London.

LEVI, L. (1972) Stress and distress in response to psychosocial stimuli, *Acta med. scand.*, Suppl. 528, 1–166.

LYKKEN, D. T., and VENABLES, P. H. (1972) Direct measurement of skin conductance: a proposal for standardization, *Psychophysiology*, 8, 656–72.

MONTAGU, J. D., and COLES, E. M. (1966) Mechanism and measurement of the galvanic skin response, *Psychol. Bull.*, 65, 261–79.

REGAN, D. (1972) *Evoked Potentials in Psychology, Sensory Physiology, and Clinical Medicine*, London.

VENABLES, P. H., and MARTIN, I. eds. (1967) *A Manual of Psychophysiological Methods*, Amsterdam.

11

MEASURING AND RECORDING
PHYSIOLOGICAL VARIABLES

J. C. SHAW

The increasing interest in the phsyiological correlates of mental states has resulted in the greater use of measuring and recording apparatus in psychiatric research (Graham, 1971; Venables, 1971). Apparatus suitable for most physiological measurements is available commercially, but often it must be specially constructed, or equipment that has been made for another purpose must be used. In any case it will probably be necessary to seek the help of a technician, engineer, or physicist to get the system operating satisfactorily. These people often find it difficult to get doctors to give a definite specification of the apparatus that they require, and frequently an attempt to tie them down results in requests for too wide a range of facilities. In this chapter, the principles of measuring and recording physiological variables are discussed in a way which is aimed to help the researcher specify his requirements and understand the apparatus designer's problems. Particular techniques or apparatus will not be described because this would require detailed technical knowledge and this information can be obtained from appropriate handbooks, e.g. Venables and Martin (1967), Geddes and Baker (1968), Greenfield and Sternback (1972).

A physiological response manifests itself as a physical change and it is this change that any measuring apparatus is required to record. The changes it is commonly required to measure are of pressure, volume, temperature, displacement, and electrical activity, though there are many others. The most convenient way of measuring them, if a permanent record is required, is by electronic or electrical apparatus. The main feature of the apparatus is that it converts the physical variable to an electrical one which is then amplified and applied to a recorder. The variable quantity is usually termed a signal when its temporal variation is of interest. The apparatus amplifying, recording, or otherwise modifying the signal is referred to as a measuring channel. Thus four variables will require four channels, though each of these may have differing characteristics.

To understand something about the characteristics of a measuring channel it is necessary to know something about the following three elements: the transducer, amplifier, and display unit.

The transducer converts the physical change to an electric change which can be processed by the remaining elements. Usually the temporal variation of the electrical change will follow in a linear manner that of the physical variable. Ways in which this linear relationship does not hold will be discussed later. In the case where the physical variable to be measured is already in the form of an electrical signal, as with the electroencephalograph (EEG) or electromyogram (EMG), the subject is connected to the apparatus by electrodes; the electrodes are then included within the class of transducers.

An amplifier controls, and where necessary increases, the sensitivity of the system. If high sensitivity is required, an amplifier will have several stages of amplification and the means for controlling the amplification or other properties of the system may be sited between stages.

The display unit enables the amplified signals to be observed. It may consist of either a simple meter having a scale and pointer, a cathode ray oscilloscope (CRO), or, more usually, a recorder so that one or more signals can be graphed. The recorder may be of the ink writing type in which case the variable is graphed directly on a moving chart, or of the indirect writing kind which requires a camera to film the graph appearing on the cathode ray oscilloscope screen.

Electrical measuring and recording systems have several advantages:

1. Any physical variable may be converted to an electrical signal having a similar temporal variation.
2. Electrical recorders having several channels are readily available. For example, EEG and electrocardiograph (ECG) recorders may be used for recording quite different variables. The characteristics of these two types of apparatus differ, however, in a way that will be discussed later. This is why it is necessary to have some understanding of the characteristics of measuring apparatus and be able to specify the characteristics of the signal to be measured so that the apparatus and signal may be correctly matched.
3. The characteristics of an electrical system are relatively easily controlled.
4. Electrical signals can be quantified in a number of ways.

In recent years there have been three main developments in the design of apparatus suitable for physiological measurement. Firstly, the use of transistorized and integrated circuits has resulted in smaller and more reliable instruments. Secondly, modular systems of construction have been introduced. This means that each functional unit of a measuring system—amplifier, stimulator, integrator, etc., is constructed as a separate unit which is fitted into a main frame designed to take many such units. The main frame may have some facilities common to all units, for example power supplies. The advantages of a modular system are that the modules can be changed to match a particular investigation, faulty modules can be rapidly replaced, and a modest system can be extended as finance becomes available. Several physiological measurement systems using this principle are available commercially.

The third change is the introduction of digital methods of measurement and display, whereas previously only analogue methods were used. These new methods are usually associated with general purpose digital computers, but are also used for devices designed for more specific applications. Thus the familiar electric meter consisting of a scale and pointer, i.e. an analog system, is being replaced by digital indicators which display the measured value as numerals.

Electrical measuring systems are costly; and they require a certain degree of expertise to make them work efficiently. So there are also practical and economic reasons why the research worker needs to grasp the principles of electronic recording.

SPECIFYING THE SIGNAL

The properties of the signal to be measured may be very simple—the number of times a particular feature occurs, for example. However, if the signal has to be amplified and displayed first, more detailed properties of the signal must be taken into account. The processing must be done with apparatus having 'hi-fi' characteristics, otherwise the properties to be detected will be distorted or eliminated. Therefore it is necessary to specify certain properties of the signal to be measured so that the apparatus with suitable characteristics may be chosen.

The signals are variations of amplitude with time and they can have a variety of different forms, but they usually consist of fluctuations of amplitude on either side of a mean value. This mean value is usually zero, but even when it is not the characteristic of the apparatus may make it so. This is because most apparatuses are designed to respond to fluctuations of amplitude rather than to steady amplitude values. It is easier to make apparatus in this way when the sensitivity required is large. In many instances the recorded patterns defy description since no part of the graph exactly matches another, the EMG for example. In other cases, such as the finger pulsatile volume change, a regular pattern is present which varies only in amplitude and perhaps in cycle time. The form differs nevertheless from other regular patterns such as the ECG. Another point illustrated by these examples is that with the EMG many waves of the pattern occur in one second of time but the finger volume change is much slower, just over one cycle of the change occurring in a second. The frequency of amplitude fluctuation in the EMG is much faster than with the other variables.

Patterns of this kind may be quantified and described in a number of ways (Cooper *et al.*, 1974); one is of particular value—harmonic or frequency analysis, also known as Fourier series analysis.

Any kind of measurement is done by reference to a unit of measure appropriate to the particular property of interest. Thus height is always measured in terms of a unit of length, weight in terms of a unit of weight, and so on. Similarly the complex waveforms usually present in physiological signals may be measured in terms of a unit of waveform. The unit waveform commonly used is called a sine wave. It is a continuous amplitude fluctuation with a shape that can be mathematically defined. Unlike the more familiar units, it has three parameters instead of one. These are amplitude, frequency, and phase, and are illustrated in FIG. 11.1 (*a*), which shows one cycle of a sine wave. Amplitude is the magnitude from the baseline to a peak or trough of the wave. The peak-to-trough (sometimes called peak-to-peak) amplitude is just double this. Frequency is the number of complete cycles of the wave that occur in one second—measured in cycles per second or Hertz (Hz).

Phase is a more difficult concept. If a point on the base line is

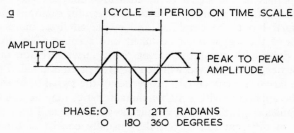

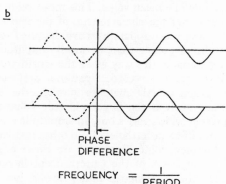

FIG. 11.1. (*a*) The sine wave and its parameters.
(*b*) Two sine waves having the same frequency,
but differing in phase by 45° ($\pi/4$ radians).

designated as zero time, the phase of the sine wave is that proportion of the period of the wave preceding it. Phase is measured in units of angle, the period of the wave being scaled as 360 degrees (2π radians) as in FIG. 11.1 (a). In FIG. 11.1 (b) the sine wave at (i) has zero phase, that at (ii) has a phase of 45° ($\pi/4$ radians). This is also the phase difference between these two waves. Phase difference expressed in this way is a constant for any particular pair of waveforms. If two waves are of differing frequency, their phase difference cannot be specified, only the phase of each individual wave is measurable. Similarly phase difference may be measured for two complex waves having identical shape and frequency, but cannot describe the relation between complex waves which differ in either shape or frequency.

Harmonic analysis is best understood by considering its inverse—harmonic synthesis. If sine waves differing in frequency are added together, more complex waves result whose shape depends on the amplitude and phase of the components. A familiar example is a musical chord. The chord of C major is a complex sound made up of the separate pure tones of the notes C, E, G, and C. Another example is shown in FIG. 11.2, the synthesis of a finger volume pulse wave.

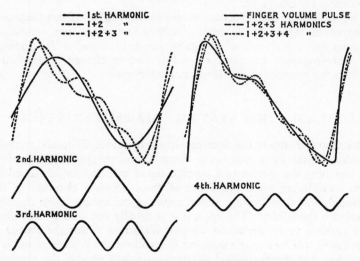

FIG. 11.2. Synthesis of one cycle of a finger pulse volume wave by addition of a number of component sine waves.

Note that the slowest component has one cycle in the time interval of the resultant signal—it is called the fundamental or first harmonic. Other components have frequencies which are integral multiples of this fundamental and are said to be the first, second, third harmonics, etc. Harmonic analysis is just the inverse of this—given a complex waveform, the harmonic components are found. There are many ways of doing this; by manual measurement (Manley, 1950) or by the use of electronic wave analysers or digital computers. It is not meant to imply that harmonic analysis has to be carried out on every physiological signal being measured. It is introduced here to give some insight into what features of signals are important in determining how they are to be measured.

The sine wave components of a given length of signal, e.g. EMG trace can be found. Whilst these components may differ in amplitude, frequency and phase from those required to synthesize another part of the trace, it can be shown experimentally that the component frequencies of EMG traces will always lie within a certain range of frequencies. Similarly, the patterns of other physiological variables will have a range of frequencies from which they can be synthesized, the range depending on the form of the variation. This does not mean that a particular range of frequencies is unique for a particular variable. For example, the range of component frequencies of the EEG overlap those of the EMG at one end of the scale and of the finger pulsatile volume at the other end.

Signals having many fluctuations per second will have faster frequency components than signals having only a few waves per second. It follows that a high rate of change of amplitude signifies the presence of fast frequency components, a low rate of change of amplitude reflects the presence of slow frequency components.

MEASURING SYSTEM CHARACTERISTICS

The characteristics of the elements—transducer, amplifier, and recorder —which make up a measuring channel, and the problems involved in matching the system to a specific signal will now be discussed by first considering some properties of these separate elements of the channel, and then looking at the result of connecting them together and with the subject. The apparatus is usually required to reproduce the variable to be measured without distortion. Thus the record of the EMG will be a graph showing fluctuations about a mean and it is required that these graphed fluctuations follow exactly the temporal variation of electrical activity of the muscle being measured.

The first requirement for accurate reproduction of a signal is that the apparatus has sufficient sensitivity to measure all the important features of the variable. Unfortunately, if a high sensitivity is asked for the complexity and cost of the apparatus will increase, its reliability may decrease and the apparatus may be sensitive to interference signals.

One should therefore avoid specifying high sensitivity simply to cover up ignorance about the details of the signal which determines this.

The second requirement is that if the element, e.g. amplifier, of a measuring channel is to reproduce faithfully a given signal, it must have the same effect on all the frequencies in the range from which the pattern could be synthesized. We have seen how the rate of change of amplitude of a signal depends on its frequency components, so the elements must have a sensitivity independent of the rates of change of amplitude appearing in the signal. We have to know about this because different kinds of apparatus are selective to different ranges of frequency.

You could not, for example, use an electroencephalograph recorder to record accurately the electromyogram pattern. This is because the frequency components of the EEG are all below 100 Hz whereas those of the EMG are in the range 40–1,000 Hz. The pen recorders of the EEG machine will not respond to these rapid frequencies. However, some indication of EMG activity will be recorded on an EEG machine, because the components between 40 and 100 Hz will be reproduced, and this may be sufficient for many purposes, provided it is realized that these components may not represent the whole picture. This dependence of sensitivity on frequency is most easily illustrated by means of frequency response characteristics, and a typical one for an amplifier is shown in FIG. 11.3. It is seen that the sensitivity is constant for a certain range of frequencies and decreases for frequencies above and below this range. The range of frequencies between those for

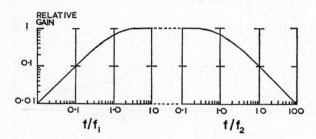

FIG. 11.3. A typical frequency response characteristic. The abscissa represents the ratio of frequency at which the gain is 0·707 of its maximum value.

which the sensitivity is 0·707 of its maximum value is known as the band width or pass band of the amplifier, and will be different for different types of amplifier.

The frequency response characteristic is measured by applying a signal of constant amplitude, varying its frequency, and noting the amplitude of output. The ratio of output to input of an amplifier or other element of the system is called the sensitivity, scale factor, or gain of the element. Sometimes it is less than 1 and may then be called the attenuation factor.

The frequency response characteristic is a measure of what is called the steady state response, and this is most useful for understanding the way in which the apparatus responds to continuous signals. There is another type of characteristic which is complementary to it and which is sometimes even more useful. This is called the transient response; it shows how the element responds to a sudden change in signal amplitude. As an example of this if the bob of a stationery pendulum is suddenly struck, it will oscillate several times before coming to rest again. This oscillatory motion does not follow a continuously applied force having a similar temporal variation, but is something which continues after the initiating force ceases. This is the transient response and we see it is a response determined by the pendulum rather than the disturbance applied to it. The period of oscillation of the pendulum is independent of the size of the force which initially disturbed it.

The importance of this can be illustrated by a specific example—the recording of the skin resistance response (srr) to a sudden stimulus using a recording galvanometer. The latter is a simple recorder consisting of a voltage- or current-sensitive meter which marks continuously on a chart driven by a clockwork or electric motor. Typical srr responses are shown in Fig. 11.4.

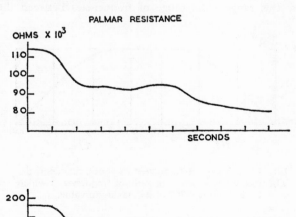

FIG. 11.4. Two examples of the skin resistance response.

To record this change faithfully the recorder must be able to deflect its pen at least as rapidly. In fact it may be shown that the instrument must be able to respond more rapidly than this for the change to be accurately reproduced. This is illustrated in FIG. 11.5 in which the lower trace of each pair shows three types of transient change applied to a recording instrument. The upper traces show the response of the instrument to these changes. The first change applied is a very abrupt one, an almost instantaneous change from one level to another. The recorder is seen

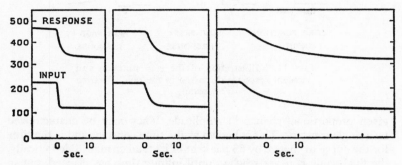

FIG. 11.5. The transient response of a recording galvanometer. See text for explanation.

to respond with a slower change of exponential shape. The next two traces are of exponential changes of increasing duration applied to the instrument, and only in the third trace does the response reproduce the input with reasonable accuracy. Even then there is a small time delay before the response starts to follow the input.

The transient response of a system or element is usually measured by instantaneously changing the amplitude of an input signal from zero to a value which is then maintained. This type of signal is called a step function. Two common forms of transient response are shown in FIG. 11.6. The element whose response is illustrated is represented by a box. (This is known as a block diagram and is a method of representation frequently used where functional properties, as distinct from the details of construction, are of interest. The block diagram of a complete channel or system would contain many boxes, one for each element, connected by lines showing the direction of signal flow.) It is seen that in one type of transient response the output follows the input immediately, but when the latter has taken up its new steady value the former returns to its original value. In the second type the output takes time to reach a new steady value. In both cases the shape of the curve is an exponential one. Exponential curves may differ in the duration of a

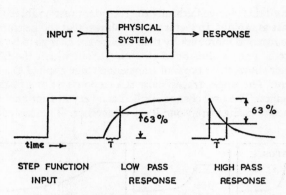

STEP FUNCTION   LOW PASS   HIGH PASS
INPUT   RESPONSE   RESPONSE

FIG. 11.6. Illustration of the step function and transient response discussed in the text. T = time constant.

given proportional change in amplitude. They may be characterized by a single constant. This is known as the time constant and is the time for the curve to change by 63 per cent of its total change. Theoretically, the final value is never reached until infinite time has elapsed, but in practice this is taken as about four times the time constant.

The term 'time constant' also gives information about the steady state response to which the transient response is complementary. Some elements have a frequency response characteristic similar to the right half of FIG. 11.3. Their sensitivity is constant for all frequencies up to a certain value, when it decreases as shown. These are said to have a 'low pass' characteristic, and have a transient response like the one labelled 'low pass' in FIG. 11.6. The time constant of such a unit gives the time for a 63 per cent change in the transient response and is also equal to the reciprocal of 2π times the frequency at which the sensitivity falls to 0·707 of the maximum. The 'high pass' transient response similarly corresponds to a system having a steady state response as in the left half of FIG. 11.4.

There is another important characteristic which gives further information about the frequency-dependent properties of the elements of a measuring system and which is complementary to the characteristics so far discussed. This is called the phase characteristic and is best understood with reference to the steady state response, which, as indicated above, is measured by applying an input of constant amplitude but varying frequency. Outside a certain range of frequencies the amplitude of the output changes as shown in FIG. 11.3. When this happens there is also a phase change between the input and the output. That is to say, for a given frequency the peaks of the output waves do not occur at the same time instants as the peaks of the input waves. Phase characteristics are shown in FIG. 11.7; the curve corresponding to a low pass system shows that peaks of the output waves are delayed in time behind those of the input, and is then said to have a lag phase characteristic. The high pass curve shows a phase advance and is said to have a leading phase characteristic. These are measured using sine waves, so that the input and output will be of identical shape, but at any instant different parts of the sine waves coincide.

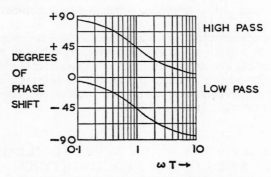

FIG. 11.7. A typical phase characteristic. T = time constant. $\omega = 2\pi f$, where f = frequency.

The result of having a large phase shift is that output waves will not be recorded in the correct time relation to input waves. Furthermore, because of the dependence of phase on frequency, the shape of the complex wave may be distorted if it has components in the range for which phase is dependent on frequency. The use of elements with suitable phase characteristics is also necessary even when the time of occurrence of events rather than correct amplitude is required. From FIGS. 11.3 and 11.7 it is seen that for a signal frequency of the order of $1/2\pi T$ the phase shift is of the order of $\frac{1}{8}$ cycle. The shift might be a second or more in the case of a respiration signal and would be a serious error in an experiment designed to measure whether a voluntary movement occurred at a particular moment of the respiratory cycle. One would have to ensure that the system had a time constant T such that the frequency of respiration is several times less than $1/2\pi T$ for a low pass system, or several times greater if a high pass system was used.

There are other ways in which the response of a system or its elements may depend on frequency or in which it may respond to a sudden input change. Some electrical systems have a steady state characteristic with a markedly increased sensitivity around a particular frequency. They behave rather like the pendulum in that a transient input will result in an oscillatory response. A mechanical example is the following. The overnight restlessness of a patient may be measured by hanging a pedometer from the bed to record the number of movements during the night. To increase the sensitivity the pedometer is hung from a spring. Such an arrangement has an oscillatory transient response so that the pedometer may record several counts following one heavy movement of the patient. Characteristics of this kind will obviously tend to produce severe distortion, although they sometimes have their uses.

The type of characteristic such a system will have depends on aspects of design with which we cannot deal here. Suffice it to say that all practical systems may be classified into a small number of groups whose characteristics may be specified by suitable mathematical expressions which will give information about their steady state, transient, and phase characteristics (Trimmer, 1950).

WHAT HAPPENS WHEN SEVERAL ELEMENTS ARE CONNECTED TOGETHER

Some of the properties of the elements of a measuring channel have been examined but the aim is to know the characteristics of the complete channel made by connecting together several of these units. When two or more elements of a measuring channel are linked, interaction between them may affect the characteristics of the whole in several ways. (i) The range over which the sensitivity of the channel is independent of signal frequency will be altered and may only be that of the elements of smallest band width. (ii) The transient response will also be affected so that the time constant is altered. (iii) When elements having similar high pass time constants are connected together, the transient response may then become oscillatory. As an example consider a system designed to measure tremor in a finger, or limb. The experimenter will be interested in low frequencies, and will need a transducer and amplifier responsive at frequencies down to 2 Hz or less. A suitable amplifier for these frequencies would be one with high pass characteristics having a time constant of 0·3 seconds. If a transducer is chosen that also has a high pass time constant of 0·3 seconds then individually each element will have a sensitivity at 2 c/s which is 93 per cent of the maximum. The sensitivity of the linked system at this frequency, however, would be 86 per cent of the maximum, and the time constant 0·15 seconds. The combined unit therefore has appreciably less sensitivity, and a lower time constant. Moreover, its transient response will also have a low-amplitude oscillatory wave with a period of about 2 seconds which might be mistaken for part of the tremor pattern. To avoid this latter difficulty, one of the elements would have to have a time constant very much longer than 0·3 seconds.

(iv) The phase characteristic of the overall system is found by adding together the phase shifts of the individual stages at each frequency.

(v) One unit may 'load' another unit so that the combined characteristics are not a simple function of the two separate ones. For example, the gain of an amplifier having two separate amplifying stages might be expected to be the product of the stage gains, but the loading effect may make it less than this. A transducer may also load the subject in such a way that the variable to be measured may be altered. This effect is dependent on how much energy a unit extracts from the preceding unit (or subject) to which it is connected. The following examples may help to clarify this.

Consider again the measurement of palmar skin resistance as an indicator of autonomic response. The current flowing in an electrical conductor is proportional to the applied electromotive force and inversely proportional to the resistance of the conductor (Ohm's law). Biological tissue is an electrical conductor, so if a battery is connected to the palm of the hand, a current will flow and may be indicated by a meter connected in the circuit. A change in the palmar resistance resulting from an autonomic response will then be indicated as a change of current. But a meter itself has resistance so that the current indicated will be lower than that due to the palmar resistance alone. Thus for the meter to have a negligible effect on the current to be measured, its resistance must be extremely small compared with the resistance of the circuit in which it is placed. The resistance a measuring device presents to a circuit to which it is connected is called its input resistance. The effective resistance of the circuit to which it is connected is called its output or source resistance—'effective' resistance, because in a more complex circuit this resistance may be due to the combined effect of several components. The proper understanding of these terms requires a knowledge of simple electric circuit theory (Hill, 1973; Donaldson, 1958a).

With the palmar resistance measurement previously mentioned, the input resistance of the measuring device must be much smaller than the output or source resistance of the circuit being measured.

A changing current has a stimulating effect on the skin, however (Rothman, 1954). This can be avoided by keeping the current through the palm small and constant. In this case the voltage across the palm is measured. By Ohm's law it will be proportional to the palmar resistance. The voltage measuring device—which may be a simple meter or a more complicated system having an amplifier and a recorder—will now be connected in parallel with the palm. Since we wish to keep the palmar current constant, only a negligibly small current must be deflected through the measuring device, though it must receive some energy from the circuit it is measuring if the instrument is to function. In this case the input resistance of the measuring instrument must be much larger than the output or source resistance of the source of variation to which it is connected. This example has been used to illustrate a general principle, although it is not necessarily the preferred method of srr measurement (Lykken and Venables, 1971). Whenever two elements of a channel are connected together, or connection is made to the subject, there must be a negligible interchange of energy. Otherwise the characteristics will be altered, sensitivity will be reduced, and indicated values will not truly represent actual values. We see that to avoid any alteration of characteristics when voltage is the variable of interest, the input resistance of the measuring instrument must be larger than the source resistance of the variable to be measured, and vice versa when current is of interest.

The term impedance is often used in this context in place of resistance. This is a more general term which applies to other ways in which electrical circuits may interact and which may also apply to systems which are not electrical. Consider again the measurement of changes in finger volume. As far as the physical variables are concerned, the finger may be regarded as an elastic mass in which are vessels containing fluid. The pressure changes in the vessels cause them to expand and contract, resulting in parallel changes in volume of the whole finger. Now suppose we enclose the finger in a rigid sealed container or cup. If it surrounds the finger without any air space, then the finger can no longer change in volume; if there is a small air space, the finger can increase its volume but the resultant increase in pressure in the cup will prevent the finger volume change being as great as if the finger was unrestricted. For the finger volume change to be unaffected by the cup, the air space must be large enough for the increase in air pressure to have an insignificant effect. The volume change may be converted to an electrical change by a suitable mechano-electrical transducer. This could be a metal diaphragm in the end of the cup which is displaced by the change in volume and in doing so alters some parameter of an electrical circuit. The force required to move the diaphragm is produced by an increase in pressure in the air contained in the cup due to a change in its volume. From the above account it is apparent that this volume change must be small. The diaphragm must therefore respond to a very small force.

If, in fact, the air space was made small enough and the diaphragm stiff enough to prevent changes in volume of the finger, the transducer would measure force which would be proportional to the pressure in the vessels in the finger, i.e., blood pressure. For volume measurement the transducer must present a low impedance and for pressure change a high impedance to the source of the variable to be measured. An exact analysis of the transducers can be carried out using the same techniques as those used for electrical circuits by converting mechanical variables to their electrical analogues (Johnson, 1944; Machin, 1958; Burger, 1957; Geddes and Baker, 1968).

SOME TYPES OF SIGNAL MEASUREMENT

The discussion in the previous sections was concerned with the problem of matching apparatus to the characteristics of the signal to be measured and considered ways of describing the signal in terms of its frequency components. In practice quite simple features of the signal may be of interest. The simplest measure of a signal is its average amplitude. For example it may be of interest to assess the efficacy of a particular drug as a tranquillizer by measuring its effect on the tonic EMG activity of the limbs derived from surface electrodes. The EMG is a very variable signal having a pattern which is random in the sense that it never repeats exactly. Its amplitude at one point is therefore meaningless and the average over the interval of interest must be obtained.

With the usual type of electronic physiological amplifier, an amplified signal like the EMG will have a zero mean value. This is because on average the amplitude of the signal fluctuates an equal amount in the positive and negative direction with respect to the base line. An average amplitude measure must therefore be obtained in some other way. One way is to derive the mean amplitude deviation or absolute amplitude. This is a measure which does not take the sign of the amplitude into account, all the negative deflections being regarded as positive. It is done electronically by first rectifying the signal.

The mean amplitude deviation is sometimes called the abundance or quantity of activity. It can be measured (after rectifying the signal) by an electronic integrator. The process is then called integration—giving the measure an unnecessary air of complexity. Integration is equivalent to measuring area, in this case the area bounded by the rectified signal and the base line. This area is equal to the mean amplitude of the signal multiplied by its duration. This is obvious for the case of a rectangular signal as shown at (a) in FIG. 11.8, but is equally true for the signal at (c) which could be an EMG signal after it has been rectified.

A convenient way of measuring mean amplitude deviation is to reset the integration value to zero every time it reaches a predetermined level or threshold value (Shaw, 1967). The number of resets will then be proportional to the area under the rectified signal and so to its mean

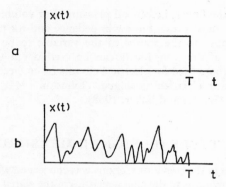

FIG. 11.8. In both (*a*) and (*b*) the area bounded by the signal and the axes is equal to the product of the mean amplitude of the signal and its duration *T*.

amplitude deviation. The resets are easily indicated on an ink recording and can be counted. Alternatively the resets can be totalled and indicated digitally by an electronic counter. Combined integrating counters for this purpose are available commercially.

This technique and modifications of it have been used to measure gestural activity as well as muscle tone (Pierce and Shaw, 1965).

At the other end of the range of measurement possibilities is the determination of the frequency components by harmonic analysis referred to above. This may give a more detailed quantitative description of the signal although it is not so easily carried out. Instruments called wave analysers are available for this, but they can be quite expensive. More recently digital wave analysers and digital computers are being used for this purpose. Sometimes a coarse wave analysis is sufficient. For example it may be required to monitor the EEG alpha rhythm, in which case a device called a band-pass filter can be used to remove all components of the EEG except the alpha frequencies. The remaining signal can be measured using the mean amplitude deviation to relate alpha rhythm changes to experimental conditions. A non-mathematical introduction to these methods is given in CHAPTER 8 of Cooper, Osselton, and Shaw (2nd edition, 1974).

ELECTRICAL NOISE

There is another limitation to accurate measurement which arises when high sensitivity is required. Electrical measuring systems all measure electrical current. Now an electrical current is composed of electrons, and these will have a degree of random motion in the conductor in which they arise, although their mean drift will be in a direction corresponding to the direction of current flow. If the signal to be measured is very small, it will have amplitude changes whose magnitude is of the same order as the random fluctuations of the electrons making up the current. The signal cannot then be distinguished from these random fluctuations in the recorded pattern. This unwanted component of the signal is called noise; its magnitude depends on the range of signal frequencies, i.e. band width over which measurements are required. Electron valves and transistors in particular are sources of electrical noise. The first transistor in an amplifier will be the most troublesome in this respect, since it has the largest degree of amplification following it. The noise from valves and transistors contain frequency components covering a wide range of frequencies, and unfortunately, the very low frequency components have relatively larger amplitudes. The resulting low frequency fluctuations of the noise signal is called drift. Drift may have a comparatively high amplitude (of the order of milli-volts) and introduces serious problems if it is required to amplify variables whose amplitude is small but constant, or changing only very slowly. For example, the srr response includes a voltage change of the order of millivolts as well as a resistance change. This had not been studied very much until recently because of the above difficulty. Amplifiers designed for this purpose are called DC or direct-coupled amplifiers, but they cannot be made as sensitive as band pass amplifiers. The latter have sensitivities decreasing for low frequencies (see FIG. 11.3) and are therefore not so sensitive to the noise components which produce drift.

There are other sources of unwanted signals which may be recorded along with the desired signals. These artifacts may arise from faulty apparatus or connexion to the subject or, with highly sensitive apparatus, from the pick-up of electrical disturbances from other sources —rather like interference on the radio. The pick-up will be due to electrostatic or electromagnetic induction and will usually result in signals at 50 cycles per second induced from the wiring of the electrical mains. Other sources are electrostatic from rubber-soled shoes, nylon clothing, etc. Many of these problems can be overcome by suitable screening of subject or apparatus, but it is often a difficult problem to eliminate (Donaldson, 1958b). The impression is sometimes given that problems of this kind are solved by a magical procedure known as 'earthing'. This does not necessarily mean connecting the subject to earth, but of removing what are known as earth loop currents. These are currents which flow between several earthed connexions resulting in an electrostatic or electromagnetic field, because no conductor—even the earth line—has zero resistance.

DIGITAL METHODS OF MEASUREMENT

It has already been said that digital methods are being used more and more in the design of electronic measuring devices. With the traditional techniques, called analog, currents and voltages proportional to the signal, or to whatever transformation of it is being carried out, are always present in the circuits. With digital methods this is not the case. The amplitude of the continuous current or voltage at the output of the transducer is sampled, that is measured at regular intervals. The magnitude of those samples are coded electrically (in binary number form) and stored. The required transformation is then carried out by

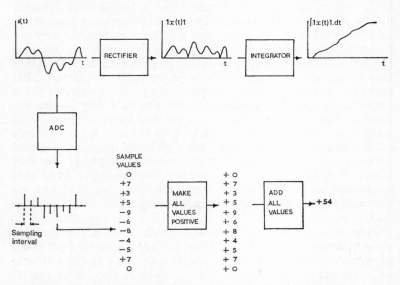

FIG. 11.9. Comparison of analog and digital methods of measuring the area enclosed by the signal $x(t)$ and the base line.

conventional arithmetic on these numbers and the result recorded or displayed as required.

The device for sampling a signal and converting each signal to a binary number is called an analog-to-digital converter or ADC. Sometimes the output is also required as a continuous function of time and to do this the stored numbers are reconverted to an analog signal using a digital-to-analog converter (DAC).

The most versatile digital devices are general purpose digital computers and these are being increasingly used for physiological measurement. Basically the computer will comprise: (1) an input system which will have one or more channels of ADC, and a teletype (electric type-writer) and paper tape reader for getting instructions and other data into the computer; (2) a store to hold the data while it is being analysed and to store the results (this can be the same teletype used for input). In addition, a set of instructions or programs, is stored in the machine; it controls the arithmetical procedures to be applied to the data, and the flow of input and output. This process is illustrated by FIG. 11.9 which compares the measurement of the area enclosed by a signal and the base line by both analog and digital methods. Dividing this area by the duration of the signal gives its mean amplitude deviation as discussed in an earlier section.

CONCLUSION

It will be apparent that the correct application of measuring equipment requires a certain level of technical knowledge and skill. Many aspects have been omitted—accepted standards of safety, for example, should always be adhered to when electrical equipment is used (DHSS, 1970) and when in doubt expert advice on this should be sought.

The principles outlined in this chapter may be applied to a wide variety of measurement problems, and may be summarized as follows. The pattern of fluctuation of the physiological variable to be measured must first be specified. This is done in terms of its frequency components, or of its time constant if it is a transient signal. The required characteristics of the complete system can then be determined, and the elements selected to give this overall characteristic. Often a complete amplifying and recording apparatus will already be available, and the problem will then be to choose a transducer with the appropriate characteristics. The recorded variable may be quantified in a number of ways and digital methods are now often used to do this.

REFERENCES

COOPER, R., OSSELTON, J. W., and SHAW, J. C. (1974) *EEG Technology*, 2nd. ed., Chapter 8, London.

DONALDSON, P. E. K. (1958a) *Electronic Apparatus for Biological Research*, Chapter 2, London.

DONALDSON, P. E. K., ed. (1958b) *Electronic Apparatus for Biological Research*, Chapter 42, London.

DEPARTMENT OF HEALTH AND SOCIAL SECURITY (1970) Safety code for electro-medical apparatus, *Hospital Technical Memorandum No. 8*, London, H.M.S.O.

GEDDES, L. A., and BAKER, L. E. (1968) *Principles of Applied Biomedical Instrumentation*, New York.

GRAHAM, D. T. (1971) Psychophysiology and medicine, *Psychophysiology*, **8**, 121–31.

GREENFIELD, N. S., and STERNBACK, R. A., eds. (1972) *Handbook of Psychophysiology*, New York.

HILL, D. W. (1973) *Principles of Electronics in Medical Research*, 2nd ed., London.

LYKKEN, D. T., and VENABLES, P. H. (1971) Direct measurement of skin conductance; A proposal for standardization, *Psychophysiology*, **8**, 656–72.

MACHIN, K. E. (1958) Transducers, in *Electronic Apparatus for Biological Research*, ed. Donaldson, P. E. K., London.

MANLEY, R. G. (1950) *Waveform Analysis*, London.

PEARCE, K. I., and SHAW, J. C. (1965) Activity measurement using the integrating and cross-over counters, *Med. Electron. Biol. Engng.*, **3**, 189–98.

ROTHMAN, S. (1954) *Physiology and Biochemistry of the Skin*, Chapter 2, Chicago.

SHAW, J. C. (1967) Quantification of biological signals using integration techniques, in *Manual of Psycho-Physiological Methods*, ed. Venables, P. H., and Martin, I., pp. 403–6, Amsterdam.

TRIMMER, J. C. (1950) *Response of Physical Systems*, London.

VENABLES, P. H. (1971) Psychophysiology and Psychiatry, *Psychol. Med.* **1**, 185–8.

VENABLES, P. H., and MARTIN, I. (1967), *A Manual of Psychological Methods*, Amsterdam.

12

PSYCHOLOGICAL TESTS

GLENN D. WILSON

MEASUREMENT IN PSYCHOLOGY

Science depends upon operational definition of its concepts, which is to say that the meaning of a phenomenon is agreed upon and understood in terms of the operations that must be performed in order to observe it. Psychology, like other sciences, also assumes E. L. Thorndike's maxim: 'Everything that exists, exists in some quantity and can therefore be measured'. Thus, if a teacher says 'Johnny is outgoing' she may well have communicated something to her colleague, but the behavioural scientist would want to know *what exactly does she mean* by outgoing?' and *by how much* does he differ from other boys on this attribute?'.

One of the main reasons for using psychological tests, then, is to ensure that the observations one makes are, if necessary, able to be repeated by other researchers. The second major function of measurement, which applies in psychology as much as other sciences, is that of providing numbers attached to objects and events in such a way that mathematical operations can be performed on them.

Four levels of measurement can be distinguished:

1. *Nominal,* in which numbers are used like names to establish identity only (e.g. numbering of football players).
2. *Ordinal,* in which the numbers are assigned so as to represent a rank-order or progression (e.g. Queue tickets).
3. *Interval,* in which the numbers carry information concerning the distances between observations (e.g. the Centigrade temperature scale).
4. *Ratio,* in which, because of the availability of a non-arbitrary zero point, statements concerning equality of ratios can be made (e.g. units of length).

Note that each level of measurement subsumes all those before it, and the kind of mathematical operations that are permissible depend upon the level that has been achieved. Most psychological tests attempt at least to achieve measurement at the interval level, where means, standard deviations, and product–moment correlations are permissible statistics.

TEST CRITERIA

Psychological tests are usually evaluated in relation to three major sets of criteria:

1. Reliability—the extent to which the same results are obtained from one testing occasion to another.
2. Validity—the extent to which the test measures what it is supposed to measure.
3. Standardization—the extent to which data are available which enable a clinician or researcher to compare his results with those obtained by other groups, or similar groups under different conditions.

The first two of these criteria are usually regarded as essential attributes of objective tests; provision of standardization data may or may not be necessary depending on the purpose for which the test is used.

RELIABILITY

The concept of reliability is used ambiguously in psychometrics, and would perhaps be better replaced by two separate concepts: (1) *Stability* refers to the extent to which subjects may be expected to obtain the same scores, at least relative to one another, on different testing occasions. It is usually estimated by the correlation between the scores obtained by the same set of subjects on two testing sessions separated by some period of time (usually at least several weeks). This is called the *test-retest reliability coefficient*. It must be assumed that the attribute being measured itself remains stable, which is not always the case (see p. 265). (2) *Internal consistency* refers to the homogeneity of the items comprising the test. It is estimated by the *split-half reliability coefficient*, which is the correlation between two randomly selected halves of the test, corrected for the fact that the number of items upon which the correlation is based has been reduced by half. A reliability coefficient based on the correlation between *equivalent* or *parallel forms* of a test incorporates elements of both stability and consistency, their proportion depending upon the *degree of equivalence* of the two forms.

Stability is probably the more important of these two kinds of reliability. Without it the test can have no validity, and the results will be meaningless. Internal consistency is not an essential characteristic of a scientific test, *nor is it even necessarily a good thing*. For example, a high internal consistency coefficient might simply indicate that the items in the test are excessively redundant.

Information concerning the homogeneity of items in a test is important, but is better obtained by *factor analysis*. A knowledge of the method is necessary for a thorough understanding of psychometrics, but is beyond the scope of this chapter; for an introduction, see Fruchter (1954) and Harman (1967). Basically, it is a statistical technique for identifying the dimensions (factors) that would account for observed intercorrelations among tests or test items.

VALIDITY

The problem of test validity concerns the extent to which the test actually measures that which it is supposed to measure. Traditionally, four types of validity have been identified: (1) *Predictive validity* refers to the power of the test to predict some future outcome (e.g. examination performance, suicidal attempts). The essential characteristic of this procedure is that the test is used to predict an outcome, and some time later the actual outcome is measured and compared with the prediction. (2) *Concurrent validity* is the extent to which scores on the test correlate with other variables already available that can be regarded as suitable criteria (e.g. teacher ratings, scores on established tests of similar attributes). This is particularly useful when the test to be validated is being considered as a substitute for a less convenient procedure. (3) *Content validity* is based upon an assessment of the extent to which the items in the test appear 'on the face of it' to be good predictors, and whether or not the item selection represents a fair sample of the behaviour domain that the test is supposed to measure. This method is typically used when an achievement test is devised to measure progress in a course of instruction. While probably adequate for this purpose, it may be questioned whether content validity is validation at all in a technical sense. (4) *Construct validity* refers to the accumulation of evidence concerning the meaning of the trait that is being measured, particularly by the experimental testing of hypotheses based on the rationale of the test. Some psychologists (e.g. Loevinger, 1957) have argued that the other methods for establishing validity may all be subsumed under construct validity, i.e. that all validation is construct validation.

Using any of these methods, the correlation between test scores and the criterion measure may be called a *validity coefficient*. It should be stressed, however, that there is no one coefficient of validity for any given test. Validity is always relative to the purpose for which the test is being used. It should also be remembered in the interpretation of both validity and reliability coefficients that the size of a correlation depends upon the amount of variance in the test and criterion scores (i.e. the heterogeneity of the sample). Thus a standard IQ test may show little validity as a predictor of performance in a university graduate course because the students are already highly selected on the variable of intelligence. Similarly, reliability coefficients based on homogeneous samples will tend to be lower than those based on a random sample of the population.

STANDARDIZATION

There are two senses in which a psychological test may be standardized: (1) *Standardization of procedure* involves the detailing of precise instructions as to how the test should be administered and raw (untreated) scores obtained. This ensures that precisely the same test is given by different testers, at different times and places. (2) *Standardization of scores* depends on the provision of *normative data* so that an individual's score can be evaluated in relation to the performance of large samples of subjects comparable in age, sex, occupation, or any other variable considered important in the situation. When an individual's score is expressed in relation to the mean and variance of a larger sample, it is called a *standard score* (e.g. modern IQ scores are based on a mean of 100 and a standard deviation of 15 or 16).

Both kinds of standardization are necessary if a test is to be used for individual assessment. For this purpose it is necessary to know how the individual stands in relation to others. The researcher, however, is often concerned only with covariance (correlations) *within his own sample*, and therefore has no need for information concerning the performance of other groups on his tests. As regards the testing procedure, it may be convenient for the researcher to report that he followed the instructions in the test manual, but he is in no way obliged to do so provided that his actual procedure is fully detailed. Thus, while standardization of procedure and scoring are important for some purposes, they need not be regarded as essentials of scientific testing in psychology.

Following these general considerations we will now outline some of the areas within which psychological tests have been applied and some of the widely used instruments within each of these areas. This is necessarily a very brief review; for a fuller account see Anastasi (1954), Cronbach (1960), or Anstey (1966).

TESTS OF ABILITY

GENERAL ABILITY (INTELLIGENCE)

The discovery that mental abilities tend to be reasonably highly intercorrelated has led to the development and widespread use of tests of general intelligence. In theory, every problem that may be used as an IQ test item measures some degree of general ability and some degree of more specific abilities (e.g. verbal fluency, perceptual speed, memory). If the specific abilities are treated as part of the error that operates in any testing situation then it is possible to achieve a fairly pure measure of general mental ability by choosing such a wide variety of items that the specific factors cancel out when the total score is calculated. In fact, the most widely used measures of intelligence lean towards verbal and numerical abilities because these have been found most useful in the prediction of academic performance.

Perhaps the best known measure of general intelligence is the *Stanford-Binet Scale* (Terman and Merrill, 1959) which has been revised several times since its original appearance in 1916. This test must be administered individually to each subject and takes more than an hour to complete. Based on the work of the French physician Alfred Binet, the S–B Scale originally made use of the concept of *mental age*. A person's performance on the test problems would initially be scored in terms of the age at which the average person would achieve his level of performance. The mental age would then be expressed as a ratio of chronological age and multiplied by 100 to give an intelligence quotient (IQ). The 1960 revision of the S–B Scale, however, like most other modern tests, uses a standard scoring system (a mean of 100 and an SD of 16). The S–B Scale is still widely used around the world. It may be applied to all age groups from about three upwards but it is probably most suitable for school-age children.

Increasingly popular as rivals to the S–B Scale are the *Wechsler Adult Intelligence Scales* (WAIS) and the *Wechsler Intelligence Scale for Children* (WISC). Besides giving an overall IQ score, the Wechsler tests provide separate *verbal* and *performance* IQ scores and scores on a variety of subtests making up these scales. The verbal scale includes tests of *information*, *comprehension*, *digit span*, *similarities*, *arithmetic*, and *vocabulary*, while the performance half includes *picture arrangement*, *picture completion*, *block design*, *object assembly*, and *digit symbol* tests. The Wechsler scales have an advantage over the S–B Scale in that grouping similar items together rather than distributing them randomly makes for simpler (and quicker) administration. Also, examination of the profile of sub-scores often gives useful information additional to the overall IQ score. For example, a performance score markedly higher than the verbal score might indicate an educational handicap. Wechsler also suggests that certain kinds of brain damage can be diagnosed on the basis of the sub-test profile, although the evidence for the validity of this procedure is equivocal. Full details of the test and recommendations regarding the interpretation of scores can be found in Wechsler (1958).

While the Stanford-Binet and Wechsler tests are virtually unrivalled as *individual* IQ tests, a variety of other scales are widely used for the measurement of general ability in the *group* setting. The *Otis Quickscoring Mental Ability Tests* (1954) are widely used to predict school achievement, particularly in the US. These consist of an assortment of verbal and numerical problems, and are speeded, with a time limit of 30 minutes. In Britain the *Raven Progressive Matrices* (1956) are popular for group testing of IQ. Since IQ's derived by this method are non-verbal, the *Mill Hill Vocabulary Scale* is often used in conjunction with it, and the two tests are now published on the same form. To some extent the two scores yielded by this combination can be regarded as providing similar information to the verbal-performance comparison with the Wechsler scales.

A number of tests of *infant intelligence* have been studied, although they have generally been found to be poor predictors of school-age test performance. Basically, these scales are designed to determine whether the child is displaying normal sensorimotor development for his age through observation of various specialized behavioural abilities such as vertical eye co-ordination, discrimination of strangers, lifting a cup by the handle, or making a tower out of two blocks. Validity of such indices as measures of intelligence is limited not only by their dubious relationship to abstract thinking, but also by the unreliability of the observations themselves. The momentary attentiveness of young children fluctuates rapidly and their maturation tends to proceed in spurts. We also have to consider the possibility that infantile prowess is *negatively* related to adult intelligence. (After all, infant monkeys are generally better co-ordinated than human babies for the first year or two.)

A rather novel approach to the measurement of intelligence in slightly older children is that adopted by Goodenough (1926) in the *Draw-a-man* Test. The child is simply asked to draw a man to the best of his ability, and the drawings are scored on the basis of the accuracy of body structure, facial details, clothes, etc. Similar techniques (e.g. House-Tree-Person Test) have been used for investigating personality dynamics as well.

We have noted that although the concept of general intelligence ('*g*') remains useful in psychological test theory, it is sometimes valuable to distinguish different types of intelligence, such as verbal versus performance IQ's. Two other distinctions are worthy of note. The first important distinction that may be made is that between *speed* and *power* in performance on ability tests. Some tests, such as the Otis, are strictly timed, and the score is highly dependent on the number of items that the subject is able to complete within the time limit. Other tests (e.g. the Raven) give scores that are based almost entirely on the subject's ability to solve problems of various difficulty levels regardless of how long he takes to do them. In fact, it has been argued that in the measurement of problem-solving ability we should separate three variables: *speed, accuracy,* and *persistence* (Furneaux, 1960).

Another distinction which is of increasing interest to psychometricians is that between *convergent* (conventional) intelligence and *divergent* (creative) intelligence (Guilford, 1967). To some extent these types of intelligence can be related to deductive and inductive thinking respectively. The recent interest in creative thinking is based upon the criticism that traditional IQ tests fail to tap originality and flexibility, which are probably more akin to genius. Creative intelligence is, of course, more difficult to define operationally than convergent intelligence. In the *Remote Associations Test* (Mednick and Mednick, 1967) the subject is given three superficially unrelated words and asked to provide another word that they all have in common (e.g. STOOL, POWDER, BALL, Answer: FOOT). Although permitting only one correct answer, problems of this kind are supposed to require greater cognitive flexibility than traditional IQ problems (perhaps fluency in generating hypotheses).

APTITUDE AND ACHIEVEMENT

Many standardized tests are available for predicting how well a person will do in a particular job (aptitude) and for assessing how much a student has gained from a course of instruction (achievement). As noted, aptitude tests depend upon predictive validity, achievement tests upon content validity. Otherwise, the distinction between these two types of tests is blurred; the same test can often be used for both purposes.

One of the best known aptitude tests is the *General Aptitude Test Battery* (GATB) developed by the US Employment Service. The construction of this battery was strongly influenced by Thurstone's factor analytic identification of six or seven 'primary mental abilities'. It consists of eight pencil-and-paper and four apparatus tests and gives scores on the following nine factors: *verbal aptitude, numerical aptitude, spatial aptitude, form perception, clerical perception, motor coordination, finger dexterity, manual dexterity,* and *general reasoning ability* (which is a composite of some of the verbal, numerical, and spatial tests). For a fuller description of these scales see Cronbach (1960). The GATB has been found particularly useful in vocational guidance because it enables a person to discover what occupations he is best suited to and able to aspire to. For selection purposes, more specific tests, or even job replicas, have generally been found to have greater validity.

PERSONALITY

SELF-REPORT

The most convenient and widely used method for assessing personality is the questionnaire. Some of the best-known standardized personality questionnaires and the different methods by which they are constructed will now be considered.

The *Minnesota Multiphasic Personality Inventory* (MMPI) was originally developed as an aid to the diagnosis of psychiatric disorder. The authors (Hathaway and McKinley, 1943) began with a set of more than 500 statements covering a variety of areas including psychiatric symptoms, physical health, general habits, domestic, occupational, and social affairs. Scoring keys were then constructed according to the power of each item to discriminate one 'known group' within the population from another (the method of *empirical keying*). In other words, after the pool of items had been selected, their content or apparent meaning was disregarded in favour of their actual power to discriminate different groups of people (e.g. schizophrenics versus normals). The original scales were: *hypochondriasis, depression,* and *hysteria* (the 'neurotic triad'), *psychopathy, masculinity-femininity, paranoia, psychasthenia, schizophrenia,* and *hypomania*. Today, the test is also provided with a number of 'control keys' which are intended to detect, and permit correction to be made, for various response styles such as 'faking good', evasiveness, carelessness. Experienced clinicians claim to be able to tell a great deal about an individual on the basis of his profile across all of these scales, but it is fair to say that empirical research has not always shown their confidence to be justified.

The MMPI has so many items, covering such diverse areas, that empirical keys can theoretically be developed to measure almost any attribute. All the researcher needs to do is discover which items are the best discriminators of his criterion groups, and in which direction, then a score key can be developed in accordance. Welsh and Dahlstrom (1956) cite 100 supplementary keys that have appeared in the literature since the original publication of the test (e.g. *socio-economic status, prejudice, social introversion.*)

Another widely used personality questionnaire is the *Edwards Personal Preference Schedule* (Edwards, 1954). This was originally designed to measure H. A. Murray's (1938) 'psychological needs' (e.g. abasement, achievement, affiliation, autonomy). Items are arranged as pairs of statements referring to various goals and activities, and the subject has to express his preference for one of the two. The 225 paired comparisons yield scores on 15 'needs' which may be regarded as personality traits. The scales were developed not by any empirical method but simply by content analysis of the items. This test has been found most useful in counselling, but has had a great deal of research application as well.

Other personality questionnaires are based upon a factor analytic identification of the primary personality traits. The *16 PF Test* (Cattell *et al.*, 1950) provides scores on sixteen factors such as *dominance, intelligence, emotional stability,* and *radicalism.* Unfortunately, the scales are so short that reliability is low and they are intercorrelated to an extent that suggests that fewer factors would be sufficient to describe the pattern of scores obtained. In fact, Eysenck (1972) has argued that little information is lost if Cattell's sixteen factors are themselves factor analysed and reduced to two independent, 'higher-order' factors that look much like his own factors called extraversion-introversion, and neuroticism.

The personality questionnaire most widely used in Britain is the *Eysenck Personality Inventory* (Eysenck and Eysenck, 1964) which measures these two major factors, *extraversion-introversion* and *neuroticism.* The use of orthogonal (independent) dimensions permits the specification of an individual by placing him within a two-dimensional space. The test also incorporates a 'Lie Scale' which enables the tester to assess the extent to which 'faking good' has occurred. Recently, the Eysencks have developed a new form of the test which incorporates a scale for measuring a third major orthogonal dimension of personality called *psychoticism* (Eysenck and Eysenck, 1969). Whereas Cattell treats intelligence and social attitudes as aspects of personality, Eysenck regards these as falling into separate domains which may be tapped with different tests.

OTHER-PERSON RATINGS

A second major method for assessing personality is that of providing a standard rating scale by which people who know the subject well (nurses, teachers, supervisors, parents, peers, etc.) can rate his characteristic behaviour. This technique is less susceptible to 'faking good' than the self-report method, but numerous other sources of error are known to operate. Some raters are over-generous and rate everybody towards the favourable end of the scale. The term 'halo effect' refers to the tendency for ratings of an individual on specific traits to be influenced by the rater's impression of his overall merit. Other sources of error include ambiguity of the attributes upon which subjects are to be rated, and the fact that raters usually have limited information about the people they are rating.

Some standardized rating scales are commercially available. Perhaps the best-known scales for rating psychiatric symptoms are the *Wittenborn Psychiatric Rating Scales* (1955). The Wittenborn presents fifteen short scales relating to symptoms and ward behaviour, which are organized into nine scores on the basis of factor analytic results. These dimensions are: (1) *acute anxiety;* (2) *conversion hysteria;* (3) *manic state;* (4) *depressed state;* (5) *schizophrenic excitement;* (6) *paranoid conditions;* (7) *paranoid schizophrenic;* (8) *hebephrenic schizophrenic;* (9) *phobic compulsive.* In general, these scales tend to show reasonably high reliability and low intercorrelations one with another. Note that they refer to temporary conditions (states) as well as diagnostic categories, so it is possible to use them to record changes in the illness, e.g. progress towards recovery.

Ratings of this kind are based upon haphazard observations, and are subject to observer errors such as selective perception and recall. For this reason, some researchers adopt the method of sampling behaviour in a standardized test situation. For example, children at play might be observed for brief periods in a predetermined order that is altered from day to day such that each child is observed an equal number of times and order effects are balanced for. The *time sampling* method is particularly suitable for recording objective behaviours that can be counted, e.g. number of social contacts, smiles, or temper tantrums.

PROJECTIVE MEASURES

A third major group of techniques is designed to examine personality characteristics and dynamics through the analysis of fantasy material generated in response to highly ambiguous stimulus material. The classic example of a projective measure is the *word-association test* attributed to C. G. Jung. In this test the subject is given a series of stimulus words and asked to respond to each with the first word that enters his head. Also notious as a diagnostic test is the *Rorschach Ink-blot Test*, in which the patient has to say what he 'sees' in a standard series of inkblots. The *Thematic Apperception Test* developed by H. A. Murray and his colleagues uses slightly more structured stimulus material; the subject is required to tell a story about each of a series of drawings depicting shadowy characters in various ambiguous situations and relationships. Supposedly, he identifies with one of the characters in the picture and projects his own needs, motives, and conflicts into the story that he writes.

Objective scoring methods have been attempted with projective personality tests but they have generally proved to be of limited reliability and validity (Jensen, 1958). Therefore, while these tests may have some clinical usefulness when impressionistically interpreted by a skilled and experienced clinician, they have generally not been found useful to researchers. For a detailed description and evaluation of the various projective techniques that are available see Murstein (1965).

INTERESTS

Inventories for summarizing an individual's pattern of interests are also available for research use, although their primary usefulness is in vocational guidance. The distinction between tests of interests and personality is often difficult to draw. Since interests (and attitudes) tend to reflect personality traits they can be regarded as indirect personality measures.

The *Strong Vocational Interest Blank* (SVIB; Strong, 1943) was developed on a purely empirical basis. As with the MMPI, scoring keys were constructed without regard to the content of items (which cover an enormous variety of interest and activities) but purely on the basis of observed correlations with outside criteria (e.g. successful performance in a particular occupation). The great disadvantage of this method is that a separate key is required for every potential occupation (e.g. teacher, typist, mortician).

The chief rival to the SVIB is the *Kuder Preference Record* (1956) which is based upon factor analytic identification of interest clusters. The individual obtains scores on a number of interest areas: *outdoor, mechanical, computational, scientific, persuasive, artistic, literary, musical, social service*, and *clerical*. The profile of interests is then examined to find the occupations that might be suited by it. Note that it tells nothing about the individual's ability or aptitude to undertake those occupations, merely the extent to which they might be enjoyed.

These two interest tests provide a classic example of the difference between empirical keying and factor-analytic (sometimes called 'homogeneous') keying in the construction of questionnaires. Many other tests are constructed out of a mixture of these techniques, while still others rely on no more than what might be called 'logical' keying. This approach is based on intuitive judgment and content validity rather than any statistical method.

ATTITUDES

Attitudes are also most commonly assessed by the analysis of patterns of response to questionnaires. These may be regarded as falling into two major groups: (1) *Scales that present directional statements of opinion* (e.g. 'Homosexuals ought to be publicly whipped') to which the subject responds with some amount of agreement or disagreement. Among the best-known scales of this kind are the *California F-Scale* (Adorno *et al.*, 1950) and the *Dogmatism Scale* (Rokeach, 1960). These scales continue to find widespread use in the US despite severe criticism on the ground of acquiescence response bias (Wilson and Nias, 1972; Wilson, 1973). *The Social Attitudes Inventory* (Eysenck, 1954) is much better founded, being factor-analytically based and largely controlling for response bias. This questionnaire is scored for two orthogonal factors in social and political attitudes: *radicalism* versus *conservatism*, and *toughmindedness* versus *tendermindedness*. (2) *Scales which present non-directional concepts* (e.g. 'Father', 'Death penalty') and require the respondent to evaluate them, e.g. the *Semantic Differential* (Osgood, Suci, and Tannenbaum, 1957) and the *Conservatism Scale* (Wilson and Patterson, 1970). When appropriate this item format appears to be preferable on a number of counts. Apart from the gain in economy and simplicity, there is evidence that it is less susceptible to the effects of acquiescence and social desirability response biases (Wilson, 1973). It eliminates certain sources of ambiguity (e.g. differences in the perceived point of emphasis in an opinion statement; perceived frequency implied by words such as 'seldom' and 'often') and averts logical problems for the respondent such as having to disagree with a negatively worded statement.

The classical methods for selecting items for an attitude test (e.g. the Thurstone and Guttman techniques) were concerned almost exclusively with the development of *unidimensional* scales. With the advent of the computer, they have been largely superseded by *factor analysis*, which permits the development of *multidimensional* attitude scales. For a detailed description of these methods of scale construction see Oppenheim (1966) or Scott (1969).

The *Conservatism Scale* is the most widely used attitude questionnaire in Britain and the Commonwealth countries. It has also been used in German, Dutch, Russian, Italian, Korean, and Afrikaans translations. It comprises a series of 50 catch-phrases representing familiar controversial issues (e.g. death penalty, evolution theory, striptease) to which the subject responds 'Yes', ' ?', or 'No' according to whether or not he 'favours or believes in' that concept. Originally designed to measure a general factor underlying all social attitudes (*Liberalism versus Conservatism*) the C-Scale is now keyed to measure a second orthogonal factor, *realism versus idealism*, and four oblique components of the general conservatism factor: *militarism-punitiveness, anti-hedonism, ethnocentrism*, and *religion-puritanism* (Wilson, 1973).

Caine and Small (1969) have developed a factor-based *Attitudes to Treatment Questionnaire* which gives scores indicating degrees of favourability towards three major approaches to psychiatric treatment: (1) *physical* (including drugs, ECT, and behaviour therapy), (2) *individual psychotherapy*; and (3) *group psychotherapy and community psychiatry*. The preferences of psychiatrists, nurses, and the patients themselves have been shown to be related to general social attitudes such as conservatism (Lillie, 1973).

Apart from the self-report techniques for measuring attitudes, various *disguised* or *indirect* methods have been used, the possible advantage being that they are less susceptible to contamination by social desirability and other response styles. Actually, the problem of social desirability is not very salient in the area of attitude measurement because of the evaluative nature of attitudes themselves. Whereas there is considerable agreement as to which end of dimensions such as intelligence and neuroticism is preferable, one's *own* attitudes are by definition 'good'. Nevertheless, attitudes can be inferred from their effects upon cognitive and perceptual processes (e.g. recognition and recall thresholds, binocular resolution) or performance on certain tasks involving materials relevant to the attitude object (e.g. sorting opinion statements on a scale of favourability towards an issue rather than indicating one's own agreement). The *lost letter technique* involves the distribution of letters, with or without stamps, that are addressed to people or organizations in which the researcher is interested, e.g. the John Birch Society, or Communist Party. Attitudes towards these two groups, for example, might be compared in a particular geographical area simply by counting the proportion of letters that arrive at the addresses given (the assumption being that people are more likely to forward letters to people that they like).

Various physiological measures of attitudes have also been attempted, especially autonomic responses such as the GSR (Cook and Selltiz, 1964). Such methods are not only cumbersome by comparison with the self-report method, but they usually can indicate only the *intensity* of an attitude response, not its *direction*. The recent hope that pupillary dilation/contraction might constitute a measure of direction as well as intensity now appears to have subsided (McGuire, 1969).

TRAITS *vs* STATES

Nearly all of the tests that have been described above are concerned with the measurement of fairly stable and enduring characteristics of the individual, called *traits*. Sometimes, however, it is temporary moods or conditions (*states*) that we are interested in assessing, and for this purpose different tests are necessary.

The *Multiple Affect Adjective Check List* (Zuckerman and Lubin, 1967) consists of a list of adjectives describing various feelings. There are two forms differing in the instructions to the subject. One asks him to check those adjectives describing 'how you generally feel' and the other 'how you feel now—today'. Thus the same set of adjectives can be used to measure either traits or states. In either case they are classified into three clinically relevant groups: anxiety, depression, and hostility.

A refinement of this technique for quantifying mood changes in psychiatric patients has been described by Fransella [see CHAPTER 17]. Shapiro advocates constructing a *Personal Questionnaire* for each patient out of the symptoms expressed by that particular patient. The progress of different clusters of symptoms (paranoid, depressive, anxiety, etc.) can be observed from time to time and their changes relative to one another used in the evaluation of different types of therapy.

DIAGNOSTIC TESTS

It is fair to say that psychometrics has so far contributed little to the problem of psychiatric diagnosis and classification. We noted that Wechsler intelligence test profiles may give clues to certain psychiatric conditions such as brain damage, and that the MMPI is purported to have some validity for the differential diagnosis of psychiatric conditions. Nevertheless, it has to be admitted that the impact of psychological tests has been extremely limited. (An outstanding exception is the Ishihara Test for colour blindness, which, along with similar psychophysical procedures, remains the *only* reliable and valid method for diagnosing this condition.) The *Repertory Grid Test* of Bannister and Fransella (1967) apparently does discriminate thought disorder, but probably for reasons much less theoretically interesting than the authors supposed (Frith and Lillie, 1972).

Eysenck (1960) has suggested abandoning the traditional diagnostic categories in favour of a psychometric classification based on personality traits normally distributed in the population. Thus anxiety neurotics would be classified as unstable introverts and hysterics unstable extraverts. Psychopaths would presumably be unstable extraverts who are also high on the third dimension, psychoticism. In so far as mental patients are not qualitatively different from many 'normal' people, this system has the advantage that it discards the disease model of psychiatric disorder as advocated by Szasz (1961). It is also likely to have higher reliability than the traditional system which notoriously varies according to time, culture, and the individual diagnostician. On the other hand, there are some psychiatric conditions (e.g. epilepsy) that clearly do not fall on a continuum with normal behaviour, which suggests that a diagnostic system based purely on personality traits would not have universal applicability.

CHOOSING A TEST

When a researcher has a need for a psychological test in order to define some variable or other, he should first make a search of the literature to see if any established test would suit his purpose. This not only avoids a great deal of unnecessary duplication of effort but also makes for better communication with other researchers, since they may already have some familiarity with that test and the meaning of its scores. We have listed some of the most widely used psychological tests in various areas, but only a small proportion of the number that are actually available. Some sources of information about tests are:

1. The *Mental Measurements Yearbook* (edited by O. K. Buros) which is brought up to date every five years or so, and is now in its seventh edition (1972). This lists all tests in print and gives critical reviews of those that are more widely used.
2. Textbooks designed to accompany introductory courses in psychological testing (e.g. Anastasi, 1954; Cronbach, 1960) also give a lot of useful information about popular tests.
3. The researcher can also consult the catalogues of major test publishers and distributors. In the United States some major companies are Psychological Corporation, Educational Testing Service, Science Research Associates, California Test Bureau, and the World Book Co. In Britain, the National Foundation for Educational Research (Windsor) handles most tests published in Britain and many of the more important ones from the United States.
4. For very recent tests it is often useful to consult *Psychological Abstracts*, the periodical which summarizes current literature in psychology, in case a suitable test has just appeared in a journal article.

Despite the bewildering variety of tests that are already published, it is possible that the researcher will find none entirely satisfactory for his particular purpose. The problems involved in the construction of new tests are beyond the scope of this chapter; a good summary can be found in Thorndike and Hagen (1962) and a comprehensive account in Jackson and Messick (1967).

The criteria for evaluating tests that were outlined at the beginning of the chapter may be applied to both the selection of established tests and the construction of new ones. Of these, validity is the most important, since a test cannot be valid without also being reliable to some extent.

REFERENCES

ADORNO, T. W., FRENKEL-BRUNSWIK, E., LEVINSON, D. J., and SAND-FORD, R. N. (1950) *The Authoritarian Personality*, New York.

ANASTASI, A. (1954) *Psychological Testing*, New York.

ANSTEY, E. (1966) *Psychological Tests*, London.

BANNISTER, D., and FRANSELLA, F. (1967) *A Grid Test of Schizophrenic Thought Disorder: A Standard Clinical Test*, Barnstaple, Psychological Test Publications.

BUROS, O. K. (1972) *The Seventh Mental Measurements Yearbook*, New Jersey.

CAINE, T. M., and SMALL, D. J. (1969) *The Treatment of Mental Illness: Science, Faith and Therapeutic Personality*, London.

CATTELL, R. B., SAUNDERS, D. R., and STICE, G. (1950) *The 16 PF Test*, Chicago.

COOK, S. W., and SELLTIZ, C. (1964) A multiple-indicator approach to attitude measurement, *Psychol. Bull.*, **62**, 36–55.

CRONBACH, L. J. (1960) *Essentials of Psychological Testing*, 2nd ed., New York.

EDWARDS, A. L. (1954) *Manual for the Edwards Personality Preference Schedule*, New York.

EYSENCK, H. J. (1954) *The Psychology of Politics*, London.

EYSENCK, H. J. (1960) Classification and the problem diagnosis, in *Handbook of Abnormal Psychology*, ed. Eysenck, H. J., London.

EYSENCK, H. J. (1972) Primaries or second-order factors: A critical consideration of Cattell's 16 PF battery, *Brit. J. soc. clin. Psychol.*, **11**, 265–9.

EYSENCK, H. J., and EYSENCK, S. B. G. (1964) *Manual of the Eysenck Personality Inventory*, London.

EYSENCK, S. B. G., and EYSENCK, H. J. (1969) Scores on three personality variables as a function of age, sex and social class, *Brit. J. soc. clin. Psychol.*, **8**, 69–76.

FRITH, C. D., and LITTLE, F. J. (1972) Why does the Repertory Grid Test indicate thought disorder? *Brit. J. soc. clin. Psychol.*, **11**, 73–8.

FRUCHTER, B. (1954) *Introduction to Factor Analysis*, Princeton.

FURNEAUX, W. D. (1960) Intellectual abilities and problem-solving behaviour, in *Handbook of Abnormal Psychology*, ed. Eysenck, H. J., London.

GOODENOUGH, F. (1926) *Draw-a-Man Test*, New York.

GUILFORD, J. P. (1967) *The Nature of Human Intelligence*, New York.

HARMAN, H. H. (1967) *Modern Factor Analysis*, 2nd ed., Chicago.

HATHAWAY, S. R., and McKINLEY, J. C. (1943) *The Minnesota Multiphasic Personality Inventory*, New York.

JACKSON, D. N., and MESSICK, S. (1967) *Problems in Human Assessment*, New York.

JENSEN, A. R. (1958) *The Reliability of Projective Techniques: Review of the Literature and Methodology*, Amsterdam.

KUDER, G. F. (1956) *The Kuder Preference Record*, Science Research Associates.

LILLIE, F. J. (1973) Conservatism, psychiatry and mental distress, in *The Psychology of Conservatism*, ed. Wilson, G. D., London.

LOEVINGER, J. A. (1957) Objective tests as instruments of psychological theory, *Psychol. Rep.* **3**, 635–94.

McGUIRE, W. J. (1969) The nature of attitudes and attitude research, in *Handbook of Social Psychology*, 2nd ed., ed. Lindzey, G., and Aronson, E., London.

MEDNICK, S. A., and MEDNICK, M. T. (1967) *Remote Associates Test*, New York.

MURRAY, H. A. (1938) *Explorations in Personality*, New York.

MURSTEIN, B. I. (1965) *Handbook of Projective Techniques*, New York.

OPPENHEIM, A. N. (1966) *Questionnaire Design and Attitude Measurement*, London.

OSGOOD, C. E., SUCI, G. J., and TANNENBAUM, P. H. (1957) *The Measurement of Meaning*, Urbana, Illinois.

OTIS, O. A. (1954) *Manual for the Otis Quick-Scoring Tests of Mental Ability*, New York.

RAVEN, J. C. (1956) *The Standard Progressive Matrices Test*, London.

ROKEACH, M. (1960) *The Open and Closed Mind*, New York.

SCOTT, W. A. (1969) Attitude measurement, in *Handbook of Social Psychology*, 2nd ed., ed. Lindzey, G., and Aronson, E., London.

STRONG, E. K. (1943) *Vocational Interests of Men and Women*, Stanford, California.

SZASZ, T. S. (1961) *The Myth of Mental Illness*, New York.

TERMAN, L. M., and MERRILL, M. A. (1959) *Measuring Intelligence*, Boston.

THORNDIKE, R. L., and HAGEN, E. (1962) *Measurement and Evaluation in Psychology and Education*, New York.

WECHSLER, D. (1958) *Measurement and Appraisal of Adult Intelligence*, 4th ed., Baltimore.

WELSH, G. S., and DAHLSTROM, G. W. (1956) *Basic Reading on the M.M.P.I. in Psychology and Medicine*, Minneapolis.

WILSON, G. D. (1973) *The Psychology of Conservatism*, London.

WILSON, G. D., and NIAS, D. K. B. (1972) Measurement of social attitudes: a new approach, *Percept. Mot. Skills*, **35**, 827.

WILSON, G. D., and PATTERSON, J. R. (1970) *Manual for the Conservatism Scale*, Windsor.

WITTENBORN, J. R. (1955) *The Wittenborn Psychiatric Rating Scales*, New York.

ZUCKERMAN, M., and LUBIN, B. (1967) *Multiple Affect Adjective Check List*, San Diego.

13

EPIDEMIOLOGICAL METHODS AND
THE CLINICAL PSYCHIATRIST

J. K. WING

Epidemiology is a branch of medical ecology, the science concerned with the relationships between human disease and the environment in which human beings live. The particular part of medical ecology with which epidemiologists are concerned is the distribution of diseases in human populations. Thus it is immediately apparent that epidemiology depends upon the accurate estimation of rates of disease.

DISEASE RATES

A *rate* is an estimate of the ratio between the number of people suffering from a given disease and the total number of people in the population being studied. The number of *cases*[1] newly appearing in a unit population of, say, 100,000 people, during a stated period of time, say one year, is the inception (incidence) of the disease. For example, it is estimated that about 15,000 patients were admitted for the first time to hospitals in England and Wales during 1969 and given a diagnosis of schizophrenia (DHSS, 1971). Since the population of England and Wales is estimated to have been about 49 million at this time, the annual inception rate of schizophrenia calculated in this way is 30·6 per 100,000 total population per year. This example illustrates the two basic types of methodological problem which have to be solved in all comparative epidemiological work; the problem of the numerator and the problem of the denominator.

The problem of the numerator is that of defining a case. Is a diagnosis of schizophrenia written on the Mental Health Enquiry form sufficient to define a case of 'schizophrenia'? When Kramer (1969) points out that schizophrenia appears more commonly among first admissions to American as compared with British mental hospitals, might the explanation be that the diagnostic rules are different in the two countries? Kendell deals with this question in CHAPTER 8, but it is worth mentioning here that in one comparative survey of three mental hospitals, about one quarter of all the cases labelled as schizophrenic in one of the hospitals had to be rejected after closer examination, in order to achieve

---

[1] A case is not, of course, a person, but an example of a disease affecting a person. People should never be referred to as cases.

comparability with the other two (Wing and Brown, 1970). Accepting, however, that the hospital diagnosis can be used for certain limited purposes, how far can it be assumed that all new cases of schizophrenia arising in a given population do result in admission to hospital and are thus included in the first admission statistics? Ødegård (1952) thought that nearly all cases did result in admission but things have changed greatly during the past twenty years. Several workers have estimated the numbers of newly arising cases on the basis of surveys of population samples (Dunham, 1965; Fremming, 1951) but a consideration of the numbers involved shows how difficult this is. A population of 100,000 people has to be observed over a period of one year in order to find 30 cases, if the British first admission rate is taken as a criterion. Case-registers which include all contacts with psychiatric services, domiciliary and out-patient as well as hospital, provide an intermediate sampling-frame. In Camberwell, for example, the number of people who contacted a psychiatric service for the first time during 1970 and were given a diagnosis of schizophrenia, was very little greater than the number first admitted with schizophrenia in the same year (Wing, Hailey et al., 1972). This is a situation which could easily change, but supposing we accept that the number of first admissions with schizophrenia is a useful figure to know, how much can we rely upon the designation 'first admission'? Brown, Parkes, and Wing (1961) found that 10 per cent of those entered on the record form as first admissions had in fact been admitted previously, and there was a further large proportion where nothing was entered. Rather strict rules are laid down by local case-registers to deal with such problems (e.g. Wing and Hailey, 1972). The criteria used in the national statistics have recently been made more stringent, so that the first admission rate for schizophrenia in 1970 is 17·7 per 100,000; the difference from 1969 being explained mainly by the use of the new criteria (DHSS, 1972). We may accept that the data are accurately coded, punched, and processed once they arrive at the Department of Health, but high quality statistics are by no means easy to achieve; a study of case-register method handbooks gives an indication of how the many technical problems, both major and minor, can be dealt with.

When the condition under investigation is one, like depression or anxiety state, which does not usually result in admission to hospital and in its milder forms may not even lead to contact with an out-patient clinic, neither national nor local case-registers are likely to be adequate, and recourse must be had to less selective sampling-frames such as general practitioners' list or the electoral register. CHAPTER 16 deals with the methods used in such epidemiological surveys. Whatever the condition under study, however, laying down the criteria for case-finding is the absolute basis for all epidemiological and survey work. Errors made in this process will undermine everything that is subsequently done and can make nonsense of the results. Reid (1960) observes that 'case-finding methods should have the quality of the perfect witness, in that they tell the truth, the whole truth, and nothing but the truth. Further, they must go on doing this consistently and reliably for the whole period of the investigation. If this ideal is not obtained, at least the observer should know by how much his methods fall short of it.'

If the problem of the numerator is that of case-finding, the problem of the denominator is that of defining the population under study. The numbers and the structure of a population can change very markedly over quite a short period of time. Even if census figures are accepted as reasonably accurate (and certain minority groups, the highly mobile, one-person households, etc. tend to be underreported), intercensal estimates are sometimes only very approximate (Benjamin, 1970). This is true both of populations which are changing rapidly and then unexpectedly cease to change, and of populations which begin to change although stability was expected. Moreover, change can be differential; there is a marked out-migration from some of the inner London suburbs but it affects mainly men and women aged forty to sixty-four; the proportions of children and of the elderly remain relatively constant, though there is a separate and slower tendency towards an increase in the older age-groups because of changes in the birth and death rates. It is not certain how far psychiatric patients are representative in their patterns of geographical mobility, but failure to take account of such factors could be misleading. Eaton and Weil (1955), for example, found low rates of schizophrenia among the Hutterite communities they studied but differential out-migration might have been one of the reasons for this. Murphy (1968) did not observe lower rates of first admission for schizophrenia among Hutterites admitted to Canadian mental hospitals. The problem of geographical mobility is discussed in detail in relation to first admission rates for schizophrenia by Dunham (1965). Changes in the social composition of the population are also likely to be important, since factors such as housing, employment, and marital status tend to be associated with the incidence of schizophrenia. One method of dealing with such difficulties, if sufficient information is available about two different populations in which rates are being compared, is to standardize so that the distributions of key variables are the same. Reid (1960) gives examples of this procedure.

Ordinarily, it will not be possible to study the whole of a population and a sample has to be taken (always after obtaining the help of an expert). If the sample is drawn in the proper way, and everyone in the population has an equal chance of being included, assumptions made about the sample should hold true of the total group as well. It is necessary first of all to know who is in the population; appropriate sampling-frames may be the electoral register or general practitioners' lists, though each has its snags. The technical details may be studied in the small but excellent monographs by Reid (1960) or Stuart (1964).

The inception of schizophrenia has been taken by way of example in order to illustrate some of the problems which arise in calculating rates. These problems are even more complex when we consider the other main type of rate, known as *prevalence*. This is the number of cases present in a unit population at a given time (point prevalence) or during a given period (period prevalence). Clearly, the period prevalence includes the incidence of new cases during that period together with cases beginning before the period but persisting into it. This introduces a new dimension for definition. It is traditional, for example, to include in the prevalence figures for schizophrenia all patients given that diagnosis who are resident in hospital during the period in question. Many of these were given the diagnosis years earlier and have long since lost any active symptoms of the condition (Wing and Brown, 1970). Whether they are included should depend upon the purpose of the study, not on routine assumptions. Another problem is that in-patient statistics are inadequate for estimating the prevalence of schizophrenia since most people with this disease are not in hospital but elsewhere. House-to-house surveys have produced a range of prevalence estimates depending on the breadth of the definition used for case-finding. Local case-registers may allow a more precise estimate since people who are regarded as possibly suffering from schizophrenia can be interviewed and a standard diagnostic procedure applied and those who used to be in contact with services several years previously but have fallen out of contact can also be considered. The one-year 'reported' prevalence rate for Camberwell was 296 per 100,000 total population in 1970. This was made up of 144 resident in hospital on 1 January 1970, 61 who were admitted during the year and 91 who were in contact with out-patient clinics, day hospitals, or other community services (Wing *et al.*, 1972). There is a special difficulty about interpreting the denominator when the condition under study is likely to give rise to chronic handicap. In Camberwell, for example, there are schizophrenic patients who were admitted to hospital forty years ago and who have remained resident since. Their houses may have been pulled down; their relatives may have moved away from the area. Are they still really residents of Camberwell ? Whether they are or not, to include them in the numerator gives rise to special problems of interpretation. In 1930 the population of Camberwell was 250,000. In 1970 it was 170,000. Which figure should be placed in the denominator ? The present population size is usually used but it is clear that the prevalence rate for a given area is a complex measure, not to be compared with that of other areas without considerable thought.

Another rate, known as the expectation of a disease, is a form of lifetime incidence and there are corresponding difficulties of interpretation. The expectation that any individual will develop schizophrenia during the years of greatest risk (say 15–45) is estimated to be something under 1 per cent (Böök, 1961). Difficulties in the calculation are discussed by Kramer (1961). The lifetime expectation of being admitted to mental hospital is 11·0 per cent for males and 16·6 per cent for females (DHSS, 1972).

MEDICAL VERSUS SOCIAL EPIDEMIOLOGY

Nowadays, when it is possible to claim that mental illnesses are myths, it will be immediately apparent to the reader that to define epidemiology in terms of studying the distributions of diseases is to beg a number of important questions. Beyond saying that mental illnesses are neither things nor myths, but theories, it is not feasible to expand upon the subject here. More extended discussions will be found elsewhere (Wing et al., 1973). It is, of course, possible to indulge in demarcation disputes between medicine and the social sciences but such arguments are trivial and time-wasting. Mechanic (1970) pointed out that it is not uncommon for social scientists 'to discover, on being introduced to the field of epidemiology, that this is what they have been doing all their professional lives'. To study the distribution in a population of some socially defined characteristic such as social class or marital status or poverty is not very different methodologically from studying the distribution of disease. Similarly, epidemiologists may legitimately study the distribution of suicide or drug 'abuse' or homosexuality or destitution. It would be a great mistake, however, if poverty or divorce, drug-taking or suicide were to be regarded as diseases rather than as markers for groups at relatively high risk of having or developing diseases. Barbara Wootton (1959) has some trenchant remarks upon the subject.

USES OF EPIDEMIOLOGY

J. N. Morris (1964) has described the uses of epidemiology under seven headings; the study of historical trends, the description of community health, the operational analysis of health services, the determination of individual risks, the completion of the clinical picture, the identification of syndromes, and the discovery of causes. Plenty of psychiatric examples can be found to illustrate each of these categories. For the sake of simplicity, however, the functions of epidemiology may be divided into two large groups, those concerned with the causes of mental illness (and therefore with its prevention) and those concerned with the course of mental illness (and therefore with its treatment, management, and prognosis and with the organization of services).

Genetic studies are by definition epidemiological since they are concerned with the frequency of disease in various population groups more or less related to proband cases. They illustrate very well the value of the epidemiological method in testing hypotheses by looking for differences in disease rates between defined sub-groups of a population. The technique is no different from that employed when a population sample is divided into non-smokers, cigarette smokers of varying intensity, and other types of smokers, in order to compare rates of carcinoma of the bronchus.

The direction of cause and effect cannot ever be taken for granted. If more patients with schizophrenia are found in unskilled manual occupations than expected, this may be because something about the work environment causes schizophrenia or because something about the disease causes a movement down the vocational scale even before the time of first contact with services. Other information has to be collected before the analysis can be taken further (Goldberg and Morrison, 1963). Similarly, it appears reasonable to conclude, on the basis of the observation that the highest rates of first admission for schizophrenia are from areas with the highest proportion of single-person household, that 'isolation' is a causal factor. However, it has first to be shown that the schizophrenic patients actually do come from such isolated living conditions; if not, some other factor, possibly quite irrelevant, may explain the association. Next it must be considered whether the patients moved from a family setting, into the isolated housing, some time before they were identified as being ill (Hare, 1967). Rutter (1972) has considered the similar problems which arise when analysing data concerning the relationship between disturbance in parents and disturbance in children.

The subject of prevention has received rather less attention but the use of epidemiological data on 'suicidal behaviours' to assess the value of preventive methods is discussed by Kreitman (1973).

The functions of epidemiology in looking for causes of illness are fairly well known but those concerned with the course and treatment of illness are less familiar. Completing the clinical picture is one of the most useful functions of epidemiology and there is considerable scope for its application to psychiatry. The depressions, in particular, tend to present rather different clinical pictures in general and in hospital practice and a complete view of them must have an epidemiological basis. Similarly, studies of prognosis tend to be of limited value unless they are carried out on representative groups of patients rather than on those who are referred to one particular hospital or agency or those who are thought suitable for some particular kind of treatment. This point may be illustrated by the results of a trial of preventive medication carried out by Leff and Wing (1971). Schizophrenic patients who might possibly be included in such a trial were interviewed as they came into hospital during an acute episode of illness. All those thought eligible could have entered the trial six weeks after discharge from hospital, from which point they would have been given active phenothiazine tablets or placebo. However, out of 116 eligible patients only 35 actually entered. In the trial group, follow-up showed an unequivocal superiority of active drug over placebo, although there were patients in both groups whose outcome could not be predicted by knowing what kind of tablets they had been taking. Of the patients who did not enter the trial, 11 did not do so because their consultants thought them too well to risk being put on an active drug. These patients had a good outcome in spite of receiving no medication. Another 15 did not enter the trial because their consultants thought the prognosis too precarious to risk being put on placebo. These patients had a high relapse rate although they *were* taking active medication. Thus the results of the placebo-controlled trial were seen to be relevant mainly to the middle group of patients whose prognosis was neither outstandingly good nor outstandingly poor. A similar point may be made concerning trials of injected forms of phenothiazine. The trial results apply only to those patients who continued to receive injections. In one series, approximately half of the patients who were tried on this form of medication did not continue with it (Denham and Adamson, 1971). The trial results are incomplete unless this context is known.

These examples illustrate the fact that the epidemiological approach can usefully be combined with experimental and other designs in order to provide a framework for assessing the overall significance and generalizability of results. Perhaps the most important application of the technique lies in the evaluation of health services. This is an increasingly important aspect of psychiatric research and some examples will be given in a subsequent section.

DESIGNS AND METHODS

Other chapters give details of how to design projects, how to measure the most important variables and how to handle the resulting data. There is nothing very distinctive about the way that epidemiologists operate once the basic advantages and difficulties of estimating rates have been grasped. Any design that might be used in other fields of psychiatry, including comparative statistics, natural 'experiments', subgroup comparisons, prospective and retrospective longitudinal studies, controlled trials, and combinations of these, may be used in conjunction with an epidemiological survey. The same is true of methods, which can range from participant observation or the content analysis of historical documents, through partially standardized interviewing or the use of questionnaires, to case-registers or laboratory testing. The one essential is that the aims of the project are clearly understood and stated and that the empirical techniques adopted are clearly relevant to the aims. It is only too easy to develop an impeccable routine of surveying a population, processing the data, and writing up the result without ever considering whether there is any theoretical or practical justification for the survey to be carried out at all. Wright Mills (1959) has written a hard-hitting polemic devoted to the castigation of 'abstracted empiricists' who use 'the Method', that is 'the more-or-less set interview with a series of individuals selected by a sampling procedure', the data from which are transferred to punched cards and then subjected to 'the Statistical Ritual'. Surveys should only be used when there is a worthwhile problem to be solved and no more economical or likely way of solving it can be thought of.

It is almost always sensible to try out the procedures in a pilot study before undertaking the main work. The actual working conditions should be simulated as closely as possible so that any snags likely to occur can be anticipated and the measuring instruments, organization, and processing routines thoroughly tested. This will save time, trouble, money, and exasperation.

EVALUATIVE RESEARCH

One of the most important applications of the epidemiological approach lies in the evaluation of health services. This is potentially a very large field of work, which is only just beginning to receive proper scientific attention but it is likely to expand rapidly in the future and opportunities will thereby be created, not only to produce results of direct value for purposes of planning and organizing services, but also to create and test the basic theories that are so conspicuously lacking in social psychiatry at the moment.

The chief aim of the health services is to decrease or contain morbidity, firstly in the patient, secondly in the patient's immediate family, thirdly in the community at large. Each service agency has a combination of diagnostic, therapeutic, rehabilitative, and preventive functions. Prevention is better than cure. Primary, secondary, and tertiary preventive methods are intended to be used to stop disease occurring in the first place, to detect illness at an early stage, to limit development of chronic disabilities following an acute illness and to prevent the accumulation of secondary handicaps if clinical disabilities are unavoidable. This is what is meant by the 'containment' of morbidity. Since much psychiatric handicap is chronic, many patients are likely to remain in contact with services for a long time. Fairly large numbers therefore accumulate and the development of secondary handicaps needs special attention but, if fully put into practice, these principles should ensure that morbidity is reduced as much as it can be.

In order to evaluate the success of services in achieving these aims work is required at many different levels, some of which (such as the effectiveness of management, the most effective methods of staff specialization, allocation and training, the morale of units, the communications between professional hierarchies, the comparative costs of different methods) do not fall within the scope of this chapter. What must be emphasized, however, is that in any health service based upon the principles of geographical responsibility, comprehensiveness and integration, all evaluation must be seen in an epidemiological context. How many people are in contact with existing services and what are their contact patterns? What are the needs of these individuals and their relatives? Are the services at present provided meeting these needs effectively and economically? How many of those not in touch with services also have needs? What modifications or innovations would reduce unmet need? When innovations are introduced, do they actually make any difference?

Some of these questions can be answered by collecting descriptive statistics, particularly through the use of case-registers which are deliberately tailored to the problems of local communities.

DESCRIPTIVE STATISTICS

The simplest and most limited technique of evaluation is to describe what is already going on; this provides a first basis for comparison and for monitoring changes. If carried out systematically, it may provide knowledge which cannot be obtained in any other way and reveal facts about the workings of services which are by no means obvious, even to the staff who have been running them. It is never possible to be purely descriptive. In effect, all routine statistics are judged in the context of clinical or administrative experience, against norms laid down elsewhere, or in the light of what is generally regarded as good practice in areas with services of exceptionally high quality.

Their major limitation is that the mere observation of a figure, or of a trend over time, gives no information about value. It summarizes the cumulative results of clinical and administrative decisions without indicating whether they are the right ones. For example, the paper by Tooth and Brooke (1961), describing a short-term decrease in mental hospital bed-occupancy and projecting the trend into the future, or the paper by Baker (1969), describing a psychiatric unit which appeared to manage with only 50 beds per 100,000 population, are not evaluative. They can be used to illustrate a trend but not to justify it.

Thus the first principle of all evaluative work is to be clear as to where the element of value lies. The commonest kind of 'evaluation' is to describe one's own practice (possibly, though not commonly, using a formidable apparatus of population sampling, data collection, and computer processing) and then simply to claim that one is doing better than anyone else. This is bearing witness to good works; it is not necessarily science. Evaluation must be comparative and it must be independent; description is not enough. Everyone now accepts that this is true of new pharmacological treatments; it is time that it was as generally accepted of the provision and organization of services.

The articles by Brooke (1973) and Kramer (1969) and Kramer and Taube (1973) are useful sources of up-to-date information on international and national statistics. The Statistical Report Series (now the Statistical and Research Report Series) of the Department of Health and Social Security provide annual data on the psychiatric services, mostly concerned with in-patients.

CASE-REGISTERS

A case-register is a collection of data about the contacts made by individuals from a defined area with specified social and medical services. Such a linked-record system gives the opportunity of studying the pattern of contacts made over time by individuals or groups of individuals, the patterns of contacts made with particular agencies, the changes in patterns of service use, and the relationship of all these patterns to other population indices, derived from the census or other sources.

Such a register can be used for four main purposes. The first two of these are statistical, to provide information about the people who use services and also about the services themselves. These uses come under the heading of descriptive statistics and the remarks made in the preceding section apply to them.

The third use of a register is as a sampling frame. Since it is based upon a geographically defined population and includes everyone from that population who makes contact with services, the statistics can be expressed in terms of *per capita* rates, which makes them more comparable with those of other areas, and representative samples can be drawn for more intensive study. Since all the services which a patient from the area might in practice attend are covered, the samples are not subject to the bias that arises when studying the practice of any individual hospital, clinic, or agency. This third use is the main one from the point of view of evaluation, since further studies can be carried out, using a combination of designs and methods as discussed earlier. For example, all the patients who contacted the Camberwell psychiatric services in 1968 were screened in order to discover those who have been given a diagnosis of psychosis, were aged 18–54, were not in hospital at the end of the year, and had been out of work for a year or more. The rate was 44 per 100,000 total population, itself a figure of considerable interest and significance. The patients were assessed and then followed up prospectively for two to three years. This design not only gives statistical information, it allows the initial designation of sub-groups and the formulation of hypotheses concerning factors predicting outcome. Lee Robins has provided a useful discussion of such designs (1970). Finally, those of the patients who were willing to be considered for a course of rehabilitation in a newly opened workshop were included in a controlled trial. Thus statistical, epidemiological, longitudinal, and ex-perimental designs were combined; a most powerful technique which enables the results to be generalized with much greater security than is usually possible (Wing et al., 1972).

Note that the advantages of establishing that a study sample is representative of its area can be obtained without the labour and cost of setting up a permanent register. Ad hoc procedures may be perfectly satisfactory for a given purpose. A study of, say, depressive patients newly referred to out-patient services might profitably begin by setting up a simple recording system at all the out-patient departments which treat patients from the area in question. This system would run for a specified time, at least until the intensive investigation conducted on a sub-group of patients had been completed. It would then be possible to show that the study sample was typical of all similarly diagnosed out-patients from the area, or if it was not, to specify how it differed.

The fourth use of registers is for service purposes; to feed back in-formation, for example concerning patients who have not attended a follow-up appointment.

Setting up and maintaining a register is a costly, time-consuming and highly technical procedure. The monograph edited by Wing and Bransby (1970) contains chapters by several experts running registers in the United Kingdom. Baldwin (1971) provides a technical discussion of the value of registers in providing descriptive statistics. The use of a case-register for planning and evaluating a community psychiatric service is described by Wing, Hailey et al. (1972).

THE LITERATURE

There is a large body of epidemiological research. Progress may be judged by the volumes edited by Gruenberg and Huxley (1961), Hill and others (1962), Hare and Wing (1970), and Wing and Häfner (1973), all of which contain summaries of work published during the preceding years. A very brief but useful overview of the whole field of social psychiatry is given by Ransom Arthur (1971). The best general introduction to epidemiology is by Morris (1964). On survey methodology, Moser's book (1958) is still the best. A textbook by Armitage (1971) deals with the statistics used in medical research including life tables, relative risk, and sequential methods as well as the usual parametric and non-parametric techniques. The Central Statistical Office has published a list (1972) of the principal government series and publications, and there is also a series known as *Social Trends* which provides an annual digest of some of the more interesting statistical data relating to social policies and conditions. The books already referred to by Benjamin (1970) on the population census and by Stuart (1964) on sampling are to be recommended. The two short W.H.O. monographs, by Reid (1960) and Lin and Standley (1962), deal with epidemiology as applied to psychiatry. Articles on the epidemiology of schizophrenia, which consider many of the problems that arise, whatever the condition investigated, have been written by Hare (1967) and by Wing (1972). Finally, the book by Wing, Hailey *et al.* (1972) indicates some of the advantages of applying the epidemiological method to the evaluation of a local community service.

REFERENCES

ARMITAGE, P. (1971) *Statistical Methods in Medical Research*, Oxford.

ARTHUR, R. J. (1971) *An Introduction to Social Psychiatry*, Harmondsworth.

BAKER, A. A. (1969) Psychiatric unit in a district general hospital, *Lancet*, **ii**, 1090.

BALDWIN, J. A. (1971) *The Mental Hospital in the Psychiatric Service: A Case-Register Study*, London.

BENJAMIN, B. (1970) *The Population Census: An SSRC Review of Current Research*, London.

BÖÖK, J. A. (1961) Genetic etiology in mental illness, in *Causes of Mental Disorders: A Review of Epidemiological Knowledge*, 1959. New York.

BROOKE, E. M. (1973) International statistics, in *An Epidemiological Basis for Planning Psychiatric Services*, ed. Wing, J. K., and Häfner, H., London.

BROWN, G. W. PARKES, C. M., and WING, J. K. (1961). Admissions and readmissions to three London mental hospitals, *J. ment. Sci.*, **107**, 1070–7.

DENHAM, J., and ADAMSON, L. (1971) The contribution of fluphenazine enanthate and decanoate in the prevention of re-admission of schizophrenic patients, *Acta Scand.*, **47**, 420–30.

DEPARTMENT OF HEALTH AND SOCIAL SECURITY (1971) *Psychiatric Hospitals and Units in England and Wales: In-patient statistics from the Mental Health Enquiry for the year 1969*, Statistical Report Series No. 12, London, H.M.S.O.

DEPARTMENT OF HEALTH AND SOCIAL SECURITY (1972) *Psychiatric Hospitals and Units in England and Wales: In-patient statistics from the Mental Health Enquiry for the year 1970*, Statistical and Research Report Series No. 4, London, H.M.S.O.

DUNHAM, H. W. (1965) *Community and Schizophrenia: An Epidemiological Analysis*, Detroit.

EATON, J. W., and WEIL, R. J. (1955) *Culture and Mental Disorders*, Glencoe, Illinois.

FREMMING, K. H. (1951) *The Expectation of Mental Infirmity in a Sample of the Danish Population*, Occasional Papers on Eugenics, No. 7, London.

GOLDBERG, E. M., and MORRISON, S. L. (1963) Schizophrenia and social class, *Brit. J. Psychiat.*, **109**, 785–802.

GRUENBERG, E. M., and HUXLEY, M. (eds.) (1961) *Causes of Mental Disorders: A Review of Epidemiological Knowledge, 1959*, New York.

HARE, E. H. (1967) The epidemiology of schizophrenia, in *Recent Developments in Schizophrenia*, ed. Coppen, A., and Walk, A., London.

HARE, E. H., and WING, J. K. (eds.) (1970) *Psychiatric Epidemiology: An International Symposium*, London.

HILL, D. *et al.*, (1962) *The Burden on the Community: The Epidemiology of Mental Illness*, London.

KRAMER, M. (1961) Discussion of contribution by J. A. Böök, in *Causes of Mental Disorders: A review of Epidemiological Knowledge, 1959*, New York.

KRAMER, M. (1969) *Applications of Mental Health Statistics*, Geneva, W.H.O.

KRAMER, M., and TAUBE, C. A. (1973) The role of a national statistics program in the planning of community psychiatric services in the United States, in *An Epidemiological Basis for Planning Psychiatric Services*, ed. Wing, J. K., and Häfner, H., London.

KREITMAN, N. (1973) The prevention of suicidal behaviours, in *An Epidemiological Basis for Planning Psychiatric Services*, ed. Wing, J. K., and Häfner, H., London.

LEFF, J. P., and WING, J. K. (1971) Trial of maintenance therapy in schizophrenia, *Brit. med. J.*, **3**, 599–604.

LIN, T. Y., and STANDLEY, C. C. (1962) The scope of epidemiology in psychiatry, *Wld. Hlth. Org. Publ. Hlth. Pap.*, No. 16.

MECHANIC, D. (1970) Problems and prospects in psychiatric epidemiology, in *Psychiatric Epidemiology: An International Symposium*, ed. Hare, E. H., and Wing, J. K., London.

MILLS, C. W. (1959) *The Sociological Imagination*, New York.

MORRIS, J. N. (1964) *Uses of Epidemiology*, 2nd ed., London.

MOSER, C. A. (1958) *Survey Methods in Social Investigation*, London.

MURPHY, H. B. M. (1968) Cultural factors in the genesis of schizophrenia, in *The Transmission of Schizophrenia*, ed. Rosenthal, D., and Kety, S. S., New York.

ØDEGÅARD, Ø. (1952) The incidence of mental disease as measured by census investigations versus admission statistics, *Psychiat. Quart.*, **26**, 212–18.

REID, D. D. (1960) *Epidemiological Methods in the Study of Mental Disorder*, *Wld. Hlth. Org. Publ. Hlth. Pap.*, No. 2.

ROBINS, L. N. (1970) Follow-up studies investigating childhood disorders, in *Psychiatric Epidemiology: An International Symposium*, ed. Hare, E. H., and Wing, J. K., London.

RUTTER, M. (1972) *Maternal Deprivation*.

STUART, A. (1964) *Basic Ideas of Scientific Sampling*, London.

TOOTH, G., and BROOKE, E. M. (1961) Trends in the mental hospital population and their effect on future planning, *Lancet*, i, 710–13.

WING, J. K. (1972) Epidemiology of Schizophrenia, *Brit. J. hosp. Med.*, **8**, 364.

WING, J. K., BENNETT, D. H., and DENHAM, J. (1964) *The Industrial Rehabilitation of Longstay Schizophrenic Patients*, M.R.C. Memorandum No. 42, London, H.M.S.O.

WING, J. K., and BRANSBY, E. R., eds (1970) *Psychiatric Case Registers*, DHSS Statistical Report Series No. 8, London, H.M.S.O.

WING, J. K., and BROWN, G. W. (1970) *Institutionalism and Schizophrenia*, London.

WING, J. K., COOPER, J. E., and SARTORIUS, N. (1973) *The Description and Classification of Psychiatric Symptomatology. An Instruction Manual for the PSE and Catego System*. To be published.

WING, J. K., and HÄFNER, H. (eds) (1973) *An Epidemiological Basis for Planning Psychiatric Services*, London.

WING, J. K., HAILEY, A. M. et al. (1972) *Evaluating a Community Psychiatric Service: The Camberwell Register, 1964–1971*, London.

WING, L., WING, J. K., GRIFFITHS, D., and STEVENS, B. (1972) An epidemiological and experimental evaluation of industrial rehabilitation of chronic psychotic patients in the community, in *Evaluating a Community Psychiatric Service* by Wing, J. K., Hailey, A. M. et al., London.

WOOTTON, B. (1959) *Social Science and Social Pathology*, London.

14

SOCIOLOGICAL METHODS IN PSYCHIATRIC RESEARCH

MARY P. PATTEN AND JUNE PRESS

'Not every research programme needs a survey and indeed many questions can be dealt with as satisfactorily by desk research as by fact collecting. With the social survey, as with any scientific method, part of the skill lies in knowing when to use it at all' (Moser, 1958). The truth of Moser's cautionary introduction is unfortunately rarely appreciated. The first contact that a social scientist has with a psychiatrist comes all too frequently in the form of a belated telephoned inquiry: 'I am carrying out a survey into alcoholism and housing, or obesity and social class, or psychopathy and education—how many cases do I need?', or 'Could you lend me some students to use as interviewers? I have to take over Dr. X's Clinic and I will not be able to get the survey finished for the winter edition of the . . . medical journal'.

The hasty and often ill-considered use of the social survey arises because psychiatrists are not familiar with the range of alternative methods of investigation. In this chapter we will consider some of these alternatives.

CHOICE OF METHOD—CONVENIENCE AND CO-OPERATION

It is important in selecting a method or methods for a project to choose a procedure that will fit in with clinical commitments and practical circumstances. The population survey is particularly suited to the worker or team of workers who are engaged full time in research. Some of the methods that we describe in this chapter, however, such as the routine collecting of one aspect of social data, can be incorporated into clinical practice. Other methods, such as a group interview, take up little time at the fieldwork stage. Techniques using participant observation might be planned to take place intensively in a free day or a short period of study leave. Some operational studies might be descriptions of routine work, such as the supervision of a psychiatric hostel or the teaching of psychiatry to nurses, but with the additional factor of built-in evaluation.

The only certain way of carrying out a research programme exactly as designed is to do the research oneself. But this may not always be possible. For example, it may not be appropriate for a doctor to stay on the ward at night, monitoring the nurses' contacts with the patients. He may plan to use taped group discussion, but find himself urged by relatives, patients, or nurses to do the talking. He may feel attracted by the idea of studying inter-professional conflict, using as data the disagreements that occur in ward rounds, but he may risk unpopularity. One must weigh very carefully before choosing a technique the tolerance of one's colleagues and the expected level of their co-operation, and in particular the work commitments and abilities of these collaborators.

ALTERNATIVE APPROACHES TO THE RESEARCH QUESTION AND DESIGN

Research questions can be explored in more than one way. First one must decide exactly what it is one would like to know. Very often, when a research topic is thought through thoroughly, it is seen to contain a number of sub-questions. Sometimes all these questions can be asked in one study. For example, one may have the impression that teachers who are suffering from depressive illness stay longer on the ward than do manual workers, and wish to confirm if this is so. One may also wish to know if this is true of males only, or is also the case with women factory workers and teacher, and if it is true at each age group within the main years of the working life. All these questions are of the same kind and they can be answered by making a statistical analysis of the records of the hospital or group of hospitals. This kind of information, in a numerical form sometimes referred to as 'hard' data, is adequate if the aim is to make predictions about patient turnover, bed availability and questions of this sort.

If one's interest is clinical rather than administrative, one will be chiefly concerned with why teachers apparently require a longer period of hospitalization than manual workers. The hypotheses selected will influence the methods of investigation. For example, the following hypothesis may be set up:

'There are grave financial disincentives for the manual worker if his hospital stay is prolonged. Pressure from his family to return to work in the early period of recovery accelerates his progress. The teacher is not subject to this pressure.'

This hypothesis might lend itself to a structured questionnaire administered by a social worker to the wives in each group at a certain point in the period of admission. If the hypothesis appears to stand, the material that has been collected will be of value in anticipating and modifying financial pressures where the stage of the clinical condition makes pressures of this sort undesirable, or it might lead to a different type of management in the late recovery phase of the teacher, with the introduction of pressures to accelerate recovery.

If, however, a hypothesis is selected which is concerned with attitudes and family interaction, the questionnaire which was useful in collecting the hard data on income and sick pay will no longer be appropriate. Such a hypothesis might be:

'The families of manual workers offer more encouragement to the patient to return home because they do not see themselves as being factors in the illness. The families of teachers engage in self-analysis and contemplation about the marriage, and may be more hesitant about their husband's homecoming.'

This kind of hypothesis means that one must get to know a few families very well indeed and work with them in an unstructured way, later giving structure to the data by a method known as 'content analysis'.

The direct influence of the patient's family, which cannot readily be changed, may be less interesting than the perception and reaction by nursing staff to family attitudes. The hypothesis might be that the staff are influenced by the hesitation of the teacher's wife, and themselves become hesitant even when the clinical condition is as good as that of the manual worker who is due for discharge. A study of the nursing notes together with a study of the visitors' book and day book reporting on telephone calls received by staff from visitors could be used to explore this hypothesis.

No one research method is exhaustive and each technique has its own set of hypotheses and logic of research. Some investigators use a number of different techniques in the same study to explore different facets of a situation, without necessarily attempting to interrelate the findings. John (1961) in *A Study of the Psychiatric Nurse*, used a questionnaire, diaries kept by student staff, participant observation by the investigator, and the interviewing of all grades of staff. In other instances the interrelation of sets of findings resulting from different techniques is an essential part of the research strategy; an example of this is afforded by a comparative clinical and social survey of three mental hospitals (Brown, 1962) in which the inventory of patients' possessions, a time budget of their activities, a survey of staff attitudes, and the clinical and social state of patients after a set period of time, are used as possible interrelating indices.

STAGES OF THE INQUIRY

Once the research question has been defined and a decision reached about the kind of information required, it is necessary to set up a mock study or 'pilot' to test whether the method chosen is the right one for the purpose. One value of a pilot is that alternative methods can be compared; for instance, one might compare a structured interview with a set of the same questions filled in by the patient. Some aspects cannot be known in advance, such as the likely response rate of a postal questionnaire to ex-patients. The pilot should give guidance as to whether one can be confident enough to go ahead with this method. When a questionnaire is being used, it is essential to use a pilot to identify ambiguous questions. Pilot studies of interviews may show weaknesses in the ordering of material if the interviewer cannot move smoothly from section to section. Very frequently, pilot studies show that the investigator is attempting to do too much—asking too much, observing too many people at the same time, or following cases which are too near to each other in discharge dates for practical convenience. It is always a mistake to rush into the main study when the pilot can be such a useful learning experience.

A particular technique may be useful only at certain stages of an investigation. In a study of patients' attitudes to Health Centres, the first stage was a series of group discussions to which a random selection of patients was invited. These discussions were taped, a content analysis was carried out, and from this a questionnaire constructed. This questionnaire was mailed to the main sample of patients and returned by the patients. Interviewers then went out with the questionnaire and interviewed a sample of the non-respondents (Woods *et al.*, 1973). Each phase may require its own pilot study.

Similarly surveys carried out on large populations very frequently yield statistical associations between variables, which are not meaningful until explored by other techniques. An example is the association between being brought up in a large mental subnormality hospital and severe social inadequacy in adolescence. Findings as general as this are of little use in the therapeutic field. Tizard, who works on problems of this kind, uses a range of methods to investigate the relative contribution of the mental handicap and the special environment, including intensive studies of small groups of children, surveys of children at home and in hospital (Tizard and Grad, 1961), and the design, operation, and evaluation of an experimental unit as a special environment (Tizard, 1964). One of his colleagues has observed child-rearing practices in the institutional setting and has constructed scales so that data may be elicited and classified in a manner that affords comparisons between institutions (King and Raynes, 1968).

ACADEMIC ACCEPTABILITY

An investigator may be hesitant about selecting a method such as participant observation as the only research tool, lest the paper or thesis be rejected as 'unscientific'. If we define the word 'scientific' as meaning that another observer, starting with the same aim or hypothesis, and using the same method will arrive at the same findings, then the techniques offered in this paper are acceptable. It is important, however, when using a method that is more commonly used in another discipline than in psychiatry to explain carefully the logic and relevant theory as well as the operational aspects. A good exposition of this kind in relation to the use of social ecology is given in Sainsbury's study of suicide (Sainsbury, 1955).

ANALYSIS OF RECORDS AND DOCUMENTS: TREND ANALYSIS

The method of research which presents fewest practical problems for the resident doctor is the analysis of records and documents. There is a wealth of written material in any hospital, not only case summary sheets and the fuller clinical and nursing notes, but also social workers' case histories, progress sheets from the occupational therapy department or the hospital workshop, letters to and from internal departments, to and from other hospitals, to and from general practitioners and social agencies. The administrative section keeps records which might be used to provide classification data of staff, the range and level of professional qualification, staff turnover, sickness absence rates, study leave, ward assignment, and success and wastage in training. Data of this sort offer many possibilities in studies of professional behaviour. Operational research depends on data such as bed occupancy, appointments made, kept or failed, and the drugs written up for patients. Other aspects of the work of the hospital might be investigated through study of the minutes of the Management Committee, the Medical Staff Committee, the Heads of Departments meeting, or meeting of Voluntary Workers Guild. If a study of this type will fit in with other interests and commitments, it is both politic and practical to start by seeking the assistance of the Hospital Secretary; he is in the best position to advise on the range and availability, and in some cases accuracy, of records and documents (see also CHAPTER 9).

The use of records to test hypotheses about associations between clinical and social facts, as in the case of studies of the social class of hospitalized schizophrenics, is a familiar one. Another method, called trend analysis, considers one social variable, such as years of education of the new patient, and shows whether changes occur over an interval of admissions. A similar type of study is the monitoring of a social variable, such as occupation of new patients, before and after an administrative change, such as the change in the location of an outpatient clinic.

THE MEANING AND ADEQUACY OF SOCIAL VARIABLES

Social variables are sometimes called classificatory data, or face sheet data. There are shorthand ways of saying something about the patient's style of life. They tell us to which social groups he belongs, and from what we already know about the regular patterns of behaviour and attributes of those groups, we are able to predict in a limited way how persons with his set of variables are likely to behave. The behaviour with which sociologists are concerned is not idiosyncratic behaviour, but the general patterns of social living—courtship, marriage choice, child-rearing, leisure interests, values and belief systems, purchasing and consumer behaviour—on which each individual puts a unique stamp.

Aubrey Lewis has remarked that 'All the studies of causation in psychiatric illness depend on two requirements, adequate detection and measurement of the mental disorder . . . and adequate measurement or description of social characteristics' (Lewis, 1967). There has been discussion of the inadequacy of psychiatric diagnosis as research data, and some investigators prefer to use symptoms rather than diagnosis. Although instruments exist to standardize the eliciting and classification of symptoms (e.g. Wing et al., 1967), unfortunately social variables other than sex and age are frequently too imprecise in the form in which they appear in medical notes to serve as indices of the patient's status and style of living. For example, it is common practice to group all religious affiliation, except for C. of E., R.C., and Non-conformist under the term 'other', and to include the agnostic in this category which also includes the fervent believers from minor sects. Denomination tells us little, unless we have additional data: Fichter (1954) drew up a classification system for Catholics, which included four distinct levels of practice; without such a system to use the social variable 'R.C.' is similar to saying of a patient that he is depressed, with no qualification. Also, social data other than the intimate data of personal relationships is usually limited to the situation at the time of admission, whereas clinical data is collected with the realization that personality is an ongoing process. The patient's style of living is also a dynamic process in which factors such as parental expectation, the patient's years of education, wife's aspirations, the job market, the consumer patterns of neighbours, and the ties of kinship limiting mobility are resolved in temporary equilibrium.

REFINING THE VARIABLES

Some research workers are obliged to rely on data that has been collected for clinical purposes by other people. This method is attractive because of its convenience, but this kind of data is rarely as precise as that which is collected specially for the study. With the exception of age and sex most social variables, such as 'social class', 'occupation', 'religion' are shorthand ways of summarizing a number of statements, and indeed assumptions about the patient. The particular research question may make it desirable to return to the sets of behaviour summarized in the variable. The way to do this is to think through every possible dimension of the social variable, and devise systems for classifying the relevant data.

Thus to return to a previous example, sociologists working in the field of religion have introduced a range of qualifying clauses and degrees of practice. When responses are limited to indicating the denomination of the patient, there will be very little useable information if one is interested in such factors as philosophy of life, the patient's value system, his religious practices, or his integration into a community of fellow believers or worshippers, all of which may operate independently to influence his condition. Further, there is some evidence that religious commitment varies with age and is rarely a constant factor in one individual in all phases of the life cycle.

Another example is provided by occupation. Data might include the particular types of skills used in the job, whether manual, clerical, verbal, or intellectual, and the effects or conditions of work, such as whether the job is heavy, the work dirty, tedious, or gives job satisfaction. It may be important to know the particular hours spent at work, whether it is shift work, night work, work at weekends, or 9 a.m. to 5 p.m.; the task may isolate the employee, or bring him into a work group; the amount of responsibility, co-operation, freedom, and guidance will also vary. Each occupation has its own mode of entry, relevant length of apprenticeship, qualifications, union representation, type and level of remuneration, security of tenure, and regularity or irregularity of work. Many jobs have a status within their own setting, as in the examples of the prestige of the velvet weaver in a textile town, of a coal-face worker in a mining community.

Once one has familiarized oneself with some of the sociological studies of social variables—occupation, social class, religion, education, and marital state—one is very much more sensitive to their complexity and therefore cautious about their use.

CLASSIFICATION AND ELICITING OF DATA

Classification systems in general use such as the Registrar General's Classification of Occupations, provide ready-made instruments, and it may be worth scanning sociological literature for others, particularly if it is hoped to compare the findings with either general population data, or findings from other sources. Some instruments can only be used if specific precoded questions are asked in a certain order. Scales for eliciting prejudice and personality and intelligence tests are usually of this type. One must be confident that the vocabulary and form of question will be appropriate for the particular population, and that this formal method of obtaining information will be acceptable to the informant. Many interviewees become anxious if they are asked to complete questions such as 'Complete this series . . . A.Z.X., B.A.Y., C.B.Z. . . .'. This kind of exercise is beyond their normal experience. Vocabulary tests are familiar and therefore more acceptable, but some subjects become distressed and resentful when they reach their limit, and insist that the interviewer is asking for something outside of 'common-sense'. Vocabulary is partly dependent on education, and clinical psychologists rarely rely on the result of a single test of this sort, any more than a clinician would draw conclusions from the examination of an isolated physiological function.

It is essential to consult, and ideally to work with, a psychologist if you are hoping to incorporate formal tests. He will advise about the most suitable instrument for the study, and also comment on its reliability in the particular cultural population. A question such as, 'I do not read every editorial in the newspaper every day . . . agree/disagree' (F. Scale, California) is irrelevant in a rural population, and even the wording of the M.P.I. in parts, as 'Do you often "have the time of your life" at social affairs ?' make it unsuitable for use with certain groups. Some questions which might be appropriate in a clinical interview, such as 'Are you afraid you might do something seriously wrong against your will ?' (Runwell) may be extremely disturbing when they are asked outside of the clinical situation, and particularly so if the test is self-administered or is administered by someone who is relatively unskilled.

Most standardized scales and tests are copyright, and it is necessary to obtain permission to use them; some are in a printed form ready for distribution, and may not be copied. The cost in this case may be prohibitive if the population is a large one. A few tests are restricted to use by qualified psychologists in specific situations. The 'Moray House Verbal Reasoning Tests' are examples of tests which would become useless if the questions became generally known. In other instruments there is no 'right' answer and the allocation of the subject to a 'neurotic' or 'normal' group depends on a pattern of answers. The best example of this is the Cornell Medical Index which is a series of questions about the patients' health (Brodman et al., 1951). Subjects appear to like to answer questions about their physical health and the few questions about psychological health are apparently more acceptable in a medical context than in a personality inventory. This test has been used in a variety of settings. If the research is concerned with children, there are standardized techniques for assessing development, mainly through questions asked to the mother, and there are also some symptom inventories of behavioural and neurotic symptoms in children. Investigations of this kind, even though standardized, are dependent for their reliability on skilled interviewers as it is essential to separate the child's performance from the mother's own ideas about it

An additional word of caution might be added to the effect that all screening procedures, whether medical or psychological, show that the clinically ill population is not inevitably identical with the group which shows abnormal test scores.

DEVIANT CASE ANALYSIS

The method called deviant case analysis shows the importance of the refinement and precision of variables. The deviant case is the case that does not fit in with the general theory that emerges from the testing of a hypothesis. A statistical analysis of findings in a study on success in psychotherapy may demonstrate that years of education is the important variable, but with a few patients who have had little education, psychotherapy is successful. Fresh contact may be made with these deviant cases and exposure to learning of all types systematically explored. It may emerge that 75 per cent of these patients have wives whose experience of education is superior; alternatively, 60 per cent of these patients may have held positions in trade unions, farmers' clubs, or sports teams, which may have increased the demands on them for verbal fluency.

CONTENT ANALYSIS

Classification is the main tool of content analysis, which is the method of reducing unstructured records, either written or verbal into a quantifiable form. The word 'content' is misleading in that one studies not only what is said, but also the form of the material—whether statement, demand, explanation, or question, the tone of the material and the grammatical presentation, possibly counting and classifying words. Omissions are also noted. Content analysis might be used to compare two sets of notes, such as medical and social notes, or to describe letters sent by general practitioners to the psychiatrist. Some studies have been based on the content analysis of material that has been elicited for the purpose in the form of letters, essays, and diaries.

Alternative sources of data may come from single or group interviews, which are taped and transcribed. Completely unstructured single interviews are difficult to analyse, and many respondents 'dry up' without stimulation of real conversation. Another form of taped interview is the 'Focused Interview' common in media research, in which people are asked for their reactions about each aspect of a film opening scene, choice of actors, etc. In this type of study the material required is carefully specified in advance and hypotheses are drawn up which are then tested by the findings yielded by the content analysis.

THE DIARY: TIME AND ACTIVITY SAMPLING

A diary is useful in an investigation which has a precise object, and diaries have been solicited on a wide range of subjects, including household expenditure, food consumption, accidents in the home, and minor illness. Sometimes material is collected in an interview in diary form: Brown (1966) asked relatives to recall the activities of the schizophrenic patient, working back from the day before the interview. Some diaries are filled in retrospectively by the subject, to avoid the recording influencing the activity; memory error and falsification of events are limitations of this method. A few diaries are prestructured. John (1961) asked student psychiatric nurses to use the headings Time/Task/Reason, /Diagnosis of Patient, /Conversation with Patient, /Topic Discussed, /Other member of staff involved / and Comment. In a time study of a senior registrar in a psychiatric hospital, an observer filled in the diary (Morgan, 1967). Studies of this type have been carried out in industry.

Occasionally random time sampling is used instead of continuous recording. The investigator may divide a 16-hour waking day into intervals of 10 minutes and take a sample of these 10-minute periods. The periods selected will be those he will spend on the ward observing and recording material relevant to the activity that he is studying. This method is suited to such topics as the frequency of conversations between patients and staff, or the involvement of patients in the domestic work of the ward. It is usual to repeat this kind of study over a number of days, and on different days of the week. Activity sampling is a variation of this method. In this case all the tasks on a ward are listed, and the investigator may be present at setting the breakfast table, bed making, chaplain's visit, line up for occupational therapy, afternoon medication, tea time, and lights out. He will observe what part the patient plays in initiating these activities, or assisting, or what conversation there is between patients and staff during these tasks. There would appear, however, to be more risk of influencing the situation which is being observed if the investigator appears on the ward at particular times, than if he is there all the time, as during a period of continuous observation.

OBSERVATIONS OF CLOSED ENVIRONMENTS
AND SPECIAL METHODS OF RECORDING
OBSERVATIONS

Observation is a useful tool in situations which are physically limited, as for example the closed environment of the ward, workshop, or prison. Sometimes the investigator functions as a participant observer in his capacity as doctor, nurse, officer, or even patient or prisoner. One advantage is that he has access to the interpretation of events of one set of participants. Observation is systematic, and the data are slotted into categories, which range between those concerned with physical properties—the colour of walls, design and colour of furnishings, intensity of illumination, or appearance of the patients, as outlined by Russell Barton (1959)—to secondary analysis of observed behaviour, such as the division of activity into purposive and ritualistic.

It is important that observations are precise and not impressionistic. Thus in a comparative social and clinical survey of three hospitals, the patients' possessions were marked off in an inventory (Brown and Wing, 1962).

Social interaction is more difficult to measure, but a tool of some precision is sociometry which in its simplest form is a graphical representation of staff/patient movement; this is useful in the way that a map or diagram is useful; and by scanning the data we may form hypotheses.

An example of the usefulness of the technique is the monitoring of the behaviour of schizophrenic patients in the workshop. The prediction could be tested that the isolated patient, whose movements do not show any interaction with other people, will have a lesser chance of succeeding in open industry than the patient who is initiating some contacts with his fellow workers, or who is the recipient of some visits from the supervisor.

It is often insufficient to plot movement alone. The investigator of social behaviour needs to know about the type of interaction as well as its frequency and direction, and he may use categories such as 'questioning', 'reassuring', 'aggressive', 'assertive', and 'compliant' to organize data about the type of behaviour which is taking place.

A more complicated form of sociometry is to ask patients for their preferred social interaction pattern, that is to say with whom they would prefer to sit or to work. The investigation of the psychological environment of participants is a complementary study to observation of their behaviour and may be useful in interpretation of data. Participants respond to their own perception of events which may be different from that of the observer; there is a sociological maxim to the effect that if events are perceived as real, they will be real in their consequence.

ANALYSIS OF INSTITUTIONS AND INTRA-PROFESSIONAL SITUATIONS

Observation is used both in descriptive and analytical studies. In the latter type of inquiry one may wish to explain, for example, the circumstances under which certain events occur, such as requests for sedation by patients or demands for extra staff. One would approach this study in a general way initially, talking with people, observing the ward systems, and reading any available notes of similar events in the past. A precise definition is then made of the event or factor in which one is interested, and also of the factors that will comprise the experimental variables, such as the composition of staff by rank, 'outsiders' including visitors present or expected on the ward, Management Committee members, voluntary helpers, or the particular age distribution of patients. Hypotheses are then formulated about the occurrence of the event in relation to certain combinations of these factors. These hypotheses may be tested from the data that we already possess or better, are tested in the form of prediction of future events. Examples of different types of combinations of factors may be seen in comparative situations as by comparing and contrasting several different wards. This method (called institutional analysis) is difficult in so far as the investigator is continually modifying his perceptual set, reorganizing his system of classification, redefining variables, and trying fresh hypotheses.

Experimental manipulations of behaviour through the modification of factors in the environment is a related research method, and has been used by Wing in the study of the optimum work situations for schizophrenic patients (Wing et al., 1964). In the writing up of investigations of this sort it is usual to include the failed hypotheses or failed experiments. It is therefore important to keep a record of one's thinking at each stage.

The study of temporary institutions such as the ward meeting, or of events in a temporary situation, for instance decision-making at a case conference, is accomplished by a combination of the methods already discussed. The meeting might first be observed in a general way, and a provisional classification system devised, followed by systematic observation. Content analysis of the transcription of the meeting might be accompanied by a sociometric representation of the communication pattern. The relationships of factors to each other may then be analysed.

Subsequent to the meeting, focused interviews might be arranged with the participants, to compare their reactions to the history of the same case and their views on management. An analogous method was employed by Loudon and Rawnsley (unpublished), who used conjectural case histories to explore differences in interpretation of data between groups of medical, engineering, and divinity students. In another study concerning doctors' referrals to social workers, the doctors' expectations of management of the case by social workers are compared with the social workers' plans (Reilly, 1972). Trend analysis might also be used to examine whether accommodation takes place over a period of time when people work together, and procedures such as case conferences might be introduced experimentally to test their effect on the accommodation process. For work of this kind the study of the social psychology of group behaviour, and of basic sociological concepts, will provide a good theoretical introduction.

SMALL GROUPS OUTSIDE THE HOSPITAL

The idea of studying a small group outside the hospital rather than a ward or hospital workshop is often attractive. Studies of groups which appear to have a function which is complementary to the hospital, such as Alcoholics Anonymous, or of groups which act as screening agents such as Samaritans, may prove very useful in clinical practice. Interesting work also has been carried out on groups who are suspected of containing above average levels of psychiatric morbidity. The systems used for classifying data would include structural characteristics of the group, its activities, communication system, and its manifest function or *raison d'être*. Secondary analysis of data might provide rudimentary information on the values, norms, and belief system of the members. Psychological material might be collected on the identification of members with the group and the intensity and range of the effects of membership on the participants.

ETHICAL PROBLEMS IN SOCIOLOGICAL RESEARCH

Studies of special groups or communities are not usually carried out without the permission of the participants, and even when this has been obtained, difficulties may arise at the stage of publication. If the group is in some way deviant, such as a group of unmarried mothers, alcoholics, or homosexuals, it is essential that they are protected from any adverse consequences. It is the practice to alter identifying characteristics so that anonymity is preserved; even this, however, may not be sufficient if the community can be identified because it is in some ways unique—one thinks of studies that have been undertaken of island communities, or certain institutions which have clearly distinguishing features. Sometimes a decision may have to be made not to publish a part of a study because of the harm this may do to the participants or to the community. One research project into the functioning of a named public institution accidentally brought to light the fact that one senior official was totally inadequate for the job. Publication of this material turned a private research project into a commission of inquiry, and harm was done to the individual, to the institution, and to public confidence not only in the organization but in the neutrality of University research. Sometimes problems arise when the research is carried out for an organization and there is no discussion of an agreed policy between the researcher and the society about the potential use of the findings and the form of their publication. One of us was personally caught in this situation when a voluntary organization divulged findings to the *News of the World*. If the mass media express an interest in a particular piece of research, prepare the press release for them, or insist on seeing the report before publication. Pressure from the mass media unfortunately sometimes leads to premature publication. There have been many examples of this in Northern Ireland, and the research material has become part of sectarian propaganda. In other instances, for example studies in children on the effects of stress caused by political friction, the handling of the material by the press so inflamed public concern that measures potentially more harmful than the 'troubles', such as evacuation, gained general support.

If a group or community is to be studied, a decision must be taken as to whether the members of the group will have access to the findings. This is not an easy decision, because the rights of the group have to be balanced against the possibility that the analysis and interpretation may be threatening to the equilibrium that they have achieved. In what is popularly called 'action research', the investigators offer therapeutic help so that the findings are a part of an experiment in controlled social change. Ethical problems arise continually when sociological models are used in psychiatric research, as it is not possible to ask questions or make interpretations without some change taking place. There is also the problem of the loss of public confidence which may result if records are seen to have been made available to people other than the clinicians to whom the information was entrusted. If such a possibility arises it is always desirable to seek guidance from the local Hospital Ethics Committee.

TOTAL SOCIETIES

SOCIAL ECOLOGY

One approach to the study of mental illness in relation to society at large is by using epidemiological techniques [see CHAPTER 13]. Another is by the method known as social ecology in which data which can be considered in special terms—such as the addresses of suicides, or of patients admitted to hospital—are plotted on a map and then related to the distribution of certain social variables. In a study on suicide Sainsbury (1955) compared the distribution of suicides in London to area data on persons living alone, population mobility, density of lodging houses, and other social parameters. Murphy (1954) used social ecological methods to study psychiatric illness in Singapore, his data being concerned with membership of territorially based ethnic groups.

Professional planners and social geographers have developed instruments for plotting the special distribution of demographic, physical, and even cultural data which are far more sophisticated than the methods of the early sociologists. It is advisable to seek expert advice at a very early stage, since the form in which the data are available may determine the physical boundaries of the area of study.

Yet however carefully ecological study has been carried out there is a simple logical error, known as the 'ecological fallacy', which has often vitiated the results. To assume without further evidence that a person or small group of people from a particular area necessarily share the prevailing characteristics of that region may be unwarranted; thus schizophrenics may be drawn chiefly from a city ward that has a high proportion of immigrants yet themselves be native-born. In general the social ecological technique when used alone is of greater value as a means of generating hypotheses than as a way of testing them.

SOCIAL ANALYSIS

Each method of approach to the study of the total society has its strengths and its limitations. Social analysis, which is normally used by social anthropologists, does not offer findings in a quantifiable form, as in social ecology, although quantitative methods may be used at some stages. The aim of social analysis is to show how a culture pattern, or way of living, fits together as a whole. Our treatment of mental illness may be understood in the context of our economic, religious, and family system, and our legacy of knowledge at a point in time. Most studies have selected aspects of social behaviour such as religious organizations (Loudon, 1966) or customs (Opler, 1959).

Social analysis is not a method that can be used by amateurs, and studies that have been attempted of small communities frequently lack systematic observation and classification of data based on accepted social systems; thus they are journalism and not science. A few psychiatrists, however, are qualified in sociology or social anthropology, and they not only have made theoretical contributions in the understanding of mental illness in society, but they have also given very useful practical help, as on the occasion of the evacuation of the islanders from Tristan da Cunha. The use of sociological methods in psychiatry at this level is not a matter of acquiring tools, but of having the ability to think in two languages, each with its own conceptual system.

QUANTITATIVE DATA ON ATTITUDE

One of the problems that sociologists and other behavioural scientists have had to face, because of the statistical tools that they employ, is the problem of quantifying material that would not normally be thought of in quantitative terms. Rating methods have been dealt with already in this volume with respect to the measurement of behaviour [see CHAPTER 12]. We would like now to look at the allied problem of assessing 'attitude', and we offer a brief account of some of the more widely used and accepted methods of measuring this.

The most obvious, and apparently the simplest, method of assessing attitude would seem to be to ask the subject to assess his own. He can be presented with a range of statements from which he is asked to choose those closest to his own position. One statement is presented, and a range of agreement/disagreement positions is provided, from which he selects.

Basically this is the method of most of the 'tests' of attitude. Our task is to assess how objective such self-rating can be and how much reliance we can place on the 'scores'.

With some of these tests it will be obvious that one 'dimension' of attitude is being measured. In others unidimensionality is assumed, but is not clearly demonstrable. In all attitude testing we make the assumption that in the universe under study there exists a continuum of attitude (to the subject of inquiry) on which individual attitudes can be placed, and their positions identified.

THURSTONE SCALES

One of the most commonly used of Attitude Scales is Thurstone's method of *Equal-Appearing Intervals*. The first step in this procedure is to assemble a large number of statements relating to the attitude to be investigated. These are reduced in number by discarding all those which are obviously duplicates or ambiguous. The remainder, on separate cards, are examined preferably by a panel of 50–300 judges. Each judge is required to assign each statement to one of eleven piles, the first pile being those he considers most favourable, through the sixth (statements judged neither favourable nor unfavourable) to the eleventh, which are those he considers least favourable.

The piles are then scored from 1 to 11, a median value is computed for each item-card, and, as a measure of dispersion (the extent to which the item has been placed at different points in the scale by different judges), the inter-quartile range. Statements with too wide a dispersion are discarded as irrelevant or ambiguous and the final items for inclusion in the scale are such that they will cover the entire range measured, and are equally spaced along the scale (as measured by the medians).

The resulting scale is a series of statements, usually about twenty, and the respondent is asked either to indicate those statements with which he agrees or the two or three statements nearest to his own position.

His score is the average of those items with which he has indicated his agreement.

LICKERT SCALES

In this method too the respondent is presented with a list of statements to which he is asked to react. He is asked, however, not simply to agree or disagree but to grade the strength of his agreement or disagreement usually on a five-point scale. No attempt is made in Lickert's method to cover the range of favourable/unfavourable positions in the list of items, and only items definitely favourable or definitely unfavourable are used.

The first step in producing a Lickert-type scale is to assemble a large number of statements relevant to the attitude to be studied, and considered to be clearly favourable or unfavourable. These are administered to a group considered representative of the study population with the five (or more) point scale. Usually the scoring is:

$$1 \text{ (or 5)} = \text{Strongly agree.}$$
$$2 \text{ (or 4)} = \text{Agree.}$$
$$3 \qquad\quad = \text{Uncertain.}$$
$$4 \text{ (or 2)} = \text{Disagree.}$$
$$5 \text{ (or 1)} = \text{Strongly disagree.}$$

Postive responses (approval) are scored in one direction, negative responses in the other. Those items selected for inclusion in the final list are those which discriminate best between high-scorers and low-scorers on the total scale.

SCALEOGRAM METHOD

Guttman developed a technique of Cumulative Scaling, the main purpose of which is to ensure that statements appearing in a questionnaire do in fact represent a graded progression of opinions, or in other words, that the questionnaire is a 'unidimensional' scale.

In the perfect scale the respondent will endorse all statements that are less extreme than his most extreme statement. An example of a perfect scale would be a series of questions:

1. Are you over 6 ft. tall?
2. Are you over 5 ft. 6 in. tall?
3. Are you over 5 ft. tall?

Positive answers receive a score of 1 and negative answers a score of 0.

SCALE DISCRIMINATION TECHNIQUE

This method, used by Edwards (1957), incorporates aspects of Thurstone's and Lickert's scale construction. Items are chosen and given a scale value as in Thurstone's method. The statements are then given a five- or six-degree agreement/disagreement scale as in Lickert's method. The scale is administered to a large group, and the responses analysed to discover which items discriminate highly between high-scorers and low-scorers. The resulting 'discriminatory coefficients' of the items are then plotted against their scale-value. The items included are those with the highest discrimination within their scale value.

CONCLUSION

Students who intend to incorporate attitude measurement in their research are advised to turn to some of the books listed at the end of this chapter for a description of methods and for consideration of questions of validity and reliability.

REFERENCES

BARTON, R. (1959) *Institutional Neuroses*, Bristol.

BRODMAN, K., ERDMANN, A. G., LORGE, I., and WOLFF, H. G. (1951) The CMI health questionnaire as a diagnostic instrument, *J. Amer. med. Ass.*, **145**, 152.

BROWN, G. W., BONE, M., DALISON, B., and WING, J. K. (1966) *Schizophrenia and Social Care*, Maudsley Monographs, No. 17, London.

BROWN, G. W., MONCK, E. M., CARSTAIRS, G. M., and WING, J. K. (1962) Influence of family life on the course of schizophrenic illness, *Brit. J. prev. soc. Med.*, **16**, 55.

BROWN, G. W., and WING, J. K. (1962) A comparative clinical and social survey of three mental hospitals. The Sociological Review Monographs, *Sociology and Medicine, studies within the framework of the British National Health Service*, ed. Halmos, P., Keele.

EDWARDS, A. L. (1957) *Techniques of Attitude Scale Construction*, New York.

FICTHER, J. (1954) *Social Relations in an Urban Parish*, Chicago.

JOHN, A. L. (1961) *A Study of the Psychiatric Nurse*, Edinburgh.

KING, R. D., and RAYNES, N. V. (1968) An operational measure of inmate management in residential institutions, *Soc. Sci. Med.*, **2**, 41.

LEWIS, A. (1967) *The State of Psychiatry*, London.

LOUDON, J. B. (1966) Religious order and mental disorder in a rural community in S. Wales (Personal communication).

MORGAN, R. (1967) The work of a junior doctor in a psychiatric hospital, in *New Aspects of the Mental Health Services*, ed. Freeman, H., and Farndale, J., Oxford.

MOSER, C. A. (1958) *Survey Methods in Social Investigation*, London.

MURPHY, H. B. M. (1954) *Med. J. Malaya*, **9**, 1.

OPLER, M. K. (1959) *Culture and Mental Health*, London.

RAWNSLEY, K. (1968) Social attitudes and psychiatric epidemiology, in *Studies in Psychiatry*, ed. Shepherd, M., and Davies, D. L., London.

REGISTRAR GENERAL (1965) *Classification of Occupations*, H.M.S.O., London.

REILLY (1972) in progress, Health Centre, Finaghy, Northern Ireland.

SAINSBURY, P. (1955) *Suicide in London—An Ecological Study*, Maudsley Monograph, No. 1, London.

TIZARD, J., and GRAD, J. C. (1961) *The Mentally Handicapped and their Families*, Maudsley Monographs, No. 7, London.

TIZARD, J. (1964) *Community Services for the Mentally Handicapped*, London.

WING, J. K., BENNETT, D. H., and DENHAM, J. (1964) The industrial rehabilitation of longstay schizophrenic patients, *Medical Research Council, Memorandum No. 42*, London.

WING, J. K., BIRLEY, J. L. T., COOPER, J. E., GRAHAM, P., and ISAACS, A. D. (1967) Reliability of a procedure for measuring and classifying 'present psychiatric state', *Brit. J. Psychiat.*, **113**, 499–515.

WOODS, O., PYPERAUD, and PATTEN, P. (1973) in progress, Health Centre, Armagh, Northern Ireland.

FURTHER READING

THURSTONE, L. E., and CHAVE, E. J. (1929) *The Measurement of Attitudes*, Chicago.

LICKERT, R. (1932) A technique for the measurement of attitudes, *Arch. Psychol.*, No. 140.

SCALEOGRAM METHOD

STOUFFER, S. A. (1950) *Measurement and Prediction, Studies in Psychology in World War II*, Vol. 4, Princetown, N.J.

EDWARDS, H. L. (1957) *The Social Desirability Variable in Personality Assessment and Research*, New York.

SEMANTIC DIFFERENTIAL

OSGOOD, L. E., SUCI, G. J., and TANNENBAUM, P. H. (1957) *The Measurement of Meaning*, Urbana, Ill.

FACTOR ANALYSIS

HARMAN, H. H. (1967) *Modern Factor Analysis*, Chicago.

15

INTERVIEWING IN PSYCHIATRIC FIELD SURVEYS

JACQUELINE GRAD de ALARCON AND
ANNEMARIE CROCETTI

In describing the results of any piece of research that is based on a field study, one is presenting data collected at interviews. It follows, then, that the results can only be interpreted if the quality of the interviewing is known. No matter how good the research design, how excellent the questionnaires, or how carefully planned the field operation is, the data collected will only be as good as the interviewing.

If we were discussing research in the physical sciences it would be unnecessary to stress that the investigator should be thoroughly familiar with the laboratory techniques he plans to employ in the collection of his data. He would be expected to know the problems and limitations, and it would be taken for granted that he would provide adequate training for his technicians and that continuous supervision would be maintained to ensure reliability of the data collected.

In field surveys in medicine, however, it is quite commonplace to find that the senior investigators are unfamiliar with interviewing as a research technique; they have never attempted to call on households and conduct interviews, and therefore have no realistic awareness of the problems. On the contrary, it is often taken for granted that, given a good questionnaire, almost anyone available and willing can be relied upon to collect the required data; that people who have interviewed previously are *ipso facto* good interviewers; and that people who are familiar with 'interviewing' clients or patients for purposes other than research possess the skills required for research interviewing.

Interviewing is a practical skill that can only be learned by experience—by trial and error under guidance and supervision. No amount of studying academic texts or interviewing manuals will equip the student to take part in a field survey if the practical experience is lacking. Nevertheless there are certain techniques available to the experienced research interviewer, and the purpose of this chapter is to try to describe them.

The quality of interviewing in any field survey, however, does not depend solely on the skill and experience of the interviewers. It is also related to the overall purpose, planning, and execution of the study and, in particular, to the quality of the questionnaire which interviewers are expected to administer. For this reason we have preceded our discussion of interviewing techniques with a description of some of the problems of standardization that have to be considered by the investigator who is planning an interviewing survey.

STANDARDIZATION—RELIABILITY AND VALIDITY

Interviews are conversations that are focused to obtain or give information, guidance or therapy. Their form and content depends on the purpose for which they are being used. If this purpose is to act as a research instrument in field surveys the interviews must be standardized rather than just focused. Uniform and standard procedures are a primary requisite of scientific inquiry. Unless the phenomena observed are defined and measured by standard instruments under standard conditions, their variable behaviour in different situations cannot be assessed.

However, standard procedures do not guarantee that the instruments used are appropriate. For an instrument to be appropriate it must also be valid and reliable, and standardization is only of value if the investigator has already done the best he can to ensure validity and reliability

An instrument is *valid* if it truly measures the entity that it purports to measure and not some other factor.

It is *reliable* if its findings are reproducible, that is, its measures of the same entity remain constant, even though it is being used in different places, at different times, or by different people. In assessing reliability not only the instrument itself but also the conditions under which it is used and the way in which measurements are read and recorded (i.e. the observer reliability) must be taken into account.

Laboratory instruments which measure psysiological changes in disease are independent of the subject's control. So the investigator who uses blood sugar determinations need consider only the validity of the particular procedure he employs and set up appropriate controls to ensure reliability in its administration.

As soon as measurements of complex social characteristics and behaviour are required, the task is complicated because the subject is able to influence the measurement. Except for a few measurements of physiological correlates of behaviour, such as tremor, the data consist of observation and description of individuals or groups, and of verbal communication.

Furthermore, the interview during which the data are collected is a social situation. Consequently, factors in the respondent, those in the person who is administering the instrument, and those resulting from the interaction between respondent and interviewer have to be considered in achieving validity and reliability of the observations

When a questionnaire is designed to serve as a case finding or screening instrument, in addition to collecting other data, the investigator faces a double task in striving for validity and reliability. He must not only check the individual questions for inherent validity and reliability but must test the relevant portion of the instrument as a screening device.

RELIABILITY

In using the interview as a research instrument one may view each question as one would a stimulus presented in a laboratory experiment; if one wishes to measure and compare different responses, then the stimulus must be similar each time it is given. This means that great care must be exercised each time the interviewer administers the questionnaire to ensure that the questions come in the specified order, that the probes are uniform, and that any extraneous conversation during the interview does not interfere with the nature of the stimulus.

In large-scale surveys it is usual for the interviewer to be given a questionnaire which demands standard administration of this kind. In smaller studies, however, where the purpose of the research is often to seek for rather than to test aetiological hypotheses, greater flexibility in interviewing is encouraged. The more the latitude allowed—in changing the wording of questions and using probes—the more the responsibility the interviewer bears for nevertheless maintaining the maximum level of standardization.

A *questionnaire* is reliable to the extent that the data it produces are consistent and reproducible when it is administered according to a standard procedure in similar conditions. *Interviewers* are reliable to the extent that, given a reliable questionnaire and standard conditions, they produce consistent and reproducible data.

The factors that can reduce the reliability of questionnaires may lie in the instrument itself; in the interviewing situation; and in the technique that is used for interviewing. Therefore it is impossible to test questionnaire reliability as such since the instrument, the interviewer, the interviewing process, and situation are inextricably mingled.

A question is likely to be reliable if it is clearly and unambiguously worded; the same wording is used on every occasion; it deals with factual data rather than opinions; it deals with quantitative rather than qualitative ideas; it provides answer categories that do not force choice; it specifies the time period covered; and finally, it does not involve memory but deals with current events.

Not only the wording of the questions but the order in which they are asked affects whether they are likely to be answered similarly on different occasions. For maximum reliability the same sequence should be adhered to throughout the study.

Finally, the amount of interpretation required from the interviewers either by implication or instruction will affect reliability. For example, if the question asks the respondent how he disciplines his children, but the interviewer is required to summarize the answer by making a judgement as to whether the respondent is a 'severe', a 'moderate', or a 'permissive' parent then answers may vary according to the interviewer's standards of severity of discipline

For obtaining reliability then, the ideal question is clearly worded, precisely directed, and asks for dichotomous or quantifiable answers. The questionnaire should be pre-coded; and the interviewer allowed little latitude to probe and make judgements on the spot. Built into this procedure, however, there is a serious problem: high levels of reliability can often be achieved only at the cost of sacrificing validity.

VALIDITY

The appropriate time to consider the validity of the questions included in the interview is when the questionnaire is being constructed. The formulation of each question should be based on careful consideration of how problems that may affect validity may be solved, and then to examine these issues by preliminary testing.

Once the actual field phase has begun it is possible to check validity further by instructing interviewers to probe for comprehension and frame of reference at randomly determined points in the interview. For example, in one cross-cultural study the interviewers were told to ask: 'What did you think I meant when I asked that question?' at pre-determined points in the interview.

Several factors may impede the validity of questions in the interview. The most obvious but frequently overlooked one is that the respondent simply does not possess the information asked for—he may not have it at all or he may not have it in the detail required by the question. Other major factors are: firstly, that the respondents may not understand the frame of reference of the question as formulated; secondly, that the topic may be one about which he may not wish to give a true answer; and lastly, his desire to give socially acceptable answers or ones which he thinks will please the interviewer.

An example of a question that gives rise to misunderstandings about the frame of reference is the following:

'Is your marriage satisfactory ?   No   0
                                        Yes   1
                                        Not known   2
                                        Inappropriate   3'

The intention of the investigator was to elicit responses concerned with the sexual relationship in the marriage. He expected the answer 'No' to be given if sexual relations were absent or unsatisfactory. In fact, several wives said 'Yes' meaning no sexual demands were made, others said 'Yes' meaning enough housekeeping money was given to them. Some said 'No' meaning they had no children.

Vague concepts and general summary terms such as 'satisfaction with marriage', 'interference with leisure activities', 'being a good parent', 'social isolation', 'withdrawal', etc. must be broken down into the component bits of behaviour that the investigator has in mind if he wishes to obtain valid replies.

The problem of obtaining information which is only reluctantly revealed, because it touches on taboo topics (drugs, abortion, etc.) is more difficult to cope with and requires greater interviewing skills. The interviewer may lead into the topic gradually by asking questions about more acceptable aspects of the topic, or he may decide that a matter of fact approach, taking it for granted that it is reasonable and sensible to ask questions about the topic, would best rob it of stigma and produce a true reply. He will be able to do this best if the inquiry is one which both he and the respondent think important and if the investigator has established a good reason for raising the sensitive topic. In any event, the use of judgement and taking decisions on the spot by the interviewer is likely to affect reliability.

The investigator must try to strike a happy balance between maximum reliability and maximum validity. In our opinion, to do this it is important to have some open-ended or 'probe' questions interspersed with the pre-coded questions in each questionnaire; but, above all, pre-testing every question is essential.

The investigator should remember that with many questionnaires planned for maximum reliability there are no checks on whether the respondent has in fact been listening to the questions. People very often do not listen attentively, especially to long questions or a series of questions. They are preoccupied with their own affairs and often answer what they thought the interviewer asked rather than what he in fact asked. When the entire interview schedule is nothing but a series of questions with replies circled 'YES' or 'NO', there is no way of telling if the respondent in fact did listen carefully. But questions requiring verbatim answers provide such a check.

TRAINING

Before starting out on the field work interviewers must learn the instructions and approach to respondents required in that particular survey. They will need to learn the detail of the questionnaires and how they are to be used to meet the intentions of the investigator.

Some aspects of training are general. The things that interviewers always need to know are first the significance of sampling procedures and the reasons why they must be followed exactly; second they must know how to approach people, to talk to them easily to establish rapport, and to handle questions respondents put to them. Next, they must understand the importance of always following the instrument exactly as it is constructed; they must know how to avoid explaining terms used in questions when this is not permitted, and how to probe in a neutral fashion so that they do not force the answers. They must be able to interview easily so that they can maintain a steady daily level of work. Also they must be able to read maps and record locations of households so that other people can find them. Finally, they must learn when to refer back to the investigator for help. Some problems may be handled by the interviewers taking decisions themselves and others cannot.

For example, an interviewer should be able to differentiate between having difficulties with a given question because *he* does not understand it and what it is supposed to gather, and having difficulties because the question does not make sense in the population in which he is working. He must also know whether the question presents difficulties to a whole group of respondents or is merely an isolated incident. If it is a matter of the interviewer not understanding the question properly he can usually remedy this by referring back to his instruction manual. If, however, he understands the question, but the respondents do not, then he should call this to the attention of the investigator.

To be able to complete an assignment and meet acceptable levels of reliability an interviewer must therefore be competent at all the following:

1. Acquiring familiarity with the questionnaire and interviewing instructions so that it can be handled and used with ease.
2. Organizing the day's work efficiently.
3. Finding the designated respondent.
4. Gaining access; introducing himself and gaining co-operation to conduct an interview.
5. Explaining the purpose of the survey without biasing responses.
6. Establishing the required setting for the interview.
7. Getting the respondent to feel at ease and prepared to talk freely.
8. Conducting and controlling the interview so that it follows previously determined lines as far as possible; avoiding extraneous topics and not wasting time while at the same time not restricting the information that the respondent may have to offer.

9. Recording the answers as instructed.
10. Checking the questionnaire before leaving, to make sure all points have been adequately covered; and editing it as soon as possible afterwards.
11. Leaving the respondent in such a frame of mind that any further examinations or follow-up interviews that may be required will be acceptable to him.
12. Filling out any additional forms that have been requested and noting any difficulties on locating the household, the hours that the respondent is available, and so on, so that any return visitor will have an easier time finding him.
13. Keeping in touch with the principal investigator so that he is informed about conditions in the field which may interfere with schedules.

FINDING THE PROPER RESPONDENT

The sampling instructions and training should have told the interviewer exactly how he is to go about finding the correct person to interview. However, every situation may not have been covered and it is the interviewer's responsibility to make sure that he is interviewing the proper person.

When a census or listing operation has already been done or where the named relatives of patients are being seen it will be fairly simple to find the right household. When there is no such list, however, the interviewer may himself be given the task of listing dwelling units and then, following sampling instructions, selecting the household to be included in the survey. He must be sure that he does not yield to the understandable temptation of omitting households where he expects to have trouble interviewing, or where he finds that the people are unpleasant, alarming, or difficult to reach. Above all, if he has made a mistake, he must report it.

Once he knows which households to approach, he must then locate the proper respondent. His instructions may simply be to interview any adult that happens to be home. Usually, however, the sampling procedure requires a designated respondent. This may mean that he has first to list all the members of the household in a specified order, for example oldest male to youngest male. Then he must use the sampling technique that has been given him, and conduct the interview with the selected person.

This can make for awkward situations. The people who have described the household composition may not understand why one person should be interviewed rather than another. If the designated respondent refuses while other household members agree, or if he is clearly not the one who can give the required information, the interviewer must know whether substitutes are permitted. It may be useful in this situation to conduct a second interview with the better informed respondent so long as separate questionnaires are used and both are returned to the investigator.

Quite often people want to know why they or their household came to be chosen for the survey. The interviewer should be able to explain this briefly and simply: 'I've been told to call at every tenth house; names were picked out of a hat and yours came up; we are seeing all families with two or more children'. Avoid complicated explanations about the technical aspects of surveys and sampling techniques; use simple everyday language and act in a matter of fact way as if the survey were quite usual and to be taken for granted.

It may not be possible to obtain an interview with the designated respondent for several reasons. He may have moved out of the area; be absent longer than the period of the survey; cannot be found; or be unfit or unwilling to be interviewed. The interviewer should find out all he can from neighbours, local records, shops, post offices, etc. in order to trace the respondent, and then record the information so that it can be usefully analysed. He should, for example, record the respondent's age, sex, occupation, household composition, reason for not obtaining the interview, and places and times at which it may be possible to reach him. He should note who gave him this information and try to assess the likelihood of this informant having accurate knowledge.

GAINING ACCESS TO THE INFORMANT

Once having located respondents, the interviewer has to persuade them to agree to being interviewed. If there has been appropriate local publicity about the survey beforehand this task will be made easier for him.

The approach that the interviewer takes when he first knocks at the door and introduces himself will influence the number who agree and the number who refuse.

The good interviewer will be friendly and persuasive rather than brash and overbearing. While the latter approach—entering officiously as if of right and expecting people to answer the questions as a public duty—may daunt timid and reluctant respondents into agreeing, it may well harden the resistance of a tougher character, who could be persuaded to agree by a more gentle approach. The good interviewer, who is self-confident and who is familiar with the culture and at ease with the people he is calling on, will alter his approach, often unconsciously, to the manner which will make him acceptable to the individual respondent. He will use the kind of greeting that is customary in order to set the respondent at ease and put him in a receptive mood. While not wasting too much time on polite chit-chat, the caller who passes the time of day and makes a comment on the weather, the garden, or the children, as he would in normal social exchange, is more likely to be received and talked to frankly than one who comes directly with an official request.

However, fortunately for interviewers, most people are perfectly prepared to talk to strangers if they are approached in a friendly and polite manner. The kinds of situations where reluctance is common are those where people have some reason to be suspicious of and hostile to callers. This may apply to minority, delinquent, or de-socialized groups of people. In disorganized communities wealthy people may not admit strangers for fear of violence and burglary, and poor ones may be afraid of police, debt collectors, and 'officials' of any kind. In these cases, if the interviewer cannot gain entry by himself, he will do well to write or telephone before calling or arrange to be introduced by a trusted local person.

Reluctance to admit the interviewer may also be met when the respondents are paranoid, suspicious, or litigious people. Here again, a letter or personal introduction may help, and the interviewer should always carry some means of identifying himself. This will normally be in the form of a signed letter from the head of the organization for which he works, such as: 'This is to introduce Miss X who is visiting households in [area] to carry out a health survey for this organization. Your help will be much appreciated.'

On the whole, so long as the interviewer himself is at ease, he will meet with little reluctance and will usually be able to overcome misgivings by a frank and clear statement of the purpose of his call. The better acquainted he is with the questionnaire he is using the more at ease the interviewer will be.

CONFIDENTIALITY

Respondents often need to be reassured that any information they may give will be treated confidentially and will not be reproduced in an identifiable form. Interviewers are usually asked to tell informants that this will be so; it should not be an empty phrase but be treated extremely seriously by the interviewer. People refuse to participate in a survey when they see confidentiality is not maintained.

Discretion is also essential, especially when neighbours are being approached for information about absent respondents. Here the interviewer should always be discreet, unalarming, unofficious and appear to be making friendly inquiries. He should have a stock of phrases on hand which will allow him to avoid questions asked by neighbours and other people who know about the survey.

The respondent who wants to know what a neighbour has said before answering a question himself should be told that it is impossible to remember the details of any one interview and that everything is confidential so that even if answers could be remembered they could not be repeated. It is also a good idea to point out that everybody has different and interesting points of view. This may reassure him that the data is indeed valuable and important.

Completed questionnaires contain confidential important information; they should not be left lying around in public places or in the interviewer's home or office for anyone to see.

APPEARANCE

The interviewer's appearance as well as his manner should be one which will be acceptable to respondents in the survey area. In dress he should appear unremarkable; he should try to look like any other social caller and not carry official-looking files or piles of papers ostentatiously. A notebook readily available in a pocket or handbag and a discreetly carried questionnaire in a folder should suffice. He should not approach the house until he is organized and ready to start interviewing. The interviewer who comes into a house heavily laden and fumbles through a mountain of papers while he is trying to get organized will be flustered, and the respondent will wonder whether he knows what he is doing and may therefore not treat the interview seriously.

INTRODUCING THE SURVEY AND AVOIDING REFUSALS

The training session should have taught the interviewer a standard explanation and introduction. It is important to keep to this and do as little elaborating as possible. Here again use simple everyday language and avoid complicated explanations about the purpose of the survey. Not only does it waste time but the respondent gets confused and feels it is all too much bother for him. Usually it is best just to repeat the standard introduction and then say: 'Well, now here is the first question', and proceed. If the questionnaire is well designed the first question will be of general interest and easy to answer; the respondent will have started being involved in the actual interview before he thinks of objections or decides that he does not want to take part. It is often prudent to avoid the term 'interview' in introductions and simply say something along the following lines: 'We are calling on people in this

district to ask about [the topic]. May I come in and tell you about it ?'
Most people will say yes.

People usually accept the fact that information is needed if none is available and are ready to co-operate if the topic is of any interest, concern, or relevance to them. Quite often they are delighted to receive a visit from somebody who is interested in their affairs, who solicits their opinions and listens respectfully, treats them seriously and does not argue back.

The best way for the interviewer to achieve the confidence and ease that are necessary to gain the respondent's co-operation is first, to be convinced himself that the survey is so important and worthwhile that it justifies intruding on people's privacy and, second, to be thoroughly familiar with the schedule he is going to administer. If the interviewer is confident he will not feel the need to embark on long-winded explanations, or be tempted to promise anything that he knows cannot be delivered such as saying that the purpose of the study is to help people in some way which cannot actually be done. There are two dangers in this. First, explanations and offers of help that depart from the standard agreed ones given to all respondents reduce reliability, and hence the comparability, of data from different respondents. Second it is likely to produce biased responses. The standard explanation will have been worded deliberately to try to avoid people giving answers which they think will be advantageous. An explanation composed on the spot can seldom be so carefully worked out.

The interviewer who is not convinced of the value of the survey is not only liable to affect reliability but may also encourage refusals by his own hesitant approach. This is a particular danger in surveys of bereaved or handicapped people, and where the families of mentally ill patients are being seen. A tender-minded interviewer may project his own feelings of embarrassment or distress at questioning such people on to the respondent and regard the interview as an unwarranted intrusion. Such sentimentality is misplaced. Most people with these problems are grateful to talk about them to a sympathetic yet detached listener, but shy from doing so when the interviewer appears squeamish or disturbed.

RESPONDENTS WHO CANNOT SPARE TIME

If the respondent says that he does not have time for a lengthy interview, the interviewer must try to judge whether this is genuinely because another time would be more convenient or the respondent is reluctant to co-operate at all. In the former case he should make a firm appointment. In the latter he should try to persuade the respondent to see him there and then, saying he would be grateful for whatever time the respondent can spare. Frequently people do not realize how long an interview takes once they become involved in the topic. Therefore, unless the person really has an urgent appointment it is quite often possible to take a chance on completing the interview. Should the respondent only have a short time and appear unwilling to arrange a later interview the interviewer should use that time to try to involve him to the extent of accepting a second visit.

The normal beginning of the interview will usually reassure the reluctant respondent so that he will change his mind and co-operate. If he is determined not to do so, pressure will only annoy him.

When the interviewer feels that he is going to get a refusal he must try to extract himself from the situation and leave the respondent not having made the refusal explicit. It is much harder to break a refusal once it has been given than to avoid one by postponing the interview. A second interviewer may have a better approach, may appeal more to the respondent, or may come at a more propitious time.

The first interviewer should, however, try to see whether he can understand why the refusal is about to happen, and whether he can allay whatever is causing anxiety or reluctance in the respondent. While it is useless to press too hard, an appeal to the good nature of a respondent to help to fulfil the quota of visits sometimes works when an appeal to help with the research does not.

Should a refusal be unavoidable the interviewer must give an accurate report of the circumstances in which it happened so that the investigator can judge whether there is any way in which the situation may be retrieved.

ESTABLISHING THE REQUIRED SETTING

By this we mean, first of all, getting to see the respondent alone, if this has been requested, or when necessary, seeing two respondents (for example husband and wife together); then contriving that the interview takes place at a time and a place where the respondent is free from other distractions and can concentrate on the matters in hand.

Most interviews, especially if personal matters are to be covered, require privacy, and this is sometimes difficult to achieve. Respondents who live gregarious lives will often not see the need for privacy—although their answers will be influenced by the presence of other people. For example, a respondent who will be prepared to answer questions about sexual practices when alone with the interviewer, is likely to be inhibited by the presence of his wife, and even more so by the presence of other people So the interviewer should take no notice of respondents who say: 'Oh, they can stay—I have no secrets from them', and should insist on a private interview. This applies particularly to children who insist on remaining. The interviewer should remember that children may be anxious about a stranger coming to talk to their parents—especially if it is about the health of a parent who has been sick. It is often necessary to allay the children's anxieties before the interview can proceed. Other family members may of course be anxious too. The interviewer who neglects to allay anxieties must be prepared for constant interruptions during the course of the interview.

Difficulties may arise when the home is crowded, when in a cold climate only one room is heated, and when family members, friends, or neighbours insist on being present during the interview. Usually a mere request to see the respondent alone may be sufficient. Or a more authoritative note may be struck: 'I will have to see you alone—will Mrs. X please excuse us?', or 'Is there somewhere we can go without disturbing the family?' Alternatively, the interviewer can plead: 'I am afraid it is too confusing [or difficult] for me if too many people are here—I can only concentrate on one at a time—can we talk now, and then if I may see Mrs. X alone after that?' (This may involve the interviewer in brief chats with people which are not necessary for the survey, but the extra time is well worth while.) As a last resort the interviewer may suggest a stroll or a drive to the informant, or arrange to see him elsewhere or at a time when other people are absent.

Situations can of course arise where it is not possible to interview the respondent without an audience. The interviewer must be prepared to judge whether insisting on privacy would cause undue tension or lose the respondent's co-operation and goodwill. If he believes it would he must then face the problem of distracting the audience so that they do not participate in the interview. Sometimes they may be helpful in reminding the respondent of facts; but when a question is aimed at getting the opinion, attitude, or the feeling that the respondent has towards a topic, it may be crucial to exclude them. The best way to deal with this situation is to visit with a colleague. Then one can distract the family while the other interviews the respondent.

The interviewer not only has to get the respondent alone, but has to try to remove other distractions from him, notably radio, television, and babies. He should not hesitate to ask to have the radio switched off, and he should find out if there is anyone else available to look after the baby.

GETTING THE RESPONDENT TO TALK FREELY

Once having got the respondent to agree to being interviewed, his sympathy for, interest in, and comprehension of the topics being pursued must be maintained. In a health survey this should not usually be difficult. It is the very rare person who does not relish the opportunity to discuss his own health. People may be reluctant at first to talk about certain topics: socially unacceptable diseases; money in some cultures; and sex in others. Many will also hesitate to reveal information which they believe may show them up as a poor provider, an inadequate parent, or deficient in some other way. However, if these topics are preceded by relatively innocuous ones, so that the interviewer has time to establish himself in the respondent's esteem as an interested and sympathetic *listener*, such reluctance will often not appear.

CONDUCTING AND CONTROLLING THE INTERVIEW

Having located the respondent, persuaded him to co-operate, and obtained his trust and willingness to talk freely, the interviewer next has to make sure that the interview procedes along the planned lines. He must establish whatever situation has been defined as suitable for the interview; he must follow his schedule according to his instructions; he must restrict the replies to the topics in hand; he must complete the interview within a limited period of time; and he must do all this while maintaining the interest and co-operation of the respondent.

FAMILIARITY WITH THE QUESTIONNAIRE

A thorough familiarity with the interviewing schedule is a prerequisite for controlling the interview so that it runs according to plan. In both structured and unstructured interviews, it is essential for the interviewer to know what topics are going to be covered; the kinds of information he is seeking to obtain; the order in which he intends to ask questions; the place where each question is to be found on the document he holds; and whether any sections of the questionnaire may be omitted in particular cases. He should be familiar with and experienced in handling and using the document before he attempts to do any of the interviews included in the survey. If his instructions are to read the question out from the questionnaire during the interview, he must still be able to concentrate adequately on the respondent's replies; he must be able to look up at the respondent without being in danger of losing his place on the schedule; and he must be able to note down the reply against the correct question and still not lose the thread of what the respondent may be continuing to talk about, even if he is busy reading the instructions or the next question.

He must know beforehand how any particular reply is to be coded and should not have to take time to consider this during the interview. He should also be prepared for those sections of the schedule where he is instructed to omit questions or to ask additional questions, depending on the answer given to the current question.

If his instructions allow him to alter the order or wording of the questionnaire to meet particular contingencies, or to interview in any manner he thinks fit so long as certain topics are covered, he must still have a plan in mind. He should have thought out beforehand the best way to cope with various informants and situations, and, while being flexible enough to recognize these, he should still be able to adhere to the plan which will allow him to complete the interview within a reasonable period of time and still cover all the topics of the interview in a way that is logical for that particular situation.

QUESTION ORDER

While keeping to the order and wording of the schedule is of course essential when a structured questionnaire is being used, even the most free and unstructured interview must be planned to some extent and proceed according to the form that the interviewer deems appropriate. If this is not done the interview will become a mere conversation whose form and content is determined by the respondent.

If the questionnaire is well written it should ease into the interview in a manner which will not alarm the respondent. This means that the first questions will deal with straightforward matters of fact which are simple to answer so that the informant gets the feeling he is competent to cope with the interview.

Quite often, when the interview is not rigidly structured and the interviewer is at liberty to choose or vary the question order, he hesitates to begin with blunt questions of fact—choosing first to try to establish a relationship with the respondent by more general discussion. This is usually a mistake. Respondents who agree to be interviewed are expecting questions about facts and opinions, and it is an advantage to both the interviewer and the respondent to get facts early on, for example household composition, income, and work and sickness histories. Both then feel that they are progressing satisfactorily, and the interviewer has a basic outline of the respondent's social situation that will help him follow subsequent references to work, and other members of the family etc. The interviewer whose instructions are to keep to a certain order and wording has a relatively simple task compared with one who is asked to cover certain topics in any order that seems appropriate. The latter situation offers many more opportunities for forgetting a topic or for neglecting to explore one aspect of a topic. We recommend that wherever the interviewer does not have to follow a questionnaire rigidly, he should never complete the interview without consulting either the schedule itself or a checklist of topics to make sure everything has been dealt with. This is quite easy to do and, in addition, provides a useful method of checking back on items to which the respondent has given inconsistent or ambiguous replies. No respondent objects to the interviewer who says, 'I just want to check through to see whether we have covered everything—you have told me all about X and Y, what about Z?' At the end of the interview, respondents frequently volunteer extra information, and this résumé of the topics covered offers a good opportunity for them to do this.

LIMITING THE RESPONDENT'S REPLIES TO THE TOPICS IN HAND

It sometimes seems to us that investigators who draw up questionnaires and instruct interviewers without themselves having attempted to conduct field interviews, too often assume that people behave as automata; reply directly and to the point when they are asked questions; listen and respond carefully; and never obtrude their own ideas, plans, and fantasies which may be completely irrelevant to the purpose of the interview. Perhaps this is because most professional people receive their interviewing experience with candidates for jobs or examinations, with students, with patients, or with clients. They see them in their own offices, and in situations where they are in a position of authority *vis-à-vis* the person who is being interviewed, and where that person is highly motivated to conform and to reply directly to any question which he may be asked.

This is an error into which physicians, when they act as investigators, are particularly liable to fall. They, more than most other professional people, hold positions of authority, and may expect the patient, in his own interest, to give frank and clear replies to their questions. However, the patient who answers obediently in the surgery is not necessarily going to do so when an interviewer comes to his home. To him, the health survey interviewer may present a fine opportunity to describe his ailments in detail; for airing his grievances about the health service; or for discussing his pet theories. Respondents may be just as beguiling and persuasive in drawing the interviewer into topics that *they* want to discuss as interviewers are, and the interviewer may have a hard time keeping to his schedule.

In our experience, by far the most difficult task of interviewing is not getting the respondent to talk, but getting him to stop talking or rather to stop rambling around the subject and keep to the point. The interviewer must have the patience to cope with this as well as the ability to cut short the respondent's irrelevant reminiscences without losing his goodwill.

While the above applies equally to both structured and unstructured interviews, the unstructured or exploratory interview requires more skill and experience to conduct. This is because the interviewer must be constantly making judgements about which topic to proceed with, while at the same time listening for and being able to follow up any clues dropped by the respondent. He must remember these clues and lead the respondent into an elaboration of them when they are likely to be relevant; and then he must be able to get him off this topic on to the next one. He constantly has to exercise a balance between encouraging the respondent to talk freely and keeping within the topics that are dealt with in the survey. Consequently there is a much greater risk of the respondent 'running away with' the unstructured interview so that it either becomes unduly extended or both parties get exhausted, the schedule is not completed, and important topics are dealt with hastily or inadequately.

The interviewer must learn how to cut off rambling replies without making the respondent feel rebuffed or under cross-examination. Having tried hard to make the respondent answer freely he should not now switch to making the respondent feel that he has to limit his answers. What can be done is to interrupt the respondent by a sentence such as: 'Oh, I see what you mean; that is very interesting; however, what I would like to ask you next is', or 'I see what you mean; I think that is going to come up later in the interview; I wonder if you would mind holding it until then'; then proceed with the next question. Another way is to say: 'You're going too fast for me, would you wait just a minute while I catch up?' Once one has 'caught up' one can simply then slip into the next question. Again one can say: 'Excuse me, I don't think I caught the last thing you said', and then simply go back further than the last thing he said, get to the last relevant part of the answer, have that repeated, and then proceed to the next question.

It is extremely important not to cut off the informant in mid-stream unless one is sure that the answer really is irrelevant; the interviewer must have the patience to wait while further relevant answers are still forthcoming.

HOW TO HANDLE THE RESPONDENT'S DIFFICULTIES WITH THE INTERVIEW

REPETITIONS OF QUESTION

In lengthy interviews the respondent may get bored and restless. When he has already discussed a topic he may be irritated to find he is asked another question about it. This may be unavoidable when the respondent prematurely introduces a topic which must be asked in its correct sequence later in the interview. The respondent is likely to think his answer should be assumed from the previous discussion and therefore the interviewer may appropriately preface the question with a remark such as: 'We have been over this before, but just to be sure I've got it right can you tell me . . . ' and proceed with the question

The interviewer himself must never assume he knows the answer to a question simply because of previous discussion and code the reply without actually asking it. One can never be certain that people really are consistent in their answers; they may suddenly remember something which changes their answer and makes it appear inconsistent with what they have said before. This applies to questions of fact as well as opinions and attitudes.

Frequently 'check questions' are built into the questionnaire. These cover the same topic from several angles to make sure that the answer one does obtain is, indeed, the correct one. Thus it may be that questions about the number of previous episodes of illness are asked in several sections of the questionnaire to make sure that the respondent has remembered them all. If he objects to this by saying, 'I've already told you', or if it is an opinion, 'I feel the same way as I said before', then the interviewer must get him to repeat the answer he gave before. He can do this by a remark such as: 'Yes of course, they seem to have repeated it here—I really don't know why. Still we had better fill it in. Can you remind me of what you said, please ?'

One of the interesting things about interviewing, however, is that most people do not remember that they have answered questions once or even twice before, and since they are involved in answering and thinking will simply give the answer again without any comment. Criticisms of the questionnaire, the types of questions asked, the form in which they are asked, or the repetitiveness occur very rarely, especially when the survey deals with illness, health, and other problems which are of great concern to most people. If the respondent does object or has criticisms to make, the interviewer should listen to them politely and give a reasonable, sensible answer, if he can think of one that will not act as a biasing kind of remark. He should never get impatient with the respondent or take the attitude that he is being awkward and uncooperative. The best and easiest way out is to blame the person who constructed the questionnaire, and simply say 'Yes, I can see why you feel this way but I have been told to ask the questions as they occur in this questionnaire'.

LOSING THE THREAD OF THE QUESTIONING

It is usual when the questionnaire passes from one topic to another for the interviewer to be instructed to introduce the new topic by a phrase such as: 'I would now like to ask you about . . .' and then mention the new topic. If no instructions are given the interviewer should still consider whether such 'bridging' phrases are necessary. If they are omitted the respondent may get confused and not understand the purport of the new questions. Should he decide they are necessary—for example when the respondent looks bewildered and has lost the thread—then he must use a bridging phrase that will not bias the answers. Naming the new topic, unless he is instructed to do so, may bias the answers. For example, if the new topic is 'Plans for retirement', and the first question (to people about to retire) is 'Where do you expect to be living this time next year', people who have had the topic labelled for them will have a different 'set' when they answer from those who do not know it is one of a series on retirement planning. The investigator's purpose may be to find out how many people spontaneously mention retirement when asked the above question. This problem may be dealt with by saying, 'Now I would like to talk about something quite different' and then read the question.

If the respondent loses the thread of the interview at any point avoid saying anything that will implicitly blame him, for example: 'I see you don't follow' or 'Don't you understand the question?' Use neutral phrases or ones that blame yourself or the questionnaire, such as 'I don't think that is very clear—shall I read it again?' or, 'I am going too fast—let me go back over that point'.

MAKING MISTAKES WHILE INTERVIEWING

While it is important for the interviewer to do his job competently, it is of course perfectly permissible for him to say 'I'm sorry, I think I've got mixed up here; just wait a minute while I look at what I'm doing'. It is much better to admit having made a mistake and to correct it immediately. The respondent will feel that what is being done is being done carefully, and of course it is understood that everybody does make mistakes. It is equally permissible if the interviewer meets a situation which he does not know how to handle to say so to the respondent and say that he will return when he had found out what he is supposed to do. This may occur during listing operations, selecting the respondent in the household, or in such cases where the questionnaire does not cover the situation which is being reported by the respondent. Interviewers often attempt to cover up when they don't know what to do. However, unless they are well trained and really familiar with the study and its purposes, they may make the wrong decision.

COMPLETING THE INTERVIEW IN THE SCHEDULED TIME

Unduly protracted interviews are completely impracticable for the purpose of health surveys. Most people are not prepared to concentrate for much more than an hour at a time, and one to one-and-a-half hours will usually be found to be the appropriate length for a survey interview with one informant. If the interviewer lets the session drag on too long by allowing interruptions, or because of time spent establishing rapport, in chatting, or for breaks for refreshment, the quality of the material will suffer.

It is sometimes necessary to accept some refreshment early in the interview, but unless the interviewer judges it appropriate to accept something early in order to establish rapport, it should be delayed until the end, when social conversation will not interfere with the progress of the interview. (Indeed, it may provide an opportunity for the respondent to come out with additional bits of information that he had neglected during the interview.)

COMPLETING ASSIGNMENTS AND WRITING REPORTS

As soon as possible after leaving the respondent the interviewer should check through the questionnaire to make sure that any notes he made are comprehensible and legible; that every pre-coded question has been filled in adequately; and that all ambiguities of recording are fully explained. Any report on the interview that has been requested should also be prepared rapidly. Reports will normally include comments on the co-operativeness, intelligence, and understanding of the respondent; difficulties during the interview; and any other relevant information that the person analysing the data might need, such as interruptions either by visitors or audience participation, or any other disturbance which made the flow of the interview difficult. Other comments may be useful. For instance, if the interviewer has reason to believe that the answers given were superficial, or given at random because the respondent was too harassed to pay attention, then this should be recorded; if the answers do not make sense, a decision to exclude the interview may have to be made.

If the interviewer has several calls to make in one day he should pause between calls to jot down notes on each interview as soon as it is completed. In this way he will avoid the possibility of confusing one respondent or one interview situation with another.

Completed questionnaires should be handed in on time; they may become soiled, damaged, or lost if interviewers leave them in their cars or homes.

AVOIDING BIAS

The investigator can do a great deal to prevent certain forms of bias by controlling publicity and by providing standardized introductions and explanations for the use of interviewers. Guarding against bias once the interview is taking place is much more difficult and may have more dangerous implications for the research, since it is seldom possible to measure the extent to which interviewers tend to bias the respondent's replies.

It is within the context of building and maintaining rapport that this bias has to be considered. Probably the task which calls for the greatest skill from interviewers, is that of striking a nice balance between establishing rapport and yet remaining detached and enigmatic enough for the respondent to talk freely without feeling impelled to take any particular line in answering questions in order that he may be approved of by the interviewer.

The way the word 'rapport' is commonly used in interviewing jargon carries subtle overtones. In therapeutic interviewing this state of rapport is often sought, so that the clients may be influenced to conform to the therapist's perception of healthy behaviour. The art of good interviewing, as practised by barristers in court, to give another example, includes the ability to make the respondent say what you want him to say—to lead him gently and imperceptibly along to agree with the kind of proposition that he might not at first have accepted. An intuitive but untrained interviewer may do this without realizing it. In survey research, however, it is to be strictly avoided.

The good *research* interviewer must be constantly aware that his presence and personality and his expectations might be imperceptibly influencing the respondent, and he should guard against revealing any indication of expected or acceptable replies. He should remember that any sign of approval or disapproval he shows (a smile, a lifted eyebrow, or an approving murmur which has not met previous replies, or any slight change of demeanour) will be sufficient to indicate to the respondent the kind of reply that is expected once rapport has been established.

The level of rapport to be aimed at in research is that of a mutual understanding and sympathy between the interviewer and the person who is being interviewed, and the ability of each to comprehend what the other is talking about. However, even this has snags. While the respondent will talk more freely and reveal more to an interviewer with whom he feels at ease and in sympathy (notably interviewers of the same sex, class, colour, and cultural background as himself), he will also endeavour to retain the sympathetic relationship by monitoring his answers in a way which will, in his judgement, please the interviewer.

Even if the respondent is not consciously trying to please the interviewer, he may still choose how he responds and what he mentions because he is reacting to the social status and role he ascribes to the interviewer. When talking to doctors for example, people tend to concentrate on medical matters, and may describe aspects of their medical history which they normally never consider. Thus the respondent may produce aches and pains if he thinks these are what the physician is interested in. Alternatively, he may play down aches and pains if he decides that they would not interest a physician. Thus under-reporting of minor conditions has been shown to be common in surveys of illnesses. For this reason it is often better if the physician or nurse do not use their titles when interviewing in the field. They should, however, be aware that their manner of interacting and their choice of vocabulary also provide clues.

The subtleties of this situation may seem somewhat over-emphasized for health survey work, but the enormous problem of bias should be well understood by all who undertake investigations in the social and behavioural sciences in order that due attention may be paid to the precautions that may be taken.

If all health surveys were exclusively concerned with collecting data about aspects of health and sickness that had no emotional connotations to the respondent, and if the investigator had no interest in attitudes, then probably the bias would be reduced. However, as practically every survey includes questions which are likely to arouse some anxiety, fear, or worries in the respondent, he will be perplexed as to how to answer these and may look to the interviewer for guidance about the 'proper' or 'expected' replies. This is particularly so when the questions the interviewer is asking refer to psychiatric symptoms or other manifestations of disease such as fits, venereal disease, or sterility which the respondent or his culture regard as unpleasant or unacceptable in some way.

Since the purpose of epidemiological surveys is to relate the manifestations of illness to other factors, the readiness of the respondent to reveal these other factors is as important as his readiness to reveal his symptoms. So here again, when the interviewer approaches topics about which the respondent is likely to be 'touchy', he must beware of seeming to encourage a socially acceptable reply. This applies particularly if he is looking for signs of social malfunctioning.

THE ABILITY TO LISTEN

Even though the interview is a conversation, it differs in an additional important aspect. In most ordinary discussions, each person is more concerned with what he is saying himself than what the other person is saying. The interviewer should be entirely concerned with what the respondent is saying. He should know his own role in the situation well enough to be able to concentrate entirely on the respondent, and not be concerned with his personal needs.

The ability to listen includes that of remaining still and relaxed. It is a quality that is quite rare in everyday life, and most respondents will enjoy the opportunity of having their every word attended to for once. The art of listening, however, is a double-edged weapon. The interviewer who possesses this art is likely to get a different response to the person who does not have it. Thus the interviewer who asks a question and then listens to the reply attentively and silently will get a more detailed reply than one who, by his very demeanour of waiting for the end of the reply to come, is clearly in a hurry to get on with the next question. A silence for even a moment after the end of the respondent's answer, can be as or more effective than a further probe. The interviewer should be well aware of the use and influence of silence.

Attentive listening will often encourage people to talk at great length, but not necessarily always to the point. The good interviewer will vary the intensity of his attention. He will remain still and silent for just that extra amount of time when the respondent touches on a topic that is important for the survey, and he will move or speak only when he has heard sufficient for his purposes. The person who is being interviewed will respond to these cues quite often more readily than he will to the words: 'tell me more about X'.

A hazard of extra-attentive listening is that while the respondent is feeling relaxed and talking freely, he may say more than he means to say and reveal personal matters that he will later regret having revealed. If this happens early in the interview, he may suddenly clam up and the interviewer will have some difficulty in getting the rest of the required information. The skilled interviewer should be able to spare the respondent from revealing personal information that he may later regret, when it is not relevant. If, however, such material is revealed, the interviewer must reassure the respondent about its confidentiality. Ideally, each respondent should be left with the feeling that he has contributed to a worthwhile enterprise, and should be willing to participate in follow-up inquiries. Follow-up inquiries are frequently necessary for checking up on interviews, and they are particularly important in mental health surveys where the initial survey is often only the basic against which changes in incidence or health status with time and changing conditions can be measured.

16

PSYCHIATRIC RESEARCH IN
GENERAL PRACTICE

DAVID GOLDBERG and NEIL KESSEL

Since the National Health Service began, studies on the prevalence, distribution, and types of psychiatric illness in general practice have been executed in profusion. The 'How many' and 'What sort' questions have largely been answered and we are now at a time when it is appropriate to embark on a different series of studies. Attention must increasingly be focused upon aetiological inquiries, upon outcome studies, upon how the doctor does his work and upon treatments and their effect. Thus we need to ask what social and medical factors are correlated with the presentation of psychiatric illness, what happens to such illnesses, what influence does the doctor's theoretical standpoint have upon his practice, and what are the results of various types of therapy which he or the larger medical and social team may carry out. These questions become more important as general practitioners increasingly become aware of the psychological illnesses of their patients and undertake responsibility for treatment.

Although replication of earlier work is always useful, the first wave of prevalence studies should give way now to a second wave of practice studies. The methods, particularly case identification and population sampling techniques, that have been forged in the early studies will remain the major devices required. However, techniques for evaluating therapy, exquisitely perfected in drug trials, will increasingly be required in general practice studies, and a knowledge of the statistical concepts involved in relating variables to each other is necessary to throw light upon problems of multiple aetiologies. Our brief in this chapter will be to concentrate on the techniques that have been used in morbidity surveys, paying particular attention to problems of case identification and of delineating the 'population at risk'. We will also point the way towards studies which examine the long-term development of illness by looking at the clinical patterns and their evolution.

General practice surveys have taken the place of expensive and elaborate psychiatric surveys of total populations and have been used to calculate prevalence, inception rates, and duration of minor psychiatric illness in the community. General practice surveys therefore have great interest for psychiatric epidemiologists, and they can be utilized both to throw light on possible associations between clinical and social variables and to study how the service functions: the latter includes the psychiatric specialist services and their relationship to general practice. Finally, general practice has been used to provide typical case material of illnesses as they occur in the community.

Unfortunately, even with this many uses to choose from, there are numerous well-intentioned studies, reaping the fruits of many hours' work, which in the end contain little of practical use to their authors, to practitioners, or to other research workers. It is, for example, of little use to be told that a given doctor finds a particular inception rate of a psychiatric condition, unless this rate can be compared with some other rate. Unless the same investigator furnishes the two rates no comparison can be made, since it is necessary to use the same criteria for what constitutes a case (the numerator) and for the population at risk (the denominator) in order for the comparison to be valid.

No research comes to any good unless a question is formulated and, sad as it may seem, the fact is that nine-tenths of the questions that one can think of either cannot be answered, or can be answered in half a day well spent in a library: that is to say someone else has answered them. The art is to pose a question that can be answered, and whose answer is neither already known nor self-evident.

INCIDENCE AND PREVALENCE SURVEYS

Many early surveys report on the work of individual practitioners and essentially consist of statements of the supposed prevalence of psychiatric disorder in that practice. Kellner (1963) reviews no fewer than twenty-five surveys in Britain alone, with widely varying consultation and prevalence rates from one survey to another. A recent computer search of the literature (Medlars, 1973) shows that there have been many more since then. Doctors who undertake such surveys are inevitably self-selected, and this fact alone is likely to influence the reported prevalence rates because of the phenomenon of 'patient recruitment'. Varying diagnostic standards and varying classifications will account for different findings. In addition, morbidity may be measured in different ways so that the various sorts of prevalence and consultation rates are confused, and the practice populations may be demographically different. Standards of recording vary with the motivation and work-load of the individual investigator, and if extra workers are enlisted to help with the analysis of data the sources of error may increase.

One solution to this problem has been the multi-practice survey, either for psychiatric morbidity on its own (Watts et al., 1964; Locke et al., 1967) or as part of a general morbidity survey (Logan and Cushion, 1958; Taylor and Chave, 1964; Shepherd et al., 1966). If steps are taken to ensure that the collective practice populations are representative of the general population about which generalizations are to be made, the bias of skewed populations is reduced but the other problems are by no means solved.

It is usual to find large differences between the rates of individual practitioners in these surveys: for example, there was a ninefold difference between the lowest and the highest rate in Shepherd's survey while in the Prince George's County Survey the rate varied between 0 per cent and 44 per cent (Locke *et al.*, 1967). It is usual to compute a mean rate from these widely varying figures, which assumes that the physicians whose rates are too high will balance out those whose rates are too low. This is, of course, an unjustifiable assumption, for even the highest reported rate might be an underestimate. Another point concerns the quality of the basic data. While it is possible to exclude practitioners whose record keeping is obviously inadequate—Shepherd excluded four practices on this basis—it is very difficult for the investigators to apply more than crude quality control checks on the data.

General practitioners may be used as important key informants in a particular form of community survey carried out by a psychiatrist. The method was originated by Klemperer (1933) in Munich, and was used both by Freming (1951) for his survey on the island of Bornholm, and by Helgason (1964) for his survey of psychiatric illness in Iceland. In this method a cohort of patients born perhaps sixty years earlier is followed by an exhaustive search of all public records. The research psychiatrist discusses each patient in detail with his general practitioner, who therefore becomes the key informant for minor psychiatric illness. The method can, of course, only be used in populations that are residentially stable, and an obvious limitation of the method is the unavailability of the general practitioners who dealt with the patients when they were young, which must produce a loss of information. In some of the studies just quoted, hospital records were still available, but accounts of minor morbidity were missing. In the Bornholm study, for example, the psychotics outnumbered the neurotics by almost 2:1.

A variant of this design which escapes these objections is where the research psychiatrist discusses current cases with the general practitioner. Jones (1962) carried out a one-year period prevalence survey of psychiatric disorder in Anglesey by visiting every general practitioner on the island and discussing their entire collection of cases with them. Kessel (1960) discussed a 10 per cent sample of a practice with the general practitioner: the sample was chosen by taking patients aged 15 years and over whose surnames began with four randomly chosen letters (A, B, U, V). While Jones found a prevalence for all psychiatric illness of only 3–4 per cent, Kessel found he could make prevalence estimates varying between 5 and 52 per cent, depending on what criteria were used to define 'a case'. The former figure was obtained by using the 'mental, psychoneurotic and personality disorder' category of the ICD, while the latter figure included all patients who presented psychological symptoms, patients with illnesses where physical factors did not appear to play a causal role, and patients with so-called psychosomatic diseases.

NUMERATOR PROBLEMS

Most of the problems described so far are concerned with the wide variations that exist in defining a case. It is reassuring to note that when one considers only those surveys by practitioners who were either already trained as psychiatrists or who subsequently became psychiatrists (Bremer, 1951; Hewetson *et al.*, 1963; Kellner, 1963; Herst, 1965; Goldberg and Blackwell, 1970) the variation between observers is considerably less, although once more the various rates cannot strictly speaking be compared with one another.

The classification adopted by the investigator will greatly influence the reported rate. It is wiser to use a classification that does not depend on making a firm diagnosis in each case: the College of General Practitioners' Research Committee (1958) found that firm diagnosis could only be made in just over half the cases seen and the range between individual practitioners was very wide (26–72 per cent). Mowbray *et al.* (1961) used a classification that ranged from 'physical illness' to 'psychiatric cases':

1. Physical illness
2. Psychological factors in physical illness
3. Psychosomatic illness
4. Psychiatric case
5. Personal problem
6. Other

This classification was found acceptable by fifteen general practitioners, and an adaptation of it was used by Goldberg and Blackwell (1970):

1. Entirely physical complaints or illness
2. Physical illness in a neurotic personality
3. Physical illness with an associated psychological disturbance
4. Psychiatric illness with somatic symptoms
5. Unrelated physical and psychiatric illness
6. Entirely psychiatric illness
7. Parents of sick children
8. Other; not ill; unclassifiable

This classification seems to work quite well in general practice. It avoids the difficulties attached to the notion of 'psychosomatic' illness, and could, if necessary, be condensed to a five-way classification.

Even when a satisfactory classification has been adopted, great difficulties are usually experienced in deciding when a psychological disturbance should be regarded as 'clinically significant'. Shepherd (1972) defines a psychiatric case in general practice as 'an individual whose symptoms, behaviour, distress, or discomfort leads to a medical consultation at which a psychiatric diagnosis is made by a qualified physician'. Although such a criterion has the advantage of being simple and workable, it leaves a lot of questions unanswered. It is apparent that different individuals will define themselves as 'ill' at widely different symptom levels, and it seems wise to distinguish between level of symptoms, and what Mechanic (1962) has termed 'illness behaviour':

It is plain that symptoms are differently perceived, evaluated and acted upon (or not acted upon) by different kinds of people and in different social situations. Whether because of earlier experience of illness, because of differential training in respect of symptoms, or because of different biological sensitivities, some persons make light of symptoms, shrug them off, and avoid seeking medical care. Others will respond to little pain and discomfort by readily seeking care, by releasing themselves from work and other obligations, and by becoming dependent on others.

SCREENING TESTS

One way of avoiding the errors introduced by the differing criteria of individual practitioners is by using a standardized screening questionnaire. One of the earliest to be used on a systematic basis in general practice was the Cornell Medical Inventory (Shepherd et al., 1966) . While this was found to correlate poorly with the general practitioner's assessment of whether or not the individual was a psychiatric case (biserial correlation over fourteen practices = $+0.19$), a modification of the Inventory by Rawnsley (1966) has recently been shown to correlate much more highly with interview by a research psychiatrist. Thus Kedward (1969) obtained a correlation of $+0.64$ between Rawnsley's modification of the CMI and a structured interview by the research psychiatrist of 100 psychiatric cases drawn from general practice, and Ingham et al. (1972) report biserial correlations varying between $+0.51$ and $+0.83$ between CMI score and psychiatric assessment of various community groups in a recent survey in South Wales. Although the CMI has been the most widely used screening questionnaire in general practice (see also Brown and Fry, 1962; Herst, 1965), its main shortcomings are firstly its tendency to miss cases (low sensitivity) and, secondly, the stability of the scores over time, which suggests that the test gives more information about personality than about current illness.

The General Health Questionnaire (Goldberg, 1972) consists of sixty items dealing with current symptoms and difficulties, and was specifically designed for use in a general practice setting. It can usually be completed by patients as they wait to see a general practitioner, and is intended for use as an aid to case identification, and also as a research tool. It furnishes a single score between 0 and 60 which correlates quite highly ($r = +0.80$) with an independent assessment of the severity of a respondent's psychiatric disturbance. The questionnaire has four distinct research uses. First, it can be used to compare the amount of non-psychotic psychiatric disturbances in two populations by comparing the means and standard deviations of scores in each population. Second, psychiatric disturbance as assessed by a score on the questionnaire can be correlated with other clinical and social variables in a population. Third, a group of patients can be tested on different occasions in order to follow changes with time. Finally, the questionnaire can be used to assess the point prevalence of minor psychiatric illness in cross-sectional studies, and in this case should ideally be the first part of a two-stage process of case identification—the second stage being a clinical assessment by a psychiatrist using a standardized psychiatric interview [see CHAPTERS 13 and 16].

With any screening questionnaire it is necessary to know how many cases the questionnaire misses ('sensitivity') and how many normals it misidentifies as cases ('specificity') (Wilson and Jungner, 1968). These two characteristics are independent of prevalence of disease in the population, and are illustrated by the following data:

TABLE 16.1

High scores on screening questionnaire	False Positives n = 13	True Positives n = 89
Low scores on screening questionnaire	True Negatives n = 94	False Negatives n = 4
	N = 107	N = 93
	Clinically normal at Interview	Psychiatric cases at Interview

$$\text{Sensitivity} = \frac{\text{Number of cases with high scores}}{\text{Total number of cases}} = \frac{89}{93} = 95 \cdot 7\%$$

$$\text{Specificity} = \frac{\text{Number of normals with low scores}}{\text{Total number of normals}} = \frac{94}{107} = 87 \cdot 8\%$$

Two other measures—hits-positive rate and overall misclassification rate—are dependent upon prevalence, but they can be calculated in a given population of known prevalence providing that the sensitivity and specificity are known for the questionnaire concerned. These measures are more fully discussed in the Appendix.

Other screening tests for general psychiatric morbidity which have been used in a general practice setting include the Health Opinion Survey (Semmence, 1969) and the Symptom Check List (Goldberg et al., 1973). Investigators looking specifically for depression have used the Beck Depression Inventory (Salkind, 1969), the Wakefield Self-Assessment Depression Inventory (Snaith et al., 1971), and the Zung Depression Scale (Popoff, 1969). Kellner and Sheffield's (1967) Symptom Rating Test also works quite well as a screening test, but is probably best used to assess change in neurotic symptomatology in therapeutic studies.

A TWO-STAGE MODEL FOR CASE IDENTIFICATION

Despite quite marked differences between them, all the screening tests work reasonably well (Goldberg, 1972). However, none of them is trustworthy enough to supplant clinical assessment by an expert. Their main use lies in identifying patients who are probably disturbed, and leaving the task of making final assessment to a clinician using a standardized psychiatric interview. A suitable interview for general practice studies has been designed at the General Practice Research Unit of the Institute of Psychiatry: this can be used to provide a profile of twenty-two symptoms and signs of illness, or an empirically derived 'overall severity score' (Goldberg et al., 1970). Investigators who wish to assess the severity of depression or anxiety in identified cases might use the appropriate Hamilton Scale (Hamilton, 1959, 1960).

DENOMINATOR PROBLEMS

Comparison of rates, as we have said, is crucial to most work in the general practice field and this always involves the division of a numerator by a denominator. The denominator in epidemiological studies represents a population at risk—represents it by including the whole population or a defined sample of it. For the rate to be accurate, we need to know the population at risk as precisely as we need to know the number of cases from which it is drawn. For other workers to make use of the rate, we also need to have a description of that population.

General practitioners know approximately the number of people on their practice lists and the Executive Council can tell them accurately for the care of how many people they have been paid. It is not always possible to give realistic figures for the list of single practitioners working in a group practice, and therefore the whole practice usually has to agree to co-operate in a survey where rates are sought. Even with total numbers for the practice, there are errors involved since people will have moved (approximately 10 per cent in any one year in urban areas), because people are born and die, and because a host of small errors creep in.

In Great Britain, the sex distribution of the population on a general practitioner's books can be found, albeit laboriously, by counting the red envelopes (male) and the blue ones (female) in which the NHS records are filed. The age distribution can only be found by reading it off the individual record card envelopes and it will only be found on these if someone has at some stage entered the date of birth. Letters from hospitals sometimes yield this information if it is missing. For this reason it is often a good start to try to find a practice which already has an age and sex register.

Almost always one will only want to work with a sample, not the whole practice. This may be specially selected so as to comprise certain groups only, for example working men, housewives, the elderly, frequent attenders, single women, and so forth, or one may wish it to be representative of the entire practice. For the latter purpose, a random sample is best. The rule for a random sample is that everybody in the population has an equal chance of being in the sample. There are certain permissible short cuts which may fairly be used because they involve little error. A 10 per cent sample, for instance, may be drawn by thinking of a number between one and ten and taking that case note in the alphabetical file and every tenth thereafter. If one is trying to sample attenders a simple device that will yield near enough a 10 per cent sample is to take everybody born on the 3rd, 13th, and 23rd of the month. What is not permissible is to decide on a sample size rather than on a sample percentage and to stop when one has, say, 200 individuals, because it breaks the fundamental rule concerning equal opportunity of selection.

For further information about sampling techniques in general practice, readers are referred to Moser (1958). Sampling in relation to general practice studies is discussed by Kessel (1962). Since the correct drawing of sample is crucial it is as well to seek expert advice before committing oneself to any method. An inaccurately worked out denominator can weaken the value of research findings nearly as much as a

loosely defined numerator. Sample size is another important consideration. It is inefficient to use a larger or a smaller sample than your problem requires for its solution. Samples are often chosen on a 'think of a
round number' basis. This has little to commend it. Once again,
experts should be consulted.

SOME FIGURES FOR PREVALENCE AND INCEPTION RATES

There has been a wide variation in the prevalence and inception rates of
various published surveys, mainly due to different methods of counting
the numerator. Thus Logan and Cushion (1958) carried out a general
morbidity survey in 106 practices, and produced prevalence rates for
psychoneuroses of 45·7/1000 and psychoses of 2·2/1000. Watts et al.
(1964) carried out a survey in 261 practices and confined their attention
to mental illness, and produced a prevalence for all mental illness of
9/1000 at risk. These figures are so much lower than those usually
accepted that it seems likely that they are an artefact of the survey
method adopted. Shepherd et al. (1966) surveyed 46 London general
practices by drawing a 10 per cent random sample of each doctor's list
and putting survey recording forms inside each patient's NHS wallet.
This method ensured that on any given surgery the practitioner would
only be required to give information about 10 per cent of the patients
he saw, and also that he would give information at the time of the consultation rather than later, when memories might have faded. Because
it was a general morbidity survey the practitioner had to give information about a survey patient irrespective of whether or not he considered
that he was psychiatrically disturbed: in some other surveys the doctor
had to answer detailed questions only when he considered that the
patient was a psychiatric case, so that he may have been tempted to
declare a patient 'well' when he was in doubt, or when time was short.
These workers (Shepherd et al., 1966) produced a one-year period
prevalence for all psychiatric illness of 140/1000 population at risk,
with an inception rate of 52/1000.

There are reasons for supposing that both these figures are, if anything, low. The general practitioners taking part in the survey were in
effect detecting what has been termed 'conspicuous psychiatric morbidity', which is defined as 'an attendance during the survey year for
one or more illnesses in which an important psychiatric component had
been detected by the general practitioner' (Kessel, 1960). More recent
research with a screening questionnaire and a research psychiatrist
carrying out a second-stage case identification procedure has drawn
attention to the 'hidden psychiatric morbidity' of general practice
(Goldberg and Blackwell, 1970). Even in a general practice where the
practitioner was himself a psychiatrist, the more elaborate case finding
procedure resulted in the discovery of an extra case for every two known

to the practitioner, and more recent work indicates that in many practices the ratio of hidden to conspicuous cases is much higher (Goldberg, 1973).

Confirmatory evidence for this view comes in a follow-up study to Shepherd's original survey by Harvey-Smith and Cooper (1970). An index group of 170 patients who had been thought psychiatrically disturbed during the original survey were demographically matched with a control group of 170 patients thought to be psychiatrically normal, and both groups were followed up for three years from the original identification. The design of the survey involved the investigators in discussing each of the controls with his general practitioner and, when this was done, for no fewer than 31 patients there were striking changes of opinion: they were considered—in the light of subsequent events—to have been suffering at the time of the original inquiry from mild but long-standing neurotic conditions. During the survey year in the practices being followed up, 9,000 patients had been divided into 2,000 cases and 7,000 normals: the reappraisals reported above would have changed these figures to 3,250 and 5,750 respectively. It is of interest that in the 139 patients remaining in the control group after the 31 reappraised patients had been removed, the annual inception rate for new episodes of psychiatric illness was 50/1000: a figure very close to the original inception rate quoted by Shepherd *et al*.

LONGITUDINAL STUDIES

Studies which follow a cohort of patients from general practice are of particular value for studying the natural history of minor psychiatric illness in the community, and they also provide an opportunity for measuring inception rates over the period of the survey.

Kedward (1966, 1969) has carried out a three-year follow-up of 422 patients drawn from Shepherd's original survey who had presented for the first time with a psychiatric illness that year. Patients were followed up by postal questionnaire, by examination of their NHS notes, and by interview with the family doctor. In addition a sample of 100 were interviewed using a structured interview. Three years after index consultation, 73 per cent of the patients were free from psychiatric symptoms, and the progress of the patients at one year had indicated the probable outcome at 3 years. It appears that there are two groups of patients, one a chronic group whose illnesses run a refractory course of at least 3 years, and the other a group of good prognosis where recovery usually occurs within 6–12 months of the onset of symptoms. Goldberg and Blackwell (1970) showed that two-thirds of psychiatric disorders seen at index consultation have in fact remitted 6 months

after index assessment. Cooper *et al.* (1969) intensively studied a group
practice where the clinical assessments were known from other studies
to be reliable over a period of 7 years. The findings of their survey
concerning prevalence, inception, and duration are in accord with the
other findings of Shepherd's team.

USES OF THE LONE SURVEY

It follows from what has been said that surveys which merely express
psychiatrically disturbed patients as a percentage of consecutive
attenders cannot be used to calculate prevalence and inception rates,
since there is no denominator. Some lone surveys such as Bremer
(1951), Llewellyn-Thomas (1960), Primrose (1962), and Kellner
(1963), established the denominator accurately and express psychiatric
disorder as a proportion of those patients currently under care; this is
much more satisfactory and each of these studies is as good as its own
numerator, i.e. its case-identification technique.

Lone surveys can, however, be used to answer more specific questions
about minor psychiatric illness. They are perfectly appropriate for exploring morbidity among groups of patients within the practice, since
the same diagnostic standards are applied to each group. Hardman
(1965) compared psychiatric morbidity in two areas within his practice:
a new housing estate and an older established community. No differences were found, despite an otherwise uniformly higher consultation
rate for other diagnostic groups for patients from the housing estate.
Kellner (1966) explored the relationship between inceptions of neurotic
ill health and physical illness over a 2-year period, and found that the
former were observed more often during convalescence from a physical
illness than at other times. Kreitman *et al.* (1966) used a more elaborate
method to study the relationship between psychiatric and somatic
illness in a single practice over a minimum period of 7 years: they
failed to find any evidence for 'clusters' of heterogeneous illnesses in
Hinkle and Wolff's terms.

OPERATIONAL STUDIES

Having discovered the quantity and distribution of morbidity, one of
the tasks of the epidemiologist is to discover how well the medical services meet the existing needs. Kaeser and Cooper (1971) studied a one
in seven sample of referrals to the Maudsley out-patient clinic over a
six months' period by interview with the general practitioner at the
time of the referral and follow-up interview with the patient three
months later. It was found that in the main the general practitioners

wanted the hospital to take over clinical responsibility, the demand for consultant advice being relatively small. The majority of patients attended two or three times only and underwent no specialized technical procedures of the sort that would have justified hospital referral. The practitioners' responses to the follow-up inquiry showed that they were rather better satisfied than the patients with the outcome of referral, which 'suggests that the referral process may be working more effectively as a means of disposal than as a step in securing effective treatment . . . the overall impression was less one of dissatisfaction than of inadequate communication between patients, general practitioners, and hospital psychiatrists.'

A complementary study by Hopkins and Cooper (1969) examined the referral process from the general practitioner's viewpoint by using a postal follow-up questionnaire sent to every patient referred to a psychiatrist over a 4-year period. Of the 115 patients referred, 18 per cent were never seen by the out-patient department, and of those that did attend, 37 per cent lapsed from treatment and no fewer than 58 per cent were regarded as unimproved by the psychiatrist seeing them. Psychotic patients were most likely (30 per cent unimproved) and character disorders least likely to be helped (79 per cent unimproved): psychosomatic disorders and neuroses were intermediate.

Another kind of study endeavours to examine general practitioners' work habits and attitudes by interviewing a large sample of general practitioners. Harwin et al. (1970) chose a particular area—the London Borough of Croydon—and as far as possible interviewed all the general practitioners within it on their experience of the local psychiatric services and their attitudes towards co-operation with social workers.

Several investigators have studied departures from the traditional relationship between psychiatrist and general practitioner (Gibson et al., 1966; Brook, 1967; Lyons, 1969) where the psychiatrist visits the general practitioner and either sees selected cases in the surgery or discusses cases with him. Although all these studies emphasize advantages of the various arrangements described, no one has so far investigated the effects of such an arrangement on the overall running of the service.

GENERAL PRACTICE USED TO 'COMPLETE THE CLINICAL PICTURE'

There have been surprisingly few studies investigating the social correlates of chronic psychiatric disability in the community, although a pilot study (Sylph et al., 1969) has been described in greater detail (Cooper, 1972). This study individually matched a group of 81 patients with chronic neurosis with 81 patients without such a handicap drawn from current surgery attenders. Each patient was assessed independently by a research psychiatrist and a social worker, using structured interviews. It was found that the index group did indeed have significantly more social difficulties, and that the differences appeared to extend into all areas of the patients' life activities. Even though the samples were matched for social class, there were differences between the groups for housing conditions and household income.

Fahy et al. (1969) studied depressed patients drawn from 8 general practices in order to find how depressions as they occur in the community can best be classified. A research psychiatrist interviewed 133 patients and accepted 126 as depressed. The investigators then used a principal components analysis to reduce the 52 variables recorded at interview to 28 variables, and a subsequent analysis revealed 6 covariant clusters of patients, of which four were considered in further detail, and were found not to replicate traditional clinical nosology. In this study, general practice was used to obtain a sample that would represent depression as it occurs in the community more accurately than the highly selected sample seen by hospital-based psychiatrists.

General practice is also used as an arena for drug studies, and a study by Porter (1970) provides an example of a useful within-practice comparison of the ecological distribution of depression, as well as a therapeutic trial of imipramine (which failed to show it was better than placebo). In the earlier part of his paper he shows that depression is more common in resettled families with housing problems and less common among the indigenous population who had been there more than 10 years. Other investigators to have reported drug studies include Wheatley (1967); Donald (1969); Hesbacher et al. (1970); Blashki et al. (1971); and Clift (1972).

GROWING POINTS

We said at the outset that many questions relating to psychiatric morbidity in general practice had already been answered. We know a lot about the types of patients who present and their numbers and there is little point in further studies which only relate to these matters. There are, however, a number of growing points which are opportune for study now.

From the strictly epidemiological point of view, it would be appropriate to study the reasons for inter-practice variation. We have seen that some practices report high morbidity figures and others much lower rates. Even when these figures are adjusted to apply to similar numerators and similar denominators, large differences persist. It has been assumed, using Occam's razor, that variation in doctors' sensitivity to psychological symptoms and their attitudes towards psychiatric illness largely account for these differences. Almost certainly this is so. Nevertheless, there may be real prevalence differences. Some contrasts spring to mind: rural : urban; new town : settled community; or high : low social mobility. It would be very useful to mount projects comparing practitioners working in contrasting areas using agreed criteria of case identification. As we have seen, there have been some ventures in this direction (Taylor and Chave, 1964; Hardman, 1965) but more are needed.

One may also consider the effect of psychiatric training. It would be worthwhile comparing the case identification rate and the treatment patterns used by doctors who have had very little psychiatric training as undergraduates, with doctors who have had an extended under-graduate apprenticeship. Since age might be a complicating factor, it would be better to compare graduates of similar age from different medical schools and one might envisage a comparison of recently graduated general practitioners from Medical School X and from Medical School Y, both working among similar populations. The effect of doctors' attitudes could be similarly examined, even simul-taneously with the foregoing. This study might be carried out fairly soon. Medical School X may be catching up fast.

Aetiological factors need to be looked at by examining the relation-ship of psychological symptoms to social variables in the population studied. Such a study is probably one of the most important exercises that could be carried out at the present, but it would need highly sophisticated techniques to arrive at meaningful conclusions and would almost certainly require a collaborative exercise.

TWO-CONDITION EPIDEMIOLOGY

Because general practitioners have information about the whole gamut of illness, general practice provides the possibility of looking at where two conditions coexist more frequently than chance would determine. If for instance the prevalence of neurosis is 15 per cent in the generality of patients aged 25–55 but was found to be 25 per cent in those in that age group who suffered from joint disease, a relationship between the two conditions would have been demonstrated. Of course, such a finding would not tell us what sort of causal relationship might exist between the two conditions but the discovery of such a relationship is important to hunches which can be tested by proper hypothesis formulation and testing. Hospital studies can never demonstrate such relationships because of the selection involved.

Insufficient study has been given to the very complex issues involved in the initiation of a consultation for psychological problems or to the converse of what leads some anxious, depressed people to keep away from their doctors. The latter is probably the more medically useful question but there are considerable difficulties in getting information about people who do not consult, although non-attenders have been studied by Kessel and Shepherd (1965). However, we should also look at those who do consult the doctor but without ever producing psychological symptoms, even though they are experiencing them. A group of such patients might be elicited by means of a questionnaire designed to reveal covert symptomatology. The former question, what leads patients to consult their doctors with such symptoms or to reveal them under questioning, is in one way easier because the right patients are readily identifiable, yet there are probably many different reasons, several operating with each patient, so the analysis will not be simple. It would be interesting to know how often the consultation is initiated at the request of a member of the family or at the suggestion of a friend or employer or how much impact psychiatric presentations in mass media may have in determining consultations. An extension of such studies would examine the cognate problem of the factors influencing referral to specialist care—psychiatric or other.

The most appropriate area for study within the general practice setting at the present time, however, is that of therapy. A considerable proportion of the nation's illness is involved and yet we know little definitively about the best ways of treating such patients. The method of study is simple—essentially it is the same as that of a drug trial. Similar patients are randomly allocated to treatments and the outcome measured for each group. Safeguards or 'blinds' will need to be drawn appropriate to each particular study. Certainly, there would be a vast financial saving to the exchequer if the indiscriminate use of minor tranquillizers, anti-depressants, and major tranquillizers was investigated in this way. Psychotherapy, supportive or otherwise, could be examined similarly and so could referral to a psychiatric clinic. It must be emphasized that for any of these studies to yield useful results they must be numerate rather than literate. Figures, not impressions, are required. These are efficacy studies; but there is also scope for efficiency studies. What effect does the use of ancillary staff have on the practitioner's time ? If patients are seen for extended consultations by regular but spaced appointments rather than at the haphazard request of the patients themselves coming when they wish to, does this represent time lost or time gained for the practitioner ? Lastly, it might be very fruitful for psychiatrists and general practitioners to collaborate in studying, again in a numerate way, the value of the psychiatrist conducting occasional 'out-patient' consultations in the surgery.

We have said that such studies are simple to execute. The difficulty, or the art, is in framing exactly an answerable question—answerable in terms of statistics and probability rather than in the speculative impressionistic terms which characterize most disquisitions on therapy.

GENERAL POINTS

All research costs effort. Much of it also costs money. Some money will always be needed for postage and for stationery. Most surveys involve a certain amount of travelling. Somehow or other these small sums can usually be found without difficulty. A more important question comes when a large amount of labour, sorting through records for example, might be avoided by the principals in research if they only could get clerical staff to carry it out. With any particular project serious thought ought to be given whether it is more economical to do it oneself or to pay for clerical labour. We mention this because the sums involved are often under £100 and there are funding bodies which by furnishing such amounts could save the doctor considerable expenditure of time on what are basically non-medical tasks.

At some stage in planning in research, the question of statistics will crop up. It is comparatively rarely that sophisticated statistical techniques will prove to be necessary in the analysis of the results, but it is true to say that the better the statistical advice one obtains at the outset, the less complicated will be the statistics that one has to use. Advice in research design and in the execution of it should always be sought. One has to be very good at research not to derive benefit from the scrutiny of a project by somebody else; and if the investigator is that good he will certainly have the sense to make sure that somebody does scrutinize it before beginning. The beginner should be prepared to seek a great deal of help until he is steeped heavily in his subject and is assured in his research techniques. We have to issue the warning that reading a chapter or even a book about research methods can do no more than fire the beginner with the desire to conduct some investigations—to ask and answer some questions—and to let him see that it is not too hard to take the plunge. We hope we may have done this in the field of psychiatric research in general practice.

APPENDIX

THE RELATIONSHIP BETWEEN THE EFFECTIVENESS OF A SCREENING TEST AND THE PREVALENCE OF DISEASE IN A POPULATION BEING STUDIED

It has already been explained in the text that while 'sensitivity' and 'specificity' of a screening test are independent of prevalence, two other

SMP

measures—hits-positive rate and overall misclassification rate—are dependent upon prevalence, and will therefore need to be calculated so that the effectiveness of a screening test can be assessed in some new setting. The *hits-positive rate* refers to the probability that an individual is diseased, given that his screening score is positive; and the *overall misclassification rate* refers to the total number of respondents misclassified by the questionnaire in the population being examined.

$$\text{Hits-positive rate} = \frac{P_1}{P_{p_1} + Q_{p_2}}$$

Overall misclassification rate $= Q_{p_2} + P_{q_1}$
where $P =$ prevalence
$\quad p_1 =$ proportion of cases with high scores (sensitivity)
$\quad p_2 =$ proportion of normals misidentified as cases (false positive rate)
and let

$\quad Q = 1 - P$
$\quad q_1 = 1 - p_1$ (false negative rate)
$\quad q_2 = 1 - p_2$ (specificity of test)

These formulae are derived from Bayes' theorem (Meehl and Rosen, 1955; Goldberg, 1972) and can be used to construct the relationship between 'hits-positive rate' and prevalence for the GHQ.

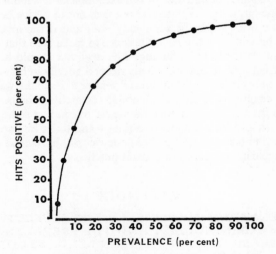

FIG. 16.1. Relationship between prevalence and 'hits-positive rate' for the General Health Questionnaire in general practice.

It is, of course, intuitively obvious that in populations with a low prevalence of disease it is more probable that an individual with a high score will be a 'false positive' than an actual case; FIG. 16.1 allows us to explore the relationship between prevalence and 'hits-positive rate' for the GHQ in general practice.

At prevalence of less than about 11 per cent an individual with a high score is more likely to be normal than ill, while at a prevalence of 34 per cent an individual with a high score has an 80 per cent chance of being a case. It is fortunate that most series of consecutive attenders at general practice surgeries contain between one-fifth and two-fifths of disturbed patients, since between these limits the questionnaire works quite well.

EXAMPLE

A general practice survey in South Manchester found that the prevalence of probable cases was 11 per cent in randomly selected patients on the list, as against 32 per cent among consecutive attenders at the practice. Data for the sensitivity of a screening test in this practice has been given in the main chapter on page 248.

The hits-positive rate for the test for the random patients was therefore:

$$\frac{11 \times 0 \cdot 957}{(11 \times 0 \cdot 957) + (89 \times 0 \cdot 122)} = \frac{10 \cdot 68}{21 \cdot 53} = 0 \cdot 49$$

while that for the consecutive patients was:

$$\frac{32 \times 0 \cdot 957}{(32 \times 0 \cdot 957) + (68 \times 0 \cdot 122)} = \frac{30 \cdot 6}{38 \cdot 9} = 0 \cdot 78$$

This means that among the random sample 49 per cent of the high scorers would turn out to be cases, while among the consecutive attenders one could expect 78 per cent of the high scorers to be cases. (It must be emphasized that since sensitivity is unaffected by prevalence, in either population 95 per cent of the actual cases will have high scores.)

REFERENCES

BLASHKI, T. G., MOWBRAY, R., and DAVIES, B. (1971) Controlled trial of amitriptyline in general practice, *Brit. med. J.*, **1**, 133–8.

BREMER, J. (1951) Social psychiatric investigation of a small community in Northern Norway, *Acta psychiat. scand.*, Suppl. 62.

BROOK, A., BLENSDALE, J. K., DOWLING, S. J., HOPKINS, J. H., POLLARD, C. J. T., and STROUD, R. A. (1966) Emotional problems in general practice. A survey of a sample of ordinary patients, *J. Coll. gen. Practit.*, **11**, 184–94.

BROOK, A. (1967) An experiment in general practitioner/psychiatrist co-operation, *J. Coll. Gen. Practit.*, **13**, 127–31.

BROWN, A. C. and FRY J. (1962) Cornell Medical Index Health Questionnaire in the identification of neurotic patients in general practice, *J. psychosom. Res.*, **6**, 185–90.

CLIFT, A. D. (1972) Sleep disturbance and dependence on hypnotic drugs, unpublished M.D. thesis.

COLLEGE OF GENERAL PRACTITIONERS' RESEARCH COMMITTEE (1958) The continuing observation and recording of morbidity, *J. Coll. gen. Practit.*, **1**, 107.

COOPER, B. (1972) Social correlates of psychiatric illness in the community, in *Approaches to Action*, ed. McLachlan G., pp. 65–70, London.

COOPER, B., FRY, J., and KALTON, G. (1969) A longitudinal study of psychiatric morbidity in a general practice population, *Brit. J. prev. soc. Med.*, **23**, 210–17.

DONALD, J. F. (1969) A study of a recognised antipsychotic agent as a tranquilliser in general practice, *Practitioner*, **203**, 684–7.

FAHY, T. J., BRANDON, S., and GARSIDE, R. F. (1969) Classification of depressive illness, *Proc. roy. Soc. Med.*, **62**, 331–5.

FREMING, K. H. (1951) *The Expectation of Mental Infirmity in a Sample of the Danish Population*, London.

GIBSON, R., FORBES, J. M., STODDART, I. W., COOKE, J. T., JENKINS, G. W., MacKEITH, S. A., ROSENBERG, L., ALLCHIN, W. H., and SHEPHERD, D. (1966) Psychiatric care in general practice: an experiment in collaboration, *Brit. med. J.*, 1287.

GOLDBERG, D. (1972) *The Detection of Psychiatric Illness by Questionnaire*, Maudsley Monographs, No. 21, London.

GOLDBERG, D. (1973) Unpublished data.

GOLDBERG, D., and BLACKWELL, B. (1970) A detailed study using a new method of case identification, *Brit. med. J.*, **1**, 439–43.

GOLDBERG, D., COOPER, B., EASTWOOD, M. R., KEDWARD, H. B., and SHEPHERD, M. (1970) A standardised psychiatric interview suitable for use in community surveys, *Brit. J. prev. soc. Med.*, **24**, 18.

GOLDBERG, D., RICKELS, K., DOWNING, B., and HESBACHER, P. (1973) in preparation.

HAMILTON, M. (1959) The assessment of anxiety states by rating, *Brit. J. med. Psychol.*, **32**, 50.

HAMILTON, M. (1960) A rating scale for depression, *J. Neurol. Neurosurg. Psychiat.*, **23**, 56.

HARDMAN, R. A. (1965) A comparison of morbidity in two areas, *J. Coll. gen. Practit.*, **9**, 226.

HARVEY-SMITH, E., and COOPER, B. (1970) *J. Roy. Coll. gen. Practit.*, **19**, 132.

HARWIN, B. G., COOPER, B., EASTWOOD, M. R., and GOLDBERG, D. P. (1970) Prospects for social work in general practice, *Lancet*, **ii**, 559–61.

HELGASON, T. (1964) Epidemiology of mental disorders in Iceland, *Acta psychiat. scand.*, Suppl. 173.

HERST, E. R. (1965) An Epidemiological Study of Psychiatric Morbidity in a suburban general practice, Unpublished M.D. thesis, London.

HESBACHER, P. T., RICKELS, K., GORDON, P. E., GRAY, B., MECHELN-BURG, R., WEISE, C. C., and VANDERVORT, W. J. (1970) Setting, patient and doctor effects of drug response in neurotic patients, *Psychopharmacologia*, **18**, 180–226.

HEWETSON, J. C., MCEWAN, J. A., and OLLENDORFF, R. H. W. (1963) The incidence of psychiatric disorders in general practice, *Practitioner*, **190**, 127–32.

HOPKINS, P., and COOPER, B. (1969) Psychiatric referrals from a general practice, *Brit. J. Psychiat.*, **115**, 1163.

INGHAM, J., RAWNSLEY, K., and HUGHES, D. (1972) A comparison of psychiatric morbidity in contrasting areas in rural Wales, *Psychol. Med.*, **2**.

JONES, A. D. (1962) Mental disorder in Anglesey, unpublished M.D. thesis, Liverpool.

KAESER, A. C., and COOPER, B. (1971) The psychiatric patient, the G.P. and the O.P. clinic, *Psychol. Med.*, **1**, 312–25.

KEDWARD, H. B. (1966) Neurotic disorders in urban practice: a three year follow-up, *J. Coll. gen. Practit.*, **12**, 148–63.

KEDWARD, H. B. (1969) The outcome of neurotic illness in the community, *Soc. Psychiat.*, **4**, 1–4.

KELLNER, R. (1963) Neurotic ill health in a general practice on Deeside, Unpublished M.D. thesis, Liverpool.

KELLNER, R. (1966) Psychiatric ill health following physical illness, *Brit. J. Psychiat.*, **112**, 71–3.

KELLNER, R., and SHEFFIELD, B. F. (1967) Symptom rating test scores in neurotics and normals, *Brit. J. Psychiat.*, **113**, 525–6.

KESSEL, N. (1960) Psychiatric morbidity in a London general practice, *Brit. J. prev. soc. Med.*, **14**, 16–22.

KESSEL, N., and SHEPHERD, M. (1965) The health and attitudes of people who seldom consult a doctor, *Med. Care*, **3**, No. 1.

KESSEL, W. I. N. (1962) Conducting a psychiatric survey in general practice, in *The Burden on the Community*, p. 13, London.

KLEMPERER, J. (1933) Zur Belastungsstatistik der Durchschnitts bevolkerung. Psychosenhaufigkeit unter 1000 stickproben massig ausgelesenen Probanden, *Z. ges. Neurol. Psychiat.*, **146**, 277.

KREITMAN, N., PEACE, K., and RYLE, A. (1966) The relationship of psychiatric, psychosomatic and organic illness in general practice, *Brit. J. Psychiat.*, **112**, 569.

LLEWELLYN-THOMAS, E. (1960) The prevalence of psychiatric symptoms within an island fishing village, *Canad. med. Assoc. J.*, **83**, 197.

LOCKE, B. Z., FINUCANE, D. L., and HASSLER, F. (1967) Emotionally disturbed patients under care of private non-psychiatric physicians, in *Psychiatric Epidemiology and Mental Health Planning*, ed. Monroe, R. R., Klee, G. D., and Brody, E. B., The American Psychiatric Association, Research Report, Washington, D.C.

LOGAN, W. P., and CUSHION, A. A. (1958) *Studies on Medical Population Subjects*, No. 14, Vol. 1, General, H.M.S.O., London.

LYONS, H. A. (1969) Joint Psychiatric consultations, *J. Coll. gen. Practit.*, **18**, 125–7.

MECHANIC, D. (1962) The concept of illness behaviour, *J. chron. Dis.*, **15**, 189–94.

MEDLARS, (1973) Psychiatric illness in general practice, *Search M.W.C.* **623/U**.

MEEHL, H., and ROSEN, A. (1955) Antecedent probability and the efficiency of psychometric signs, patterns or cutting score, *Psychol. Bull.*, Suppl., **2**, 194–216.

MOSER, C. A., (1958) *Survey Methods in Social Investigations*, London.

MOWBRAY, R. M., BLAIR, W., JOBB, I. G., and CLARKE, A. (1961) Pilot survey of psychiatric illness in general practice, *Scot. med. J.*, **6**, 314.

PAULETT, J. D. (1956) Neurotic ill-health: a study in general practice, *Lancet*, **ii**, 37–8.

POPOFF, L. (1969) A simple method for diagnosis of depression by the family physician, *Clin. Med.*, **24**, 9.

PORTER, A. M. W. (1970) Depressive illness in a general practice: a demographic study and a controlled trial of imipramine, *Brit. med. J.*, **1**, 773.

PRIMROSE, E. J. R. (1962) Psychological Illness—a community study, London, Tavistock publications.

RAWNSLEY, K. (1966) Congruence of independent measures of psychiatric morbidity, *J. psychosom, Res.*, **10**, 84–93.

SALKIND, M. R. (1969) Beck depression inventory in general practice, *J. Roy. Coll. gen. Pract.*, **18**, 267–71.

SEMMENCE, A. (1969) The health opinion survey. A psychiatric screening instrument, *J. Roy. Coll. gen Practit.*, **18**, 344.

SHEPHERD, M. (1972) Mental illness, general practice and the N.H.S., in *Approaches to Action*, ed. MacLachlan, G., p. 57–64, London.

SHEPHERD, M., COOPER, B., BROWN, A. C., and KALTON, G. (1966) *Psychiatric Illness in General Practice*, London.

SNAITH, R. P., AHMED, S. N., MEHTA, S., and HAMILTON, M. (1971) Assessment of the severity of primary depressive illness, *Psychol. Med.*, **1**, 143–9.

SYLPH, J., KEDWARD, H. B., and EASTWOOD, M. R. (1969) Chronic neurotic patients in general practice, *J. Roy. Coll. gen. Practit.* **17**, 162.

TAYLOR, S. J., and CHAVE, S. (1964) *Mental Health and Environment*, London.

WATTS, C., CAWTE, E., and KUENSSBERG, E. (1964) Survey of mental illness in general practice, *Brit. med. J.*, **3**, 1351.

WATTS, C. A. H., and WATTS, B. M. (1952) *Psychiatry in General Practice*, London.

WHEATLEY, D. (1967) Influence of doctors' and patients' attitudes in the treatment of neurotic illness, *Lancet*, **ii**, 1133–5.

WILSON, J., and JUNGNER, G. (1968) Principles and practice of screening for disease, *Wld. Hlth. Org. Publ. Hlth. Pap.*, No. 24.

17

STUDYING THE INDIVIDUAL

FAY FRANSELLA

INTRODUCTION

This is not intended to be a complete account of how to obtain meaningful and useful information about a single patient. For those who feel encouraged to look at any one method in more detail, a few texts and articles are listed at the end. The primary aim is to provide the interested researcher or clinician with some ideas of techniques that are available for the psychological investigation of individuals, with particular reference to the measurement of change.

This aim imposes two limitations on the content of the chapter. Firstly, it is about *techniques* and not tests. Thus there will be little discussion of norms or standardization samples, but there will be comment on the psychological meaning of the concepts of reliability and validity.

Secondly, there will be no reference to the application of principles derived from experimental psychology to the systematic investigation of specific symptoms or behaviours. This is not to be taken as implying the view that such approaches have no value. On the contrary, the single case investigation, tailored to the requirements of the individual and without using standard psychometric techniques or tests, has an important contribution to make. Shapiro has been one of the chief exponents on the value and importance of such single case research (e.g. 1961, 1964). In 1962, he wrote:

> The essential requirement for the use of the single case in fundamental research would seem to be that of predictive experimental control. The phrase 'predictive experimental control' means that one knows enough about a phenomenon to be able to predict how it will appear in situations in which it has not yet been observed. If one is in a position to do this, then one is in possession of observations about a process, and an observed process is unlikely to be peculiar to only one individual (Shapiro 1962, p. 123).

Examples of such experimental investigations into specific disorders are numerous (e.g. Shapiro and Nelson, 1955; Metcalfe, 1956; Beech and Parboosingh, 1962). But few have gone on, as Shapiro suggests, to investigate the generality of the 'process'.

IDIOGRAPHY OR NOMOTHESIS?

There are two general ways in which techniques can be used for investigating psychological processes in individuals. One can study the process itself in one person, or one can study this same process in numbers of individuals. The terms 'idiographic' and 'nomothetic' are attributed to Windelbrand (1904). He coined the former to describe the forms of knowledge derived from the study of an individual happening or single event and the latter for knowledge derived from the classification of a number of experiences. One is a logical extension of the other but some still need to be persuaded that the idiographic approach is scientifically justifiable.

The traditional way to study psychological functions of individuals has been to compare them to some group norm, and thus those who seek to study a person in relation to himself are in a minority. But they are not without substantial historical support. Ebbinghaus (1885) achieved fame for the mammoth task of learning some 2,300 nonsense syllables under a variety of conditions in order to investigate the processes of memory and forgetting. Freud, less systematically but none the less importantly, studied his own feelings and dreams. This led him to formulate his theory of personality structure and development. William James (1891) even defined psychology as 'the science of finite individual minds'. But he, like others, found it necessary to make generalizations about the mind. This is, of course, essential. The argument is about the validity of generalizations based on data derived from the individual.

An interesting twist can be given to this argument by showing that, in some cases, group data are irrelevant to the precise description of behaviour in the individual. To take one example from many, Baloff and Becker (1967) demonstrated that the learning curve for a single individual often bears little or no relationship to the group curve of which the individual curve forms a part. This is something to be borne in mind when using tests based on nomothetically-derived data to study an individual's attitudes.

RELIABILITY AS A MEASURE OF FAILURE TO REFLECT CHANGE

One thing that the study of individuals does (particularly if the investigation involves repeated testings) is to call into question the statistical notion of reliability. If one is studying some supposedly general personality characteristic such as extraversion, it is reasonable to expect that the scores obtained will be relatively stable over a more prolonged period. If, however, one is specifically looking at a *change* in attitudes, behaviours, or feelings, then a *high* reliability coefficient would merely indicate that there had been *no change*. If the patient had been undergoing some psychological treatment designed to bring about improvement (change), this high reliability would be an indicator of treatment failure.

If a man were inanimate, he could be expected to behave like the thermometer—the same amount of heat giving the same recording over many testings. However, man is not inanimate. If he is considered a form of motion then the use of the concept of reliability needs serious consideration.

Traditionally, the most common way to test the reliability of an instrument is to give it to the same people on more than one occasion and to correlate the two or more sets of scores. *Test–retest* reliability measures the degree to which the same relative difference between people has been preserved on the two occasions. Of course, the actual scores of the people may not remain the same. For example, it can be expected that there will be an increase in score on an intelligence test on a second administration. What is important for reliability is that the position of the subjects *relative to one another* stays the same. Any factor, such as practice, which affects all scores on a test in the same relative way raises questions about its validity but not its reliability.

In addition to the test–retest method, reliability can be assessed by the *split-half* or the *equivalent form procedures*. In the former, the scores derived from one half of a lengthy test can be correlated with those from the other half. With the method of equivalent or parallel forms one might correlate scores on two tests of anxiety, which are similar in form, content, general nature of the questions, and method of scoring. The only point of difference is the actual questions. The correlation between these two forms is a measure of the test's stability.

If there are no right and wrong answers on a test, in absolute terms, then there is another form of reliability to take into account. Two different scorers looking at the same Rorschach responses may score them differently. So wherever there is a subjective element in the scoring procedure, inter-scorer reliability has to be taken into account.

Since psychological measurement of the individual calls into question the whole concept of reliability, one might follow Mair's suggestion (1964, 1964a) that one should predict in advance where one will expect change and where one will expect stability. The only certain statement that can be made about the consistency or reliability of any of the techniques to be discussed is that no *general* statement can be made. There is considerable evidence as to the reliability of particular repertory grids and particular semantic differentials in particular situations: the former are discussed in Bannister and Mair (1968). But there is no one reliability coefficient for THE repertory grid or THE semantic differential.

Before leaving this difficult problem, it is worthwhile noting that Bannister (1960, 1962) turned the tables on the traditional notion of reliability by using it *as a measure*. He argued that not only did the type of disordered thinking found in some schizophrenics show itself as a weakening of relationships between constructs (operationally defined as low correlations), but that the schizophrenics were also inconsistent (unreliable) in the way they used the limited structure remaining.

The concept of reliability, therefore, needs to be reconsidered when techniques of measurement are used with individuals on more than one occasion. If it is important to know whether a particular technique is yielding repeatable results in a specific instance, the researcher must develop his own method for assessing this. One fact to be borne in mind is that the actual 'doing' of one of these techniques can bring about psychological change. This applies to standard tests as well, but is particularly pertinent when the person is being faced with ideas specifically related to himself and others important in his life (see Slater, 1972).

VALIDITY AS A DEMONSTRATION OF THE OBVIOUS

A test or technique may be highly reliable and yet not valid. It may give reliable scores but may not measure what it is intended to measure. Just as there are several types of reliability so there are types of validity.

FACE OR CONTENT VALIDITY

This type asks the question 'does this anxiety questionnaire seem to be dealing with anxiety—are the items related to the concept of anxiety?' Even if they are, one does not know from this whether the person scoring as 'anxiety-prone' is so in actual fact. For this one needs:

CRITERION VALIDITY

This can be of two kinds. If the scores on the questionnaire are to be related to therapists' ratings of anxiety, then one has *concurrent validity*. The scores on the test are related to something that is already known about the individual. One factor that has to be borne in mind here is that there must be good reason for thinking that the criterion measure itself is valid. However, the criterion to be used may be only available at some future date and then one is dealing with *predictive validity*. An arithmetic test is useful in so far as it is predictive of future arithmetic performance.

CONSTRUCT VALIDITY

This is of by far the greatest theoretical significance. If someone has a theory about the nature of anxiety, then the test derived from the theory is assumed to measure anxiety. If predictions are then made from the theory, the degree to which they are borne out, using the test as one of the measures, is an indication of the test's construct validity.

TECHNIQUES OF MEASUREMENT

Four techniques have been chosen for discussion, differing in degree of flexibility and personal relevance. They are Repertory Grid and Semantic Differential technique, the Personal Questionnaire and the Interpersonal Perception Method.

REPERTORY GRID TECHNIQUE

The original form of repertory grid technique, the Rep Test, was described by George Kelly in his *The Psychology of Personal Construts* (1955). The technique is directly related to his theory and was designed primarily to provide clinical hypotheses which might later be of value in the individual's psychotherapy. This technique is being used in a number of contexts, both with and without the theory. It can be argued that psychology is not so rich in ideas that it can afford to ignore any source that is potentially useful in increasing our understanding of ourselves. But others argue that theories can confuse the issue and limit the investigator in his hunt for hypotheses to account for a certain behaviour. The emphasis here will be on technique and not theory, which will be discussed only where relevant to a particular investigation.

There are several forms of grid now in use (for details see Bannister and Mair, 1968), but they all have certain characteristics in common.

1. They all involve some form of sorting procedure. In most cases *elements* (for instance cars) are sorted in terms of a number of *constructs* (for instance sportiness, status, comfort). A construct is thus a conceptual dimension with which to categorize elements. The construct *sporty/not sporty* can be used as a way of looking at makes of car. Each car (element) is categorized in terms of its sportiness. The elements can be looked at further, for example according to the degree to which they invest their owner with *status* and then the extent to which they provide *comfort*.

Constructs can either be elicited from an individual or supplied to him by the investigator. Elicitation is carried out by presenting the person with three elements (for example three makes of car) and asking him in what important way two of the cars can be seen as being alike and thereby different from the third. The answer may be in terms of status or *wankel* versus *piston engine*, but whatever emerges is called a *construct*.

2. In most cases all grids aim at establishing the relationships between the constructs (and in some cases the elements) *for a particular individual*.

3. They have no fixed content—this is determined by the purpose of the investigation.

4. All are designed so that statistical tests of significance can be applied.

5. The basic assumption underlying them all is that statistical relationships between two constructs reflect psychological relationships.

FORMS OF GRID

One form of repertory grid in common use is that involving the rank ordering of elements in terms of constructs. In a typical case the person is asked to name ten people he or she knows (these are the elements). If one of the constructs is *like me in character*, the person is asked to select the person most like him, then next most like him in character and so on until all ten people have been ranked. The same set of elements (people in this example) are thus construed in terms of all the constructs in this way.

The resulting set of rankings of the same ten elements on a number of different constructs can be analysed into clusters, into their principal components (preferably by computer, see Slater, 1964) or else by hand, using a method developed by Bannister (1960). This latter method identifies the construct that is most related to all other constructs (accounts for the most variance) as the first axis, and the second axis is the next most highly 'meaningful' construct but which is statistically independent of the first. The remaining constructs can then be plotted along these two construct dimensions [see FIG. 17.1]. The figures are correlations squared multiplied by one hundred. Thus the correlation between *as I'd like to be* and *friendly* is about 0·7.

An advantage of the computer method of Slater, is that the elements can be plotted in relation to the constructs and vice versa. This can provide very valuable additional information when the elements are personally relevant people or situations rather than, for instance, photographs. Bannister's and Slater's methods have been shown to be highly related with regard to the construct relationships (Fransella, 1965); the advantage of Slater's method is to enable one to plot the element relationships.

FIG. 17.2 shows the construct loadings of a grid plotted along the two principal components; the constructs are plotted in the 'element space'.

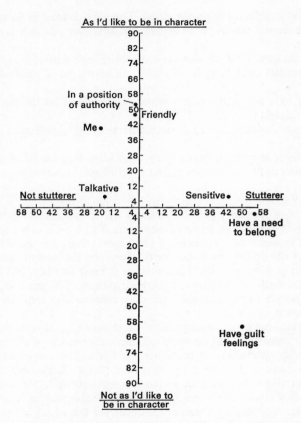

FIG. 17.1. A plot of constructs in terms of their correlations (rho² × 100) with the two main axes derived from a rank order form of repertory grid.

FIG. 17.3 gives the element plot from the same grid, that is the elements are plotted in the 'construct space'. Psychologically, there is no reason why both elements and constructs should not be plotted together, but this is invalid from the statistical viewpoint.

One method of relating constructs to elements which gets very close to semantic differential procedure is that of rating instead of ranking. For instance, instead of having the person make a decision as to who is most like him, next most like him, and so forth, he is asked to state the *degree* to which each person is like him. If a seven-point scale is used, then '1' might arbitrarily be chosen to indicate an absolute likeness and '7' a total dissimilarity, with the midpoint indicating neither likeness nor unlikeness. Bannister and Mair (1968) point out that this method allows the individual much more freedom of action than he gets with the ranking method, a freedom similar to that allowed in Kelly's original Rep Test.

Ryle and Lunghi (1970) used this rating method when demonstrating

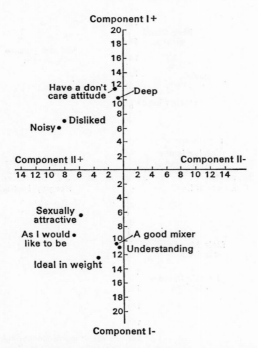

FIG. 17.2. A plot of constructs in the 'element space' derived from a principal components analysis of a rank order grid.

how the technique can be designed to focus on role relationships. Kelly's original grid was called the Role Construct Repertory Test and was aimed at analysing role construct relationships. He points out that this method for analysing relies heavily

. . . upon one's interpretation of the client's language. But we can look beyond words. We can study contexts. For example, does the client use the word 'affectionate' only when talking about persons of the opposite sex? Does he apply the term 'sympathetic' only to members of his own family or only to persons who have also been described as 'intimate'? The answers to questions such as these may give us an understanding of the interweaving of the client's terminology and provide us with an understanding of his outlook which no dictionary could offer.

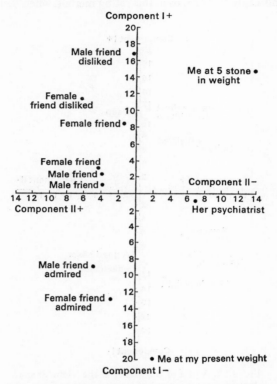

FIG. 17.3. A plot of elements in the 'construct space' derived from a principal components analysis of a rank order grid.

In their *dyad* grid, Ryle and Lunghi examine role construing by using the *relationship* between two people as the element rather than the two people as two separate elements. They point out that in most of the grid modifications, each element is given a global rating which can smother important differences. A person may, in general, be *kind*, but he may be outstandingly kind to his mother and unkind to his secretary. The emphasis here is very much of the relationship between elements and so, at the present time, Slater's method of analysis is the most appropriate to use.

SOME EXAMPLES

One of the earliest single case studies, using the rank order form of grid (Fransella and Adams 1966) was designed to obtain some insight into the 'meaning' fire-setting had for an arsonist. Six rank order grids were administered in all, each one testing a hypothesis derived from the previous one. The sixth grid [in FIG. 17.4] shows how ideas of punishment, sin, and so forth, are related to ideas of arson and how unrelated

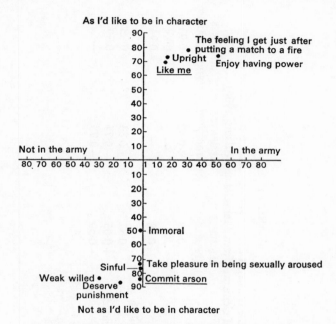

FIG. 17.4. Supplied and elicited constructs in a rank order grid of an arsonist (redrawn from Fransella and Adams, 1966).

all these things are to how he sees himself. The constructs are plotted according to the correlations they have with the main dimension (*as I'd like to be in character*) and the second, independent dimension (*in the army*). Every grid showed one particular feature; this man did not see himself as an arsonist—they are 'bad' and he is 'good'. This separation of the view of *self* from the category of person to which the *self* belongs has since also been demonstrated with stutterers (Fransella, 1965, 1968, 1972) and with alcoholics (Hoy, 1973).

The degree to which certain construct relationships remain stable over time is illustrated by the correlations in TABLE 17.1. Not only did

TABLE 17.1

Spearman rho correlations between the construct *like me* and six other constructs on occasions with two different sets of elements (from Fransella and Adams, 1966)

Construct *like me* correlates with	ELEMENTS (PEOPLE)	ELEMENTS (PHOTOGRAPHS)	ELEMENTS (PHOTOGRAPHS)	ELEMENTS (PEOPLE)
1. Like I'd like to be	+0·88	+0·92	+0·93	+0·84
2. Enjoy having power	—	—	+0·89	+0·87
3. Upright in character	+0·88	—	+0·94	+1·00
4. Have feelings like mine aroused when lighting a fire	+0·87	+0·88	+0·93	+0·89
5. Take pleasure in being sexually aroused	+0·05	−0·77	−0·39	−0·39
6. Likely to commit arson	−0·59	−0·75	—	−0·90

this arsonist maintain several construct relationships consistently over several weeks, but they remained so in spite of the use of two different types of element.

Rank order grids have also been used to monitor change in the conception of *self* as the person changes physically. Single case investigations have shown that some obese women see themselves when fat as 'bad' and themselves at a normal weight as 'good'. A similar relationship is sometimes found also in anorexic people, except that it is being thin that is 'good'. FIGS. 17.5*a* (obese) and 17.5*b* (anorexic) show how weight change and conceptual change occur together in two patients, although which is the chicken and which is the egg has yet to be determined (Fransella and Crisp, 1970; Crisp and Fransella, 1972).

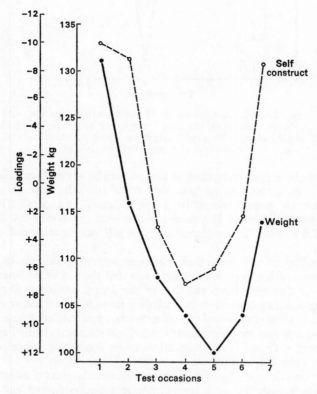

FIG. 17.5(*a*) Loadings of a self-construct for an obese woman on the major component of a repertory grid plotted along with actual weight on 7-test occasions over 15 months (Fransella and Crisp, 1970).

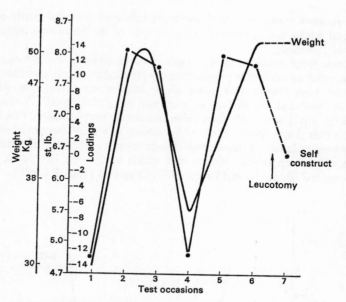

FIG. 17.5(b) Loadings of a self-construct for a patient with anorexia nervosa on the major component of a repertory grid plotted along with actual weight on 7-test occasions over 42 months (Crisp and Fransella, 1972).

What these grid plots show is that as weight approaches normality there is an accompanying 'polarization' of the self. Both the obese and anorexic patient moved from seeing herself as generally 'bad' to being generally 'good'. But relapse is common and both FIGS. 17.5(a) and 17.5(b) show how evaluation of the *self* closely mirrored weight change.

Over the last few years there has been increasing interest in group processes. At least two studies have reported the use of members of a group as elements. Each member of the group completes a grid by ranking or rating the members, including himself, on a number of constructs. Watson (1970) used the rating method and studied interpersonal relationships and the construing of individual members, while Fransella and Joyston-Bechal (1971) focused more on construing processes and their relationship to outcome.

The use of a 'group' grid can provide a massive amount of information concerning such things as therapist/patient understanding and interaction, the accuracy of a person's perception of how others construe him, changes in thought process as well as content, and much else besides. To date, studies have been limited by having to supply instead of elicit constructs so that the grids can be compared across members.

In the forms of behaviour therapy that involve the construction of hierarchies of situations, it is left to the therapist to judge whether the 'steps' in the hierarchy are of approximately equal size. A method has been described for quantifying such a procedure (Fransella, 1972). The situations in the hierarchy can be used as elements in a rank order grid and the relationships between each, in terms of, say, degree to which they arouse anxiety, can be mathematically determined. This method has not yet been validated, but such 'situation grids' offer a possible next step from subjective impression.

One elaboration of the concept of role relationships has proved particularly popular in recent years. This is the use of grids of various sorts to see the degree to which a pair of people can construe each other's construction processes. The most commonly investigated dyad is that of patient and therapist.

One of the first studies of this sort was that of Cartwright and Lerner (1963). They found that improvement was related to increase in the therapist's understanding of the patient. Landfield and Nawas (1964) have similarly looked at therapist/patient understanding and outcome. Since these early studies there have been a number of others, including single case studies, which have looked at the therapist's ability to predict the patient's grid responses (for example, Rowe, 1971; Ryle and Lunghi, 1971). By far the most substantial work in this field is that of Landfield (1971). He investigated therapist/patient role relationships in a large number of patients and eight therapists. Amongst other things, he found that the 'congruency' of the pair, in both conceptual content and organization, was significantly related to successful interaction. Also, where such congruency was low, the probability of premature termination was high.

Although grid technique is primarily for the investigation of an individual's view of his world, there is nothing to prevent one from establishing a standard form for a specific purpose. The Grid Test of Thought Disorder (Bannister and Fransella, 1967) is a case in point. A standard rank order grid was also used in a validation study in which voting behaviour was predicted (Fransella and Bannister, 1967). But such exercises are the exception rather than the rule.

OTHER FORMS OF GRID

Two other forms of grid of particular interest have been developed by Hinkle (1965). These are the *implications grid* and the *resistance to change grid*. Hinkle was concerned to define more precisely Kelly's idea of the construct. He saw its meaning identified by that which it implied, and his implications grid resulted. It does not use elements to be sorted in terms of constructs as do most other forms of grid. In this case the person is required to relate each construct with all others and note when one implies another or, in turn, is *implied by* another.

An implications grid is completed by asking which pole of each construct (*shy* or *gay*, *relaxed* or *tense* for instance) he would prefer to be described by. Then each construct is paired with every other in turn and he is asked whether a personal change from one pole to the other on one construct would involve a change from one pole to the other on the second construct. The detailed instructions can be found in Bannister and Mair (1968).

Apart from developing two additional forms of grid, Hinkle showed how it was possible to encourage a person to verbalize the implications of a construct in increasingly abstract terms. This has come to be referred to as 'laddering'.

For example, if the construct *makes good friends* versus *two-faced* and *dishonest* has been elicited from elements in the usual way, the person is asked by which pole of the construct he would prefer to be described. If *makes good friends* is preferred, then he is asked *why* he makes this choice. If he says one is *not lonely*, then *not lonely/lonely* is another construct, superordinate to the first. This process of asking 'why' is continued until no more constructs are forthcoming. Theoretically (and seemingly in practice) the higher up the construct system one 'climbs', the fewer constructs there are. Thus, if the laddering technique is being applied to several elicited constructs, they will tend to link into only one or two superordinate constructs at the 'top' of the system.

The resistance to change grid can be constructed with the same constructs as used in the implications grid. The person is asked to decide on which construct he would find it easier to change if he *had* to change on one of the pair. That is, would he find it easier to become *shy* or become *tense* if he actually preferred to be *gay and relaxed*. This form of grid has been put to little use since Hinkle's original demonstration of the relationship between resistance to change of a construct and its superordinacy (its psychological importance for the individual). He showed that the more implications or 'meaning' a construct has, the more resistant to change it tends to be. But its potential value in measuring and predicting change in psychotherapy is clear.

Very little work has been reported in which Hinckle's implications grid has been used. But two examples may serve to illustrate the type of work that can be undertaken. One is a single case study (Wright, 1970) in which the *meaning* of symptoms for a patient was investigated. This was done by eliciting constructs and then 'laddering' them. Wright showed very clearly how the patient's construing of life presented her with an insoluble dilemma and her neurotic attempt at a solution. In this study the emphasis was moved away from problems of diagnosis or symptom interpretation to problems of personal meaning and the relation of these to behaviour.

In a second example, implications grids were used to obtain both group measures and individual information in a research project on a construct theory treatment of stuttering (Fransella, 1969; 1972). The grids were modified slightly so that the implications of both poles of each construct could be studied. FIG. 17.6 shows one such grid. The ticks in line 1a indicate that the man said that *quiet* people are *like me, wrapped up in their own thoughts* and *keep themselves to themselves, confide in only a few*. A computer program for analysing such grids is

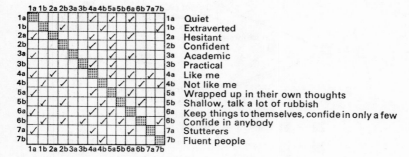

FIG. 17.6. A bi-polar implications grid with elicited constructs completed by a stutterer (see text).

lodged with the MRC Computer Unit. It provides the probabilities of obtaining the observed number of matching and mismatching ticks in each pair of lines.

An example of the type of information that such grids can give is shown in FIG. 17.7. This man was quite satisfied with himself as he was and it transpired he had only come along for treatment at the insistence of his fiancée's parents. The grid plot suggests that he was being asked to give up a great deal more than just stuttering.

These examples have been chosen to show some of the many ways in which grid technique can be used. Basically, it can provide both individual and group data, can be used as a research tool, as a test to measure some psychological variable, as a possible predictor of therapeutic outcome, as a measure of social understanding and, above all else, as a method for helping in our understanding of an individual's view of his world.

Grid technique is increasingly being used to monitor change. Although change in *content* of thinking is of interest and importance in psychotherapeutic settings, the demonstration of change in thought *process* is another possibility offered by this technique. One aim must

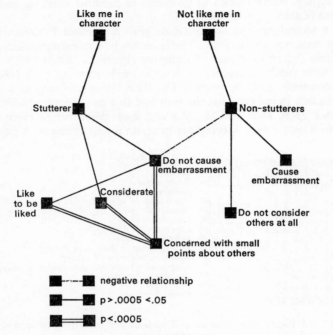

FIG. 17.7. A pictorial representation of construct relationships
derived from a bi-polar implications grid.

be to relate change in content with change in process. This should lead
to an increased understanding of the nature of the whole psychotherapeutic enterprise.

SEMANTIC DIFFERENTIAL TECHNIQUE

In *The Measurement of Meaning*, Osgood *et al.* (1957) described this
technique as a method for establishing where, in a multi-dimensional
space, a particular word will 'fall'. The word's location in this semantic
space indicates its meaning. As a first step in defining this space,
Osgood and his colleagues had groups of subjects rate several series of
concepts ('things') on a number of adjectival bipolar scales such as
good/bad, large/small, active/passive. All these ratings were then factor
analysed. This and subsequent analyses all tended to produce the same
three major dimensions.

The factor accounting for by far the greatest amount of variance in
all studies is Evaluative (for example *good/bad*), then comes Potency
(for instance *strong/weak, large/small*) and then Activity (for example

fast/slow, active/passive). These main factors define the 'semantic space' and a concept's location along each one defines its meaning.

Unlike grid technique, there is an assumption of generality of underlying factor structure. But in 1962, Osgood reported an analysis of specifically people-oriented concepts and found several other significant factors. The first three of these were described as Moral Evaluation, Rationality, and Unusualness. This called into question the validity of using scales to represent supposedly stable factors. However, in practice, people often tend to think and work in terms of the original E (Evaluative), P (Potency), and A (Activity) factors.

To analyse the meanings of concepts for an individual, one typically selects sets of seven-point scales to represent each of these three factors (usually more for the Evaluative than for the other two). The person is then required to rate each concept on each scale according to whether it is, say, relatively *nice* or *nasty*. One is not limited to Osgood's original factors however. The bipolar adjectival scales shown in Fig. 17.8 were selected to represent four factors derived from 100 people rating ten speech-related concepts on thirty scales (Smith, 1962). The factors so produced were Interestingness, Honesty, Pleasantness, and Difficulty.

Concept
My voice

RATING

	1	2	3	4	5	6	7	
Boring:	—:	—:	—:	—:	—:	—:	—:	Interesting
Lenient:	—:	—:	—:	—:	—:	—..:	—:	Severe
Honest	—:	—:	—:	—:	—:	—:	—:	Dishonest
Difficult:	—:	—:	—:	—:	—:	—:	—:	Easy
Empty:	—:	—:	—:	—:	—:	—:	—:	Full
Pleasurable:	—:	—:	—:	—:	—:	—:	—:	Painful
True:	—:	—:	—:	—:	—:	—:	—:	False
Narrow:	—:	—:	—:	—:	—:	—:	—:	Broad
Relaxed:	—:	—:	—:	—:	—:	—:	— :	Tense

Fig. 17.8. A typical form for presenting the seven-point scales of a semantic differential.

Concepts need not, of course, be represented by single words. Quite often it is necessary to use a phrase or even a short sentence to convey clearly what is to be rated. In practice, the person simply has to rate each concept on all the scales according to whether, for instance, he sees himself as *boring* or *interesting*, *lenient* or *severe*. Once the factor structure for a particular set of scales has been determined, so that it is known which scale belongs to which factor, there are two main ways of deriving scores. Osgood described how the distance between two concepts could be used as an operational definition of a difference in their meaning (Bannister and Mair, 1968, p. 123; Osgood *et al.*, 1957, p. 91). A simpler method is to take the average rating on the scales representing each factor. If there are three factors represented by a number of scales then there will be three factor scores for each concept. One method of plotting concepts in such a three-dimensional space is shown in FIG. 17.9.

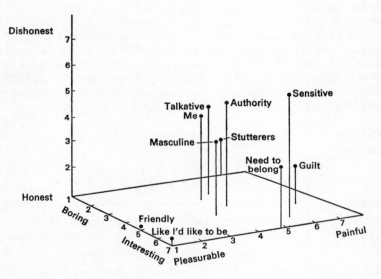

FIG. 17.9. A three-dimensional plot of concepts on Smith's (1962) three semantic differential factors for speech-related concepts.

There are some important points that must be borne in mind when considering whether to use scales representing factors derived from factor analyses of group data (e.g. Osgood's or Smith's) when investigating the individual case.

Firstly, one is not using completely idiographic data. An individual's ratings are being related to correlated data derived from large numbers of people. The individuality has been ironed out to a considerable extent. Just as it has been shown that an individual's learning curve sometimes bears no resemblance to the group's learning curve, so this has been demonstrated for the semantic differential scales (Bannister and Fransella, 1971). On the other hand, Marks and Gelder (1967) carried out principal component analyses on semantic differentials of each patient they were studying. They found that for the Evaluative factor, the sum of the scale scores were similar whether the scales were chosen from Osgood's original set or from the set produced by the individual's 'personal' principal component analysis. But there is no such evidence for the Activity and Potency factors.

Secondly, quite often the task facing the subject approaches the meaningless, nicely commented upon by Brown (1958) in his article 'Is a boulder sweet or sour?' Such psychological tasks face the subject with having either to indulge in fantasies about the edibility of boulders or else to give a middle-of-the-road rating. This latter does not necessarily produce grave distortions but leads to a reduction in sensitivity. This problem is solved to some extent if special semantic differentials are constructed for specific purposes, such as for Osgood's people-oriented and Smith's speech-related concepts.

Lastly, there is the problem of concept/scale interaction. For instance, the correlation between the scales SOBER/DRUNK and MATURE/YOUTHFUL range from $+0.6$ to -0.6, depending on the concept being rated. If the concept to be rated is DAWN, then SOBER and YOUTHFUL go together, but if the concept is UNITED NATIONS then SOBER goes with MATURE. In fact, at the end of his book, Osgood indicates his realization of the importance of this interaction. He concludes that it may be necessary to construct separate differentials for each class of concept being used (although he hopes this will not be the case). And again in 1962, he writes that, from the standpoint of semantic measurement, there is no such thing as THE semantic differential with rigidly defined sets of factors.

These three points lead to the possibility of divorce between the technique and the part of the theory that states that there are universal sets of factors to describe meaning. From one point of view this is an advantage as it gives the investigator of an individual's 'meaning' system greater freedom. On the other hand, it suggests that a differential must be subject to a factor or cluster analysis *for each individual*. If this suggestion is accepted, then semantic differential technique becomes a variant of repertory grid technique.

PERSONAL QUESTIONNAIRE TECHNIQUE

Shapiro developed the personal questionnaire technique because he found that existing questionnaires did not suit his research requirements:

They are general in character, that is each questionnaire has been constructed on the basis of certain *a priori* and empirical considerations, and the same questions are directed at every subject. Such questionnaires might, in the case of a given individual, miss important items, and waste time in dealing with irrelevant ones. Moreover, in keeping as close as possible to the psychiatrist's interview, it seemed necessary to make use of the patient's own utterances and formulations. It was decided to develop a technique which did this and to call it the 'personal questionnaire' (Shapiro, 1962, p. 133).

The technique has primarily been used to measure changes in a patient's feelings about his symptoms. The questionnaire consists of statements made by the patient and each statement is supplemented by additional statements to produce a grading of severity. For example, if the patient says 'I feel depressed', two additional statements might be 'I feel only a little depressed' and 'I do not feel depressed at all'. These statements are then paired so that each is presented in relation to the other (1 with 2; 2 with 3; and 1 with 3). The pairs of statements for all the symptoms constitute the questionnaire. This method also provides an indication of the patient's understanding of the task since, with three pairs of statements per symptom, inconsistencies can be spotted.

One of the main values of this technique is the opportunity it provides for the detailed monitoring of change in the patient's feeling state during the course of treatment.

To obviate one of the principal disadvantages—time required for scoring—Phillips (1968) reports the development of a computer program to process the pairs of questionnaire statements, each of which is written directly on a computer card. Phillips (1970; 1970a) has also developed two different types of scaling procedure that can be used to quantify patients' personal statements about their psychological state and to which statistical techniques can be applied for testing the significance of differences obtained over time.

Just as a semantic differential can be regarded as a variant of repertory grid technique, once the focus is on individual rather than group-based factors, so can the personal questionnaire. Slater (1970) demonstrates the similarity between techniques designed to investigate personal psychological meanings by treating personal questionnaire data as if they were in repertory grid form. This is a particularly useful paper since Slater discusses in some detail the statistical problems involved in all such scaling methods.

The reliability and validity of this technique, as with the others, call into question the traditional view of these concepts. How does one check if a patient 'has really changed' or is just being 'unreliable'? How does one check whether what a patient (or anyone else for that matter) says is a 'true' reflection of his feelings? The absence of reliability and validity data should not prevent the researcher or clinician from using this or any of the other techniques on these grounds alone. He must, however, do his best to check his findings against other data or observations wherever possible.

INTERPERSONAL PERCEPTION METHOD

In an absolute sense, this method is not concerned with individuals nor is it a technique. But the borderline between a technique and a test is sufficiently obscure to allow the inclusion of this methodological development. The Interpersonal Perception Method (Laing *et al.*, 1966) is designed to study one person's (A) views of another (B) and the 'accuracy' of these views is checked by asking B what his views are of himself and what he thinks A's views are of him.

This method is thus a faithful reflection of Kelly's notion of role (1955). In his sociality corollary Kelly states that 'to the extent that one person construes the construction processes of another he may play a role in a social process involving the other person'. The interpersonal perception method has not yet been used to investigate social behaviour and construing in relation to construct theory ideas, but the possibilities for a partnership between theory and method are clear.

The method deserves consideration because of the current interest in and emphasis upon interpersonal relations. But it is not a technique as are the others under discussion since there is no flexibility—the questions asked are standard. However, there is no reason why this should remain the case for all time.

The method is designed to measure how pairs of people construe each other at three different levels of perspective. For example, there is a wife's view of marriage, the wife's view of the husband's view of marriage, and the wife's view of the husband's view of the wife's view of marriage. From the answers wife and husband give, measures of the degree of agreement, understanding, and 'realization or failure of realization' can be obtained at all three levels.

The form the questions take for each partner at the three levels of perspective is as follows and each answer is given on a 4-point scale ranging from 'very true' to 'very untrue'.

A. How true do you think the following are?
  1. She respects me.
  2. I respect her.

3. She respects herself.
4. I respect myself.

B. How would SHE answer the following?
   1. I respect him.
   2. He respects me.
   3. I respect myself.
   4. He respects himself.

C. How would SHE think you have answered the following?
   1. She respects me.
   2. I respect her.
   3. She respects herself.
   4. I respect myself.

There are sixty such issues, representing six categories. These are interdependence and autonomy; warm concern and support; disparagement and disappointment; contentions; fight/flight; contradiction and confusion; extreme denial of autonomy. This procedure can be used not only as a basis for comparison of differences between any two people, but as a starting point for marriage counselling (or whatever the aim is) and also as a measure of the amount of change that has occurred over time. The results from this method (as with all other techniques) can also be utilized for discussion of relevant problems in the therapy setting.

The authors give some data on the method's reliability and validity, and these are sufficiently high to encourage others to experiment with the procedure. But so far there has been disappointingly little additional work.

Jahoda's comments in the Foreword of the book on the difference between this method and 'test' are equally applicable to all the other techniques mentioned.

It should be emphasized that what the authors have developed is a method for investigating dyads rather than a test in the strict sense of the term.

What one likes about a test is that it is standardized for a 'normal' population and validated against 'objective' performance criteria. The method presented here cannot claim these advantages. There exist no norms for interpersonal encounters which specify how many dyads are based on understanding each other on a particular issue, being understood by the other and realizing that one is understood, or on the various combinations of these levels in interaction. The psychological and statistical problems confronting the establishment of such norms are formidable (Jahoda, 1966, p.v).

CONCLUSION

The overlap between all these techniques is very great, particularly between the first three. But they all share at least one basic characteristic. They all ignore the traditional segmenting of man. Cognition, personality, attitudes and even perception become as one when it is argued that the meaning an individual imposes on events determines his behaviour towards those events.

REFERENCES

BALOFF, N., and BECKER, S. W. (1967) On the futility of aggregating individual learning curves, *Psychol. Rep.*, **20**, 183–91.

BANNISTER, D. (1960) Conceptual structure in thought disordered schizophrenics, *J. ment. Sci.*, **106**, 1230–49.

BANNISTER, D. (1962) The nature and measurement of schizophrenic thought disorder, *J. ment. Sci.*, **108**, 825–42.

BANNISTER, D., and FRANSELLA, FAY (1967) *A Grid Test of Schizophrenic Thought Disorder*, Barnstaple.

BANNISTER, D., and FRANSELLA, FAY (1971) *Inquiring Man: the Theory of Personal Constructs*, Harmondsworth.

BANNISTER, D., and MAIR, J. M. M. (1968) *The Evaluation of Personal Constructs*, London.

BEECH, H. R., and PARBOOSINGH, P. C. (1962) An experimental investigation of disordered motor expression in a catatonic schizophrenic patient, *Brit. J. soc. clin. Psychol.*, **1**, 222–7.

BONARIUS, J. C. J. (1965) Research in the personal construct theory of George A. Kelly: Role construct repertory test and basic theory, in *Progress in Experimental Personality Research*, ed. Maher, B., New York.

BROWN, R. W. (1958) Is a boulder sweet or sour?, *Contemp. Psychol.*, **3**, 113.

CARTWRIGHT, R. D., and LERNER, B. (1963) Empathy, need to change and improvement with psychotherapy, *J. consult. Psychol.*, **27**, 138–44.

CRISP, A. H., and FRANSELLA, FAY (1972) Conceptual changes during recovery from anorexia nervosa, *Brit. J. med. Psychol.*, **45**, 395–405.

EBBINGHAUS, H. (1885) *Uber das Gedachtnis*, Leipzig, Trans. Ruger, H., and Bussenius, C. E., 1913.

FRANSELLA, FAY (1965) The effects of imposed rhythm and certain aspects of personality on the speech of stutterers. Unpublished Ph.D. Thesis, University of London.

FRANSELLA, FAY (1968) Self concepts and the stutterer, *Brit. J. Psychiat.*, **114**, 1531–5.

FRANSELLA, FAY (1969) The stutterer as subject or object ?, in *Stuttering and the Conditioning Therapies*, ed. Gray, B. B., and England, G., Monterey Institute for Speech and Hearing, California.

FRANSELLA, FAY (1972) *Personal Change and Reconstruction*, London.

FRANSELLA, FAY, and ADAMS, B. (1966) An illustration of the use of repertory grid technique in a clinical setting, *Brit. J. soc. clin. Psychol.*, **5**, 51–62.

FRANSELLA, FAY, and BANNISTER, D. (1967) A validation of repertory grid technique as a measure of political construing, *Acta psychol. (Amst.)*, **26**, 97.

FRANSELLA, FAY, and CRISP, A. H. (1970) Conceptual organisation and weight change, *Psychother. Psychosom.*, **18**, 170–85. Also (1971) *Recent Research in Psychosomatics*, ed. Pierloot, R. A., Basel.

FRANSELLA, FAY, and JOYSTON-BECHAL, M. P. (1971) An investigation of conceptual process and pattern change in a psychotherapy group over one year, *Brit. J. Psychiat.*, **119**, 199–206.

HINKLE, D. E. (1965) The change of personal constructs from the viewpoint of a theory of implications, Ph.D. Thesis, Ohio State University.

HOY, R. M. (1973) The meaning of alcoholism for alcoholics, *Brit. J. Soc. clin. Psychol.*, **12**, 98.

JAHODA, MARIE (1966) Foreword, in *Interpersonal Perception Method*, Laing, R. D., Phillipson, H., and Lee, A. R., London.

JAMES, W. (1891) *Principles of Psychology*, Vol. I, London.

KELLY, G. A. (1955) *The Psychology of Personal Construct*, New York.

KNOWLES, J. B., and PURVES, C. (1965) The use of repertory grid technique to assess the influence of the experimenter-subject relationship in verbal conditioning, *Bull. Brit. Psychol. Soc.*, **18**, 59.

LAING, R. D., PHILLIPSON, H., and LEE, A. R. (1966) *Interpersonal Perception: a Theory and a Method of Research*, London.

LANDFIELD, A. W. (1971) *Personal Construct Systems in Psychotherapy*, New York.

LANDFIELD, A. W., and NAWAS, M. M. (1964) Psychotherapeutic improvement as a function of communication and adoption of therapist's values, *J. Council Psychol.*, **11**, 336–41.

MAIR, M. M. (1964) The derivation, reliability and validity of grid measures: some problems and suggestions, *Bull. Brit. Psychol. Soc.*, **17**, 95.

MAIR, M. M. (1964a) The concepts of reliability and validity in relation to construct theory and repertory grid technique in *Brunel Construct Theory Seminar Report*, ed. Warren, N., Brunel University.

MARKS, I. M., and GELDER, M. G. (1967) Transvestism and fetishism: clinical and psychological changes during faradic aversion, *Brit. J. Psychiat.*, **113**, 711–29.

METCALFE, M. (1956) Demonstration of a psychosomatic relationship, *Brit. J. med. Psychol.*, **29**, 63–6.

OSGOOD, C. E. (1962) Studies on the generality of affective meaning systems, *Amer. Psychologist*, **17**, 10–28.

OSGOOD, C. E., SUCI, G. J., and TANNENBAUM, P. M. (1957) *The Measurement of Meaning*, Urbana., Ill.

PHILLIPS, J. P. N. (1968) A scheme for computer scoring a Shapiro Personal Questionnaire, *Brit. J. soc. clin. Psychol.*, **7**, 309–10.

PHILLIPS, J. P. N. (1970) A further type of personal questionnaire technique, *Brit. J. soc. clin. Psychol.*, **9**, 338–46.

PHILLIPS, J. P. N. (1970a) A new type of personal questionnaire technique, *Brit. J. soc. clin. Psychol.*, **9**, 241–56.

ROWE, DOROTHY (1971) An examination of a psychiatrist's predictions of a patient's constructs, *Brit. J. Psychiat.*, **118**, 231–44.

RYLE, A., and LUNGHI, M. (1970) The dyad grid: a modification of repertory grid technique, *Brit. J. Psychiat.*, **117**, 323–7.

RYLE, A., and LUNGHI, M. (1971) A therapist's prediction of a patient's dyad grid, *Brit. J. Psychiat.*, **118**, 555.

SHAPIRO, M. B. (1961) A method of measuring psychological changes specific to the individual psychiatric patient, *Brit. J. med. Psychol.*, **34**, 151–5.

SHAPIRO, M. B. (1962) A clinical approach to fundamental research with special reference to the study of the single patient, in *Methods of Psychiatric Research*, ed. Sainsbury, P., and Kreitman, N., London.

SHAPIRO, M. B. (1964) The measurement of clinically relevant variables, *J. psychosom. Res.*, **8**, 245–54.

SHAPIRO, M. B., and NELSON, E. H. (1955) An investigation of an abnormality of cognitive function in a co-operative young psychotic: an example of the application of experimental method in a single case, *J. clin. Psychol.*, **11**, 344–51.

SLATER, P. (1964) *The Principal Components of a Repertory Grid*, London.

SLATER, P. (1970) Personal questionnaire data treated as forming a repertory grid, *Brit. J. soc. clin. Psychol.*, **9**, 357–70.

SLATER, P. (1972) The measurement of consistency in repertory grids, *Brit. J. Psychiat.*, **121**, 45–51.

SMITH, R. G. (1962) A semantic differential for speech correction concepts, *Sp. Monogr.*, **29**, 32–7.

WATSON, J. P. (1970) A repertory grid method of studying groups, *Brit. J. Psychiat.*, **117**, 309–18.

WINDELBRAND, W. (1904) *Geschichte und Naturwissenschaft*, Strasbourg.

WRIGHT, K. J. T. (1970) Exploring the uniqueness of common complaints, *Brit. J. med. Psychol.*, **43**, 221–32.

FURTHER READING

SINGLE CASE INVESTIGATIONS

DAVIDSON, P. O., and COSTELLO, C. G. eds. (1969) N = 1: *Experimental Studies of Single Cases*, Insight Book, New York.

SHAPIRO, M. B. (1963) A clinical approach to fundamental research with special reference to the study of the single patient, in *Methods of Psychiatric Research*, ed. Sainsbury, P., and Kreitman, N., London.

SHAPIRO, M. B. (1970) Intensive assessment of the single case: an inductive–deductive approach, in *The Psychological Assessment of Mental and Physical Handicaps*, London.

REPERTORY GRID TECHNIQUE

KELLY, G. A. (1955) *The Psychology of Personal Constructs*, New York.

BANNISTER, D., and MAIR, J. M. (1968) *The Evaluation of Personal Constructs*, London.

BANNISTER, D., and FRANSELLA, FAY (1971) *Inquiring Man*, London.

BONARIUS, J. C. J. (1965) Research in the personal construct theory of George A. Kelly, in *Progress in Experimental Personality Research*, Vol. 2, ed. Maher, B. A., New York.

FRANSELLA, FAY (1972) *Personal Change and Reconstruction*, London.

SLATER, P. (1965) The use of the repertory grid technique in the individual case, *Brit. J. Psychiat.*, **111**, 965–75.

SLATER, P. The measurement of consistency in repertory grids, *Brit. J. Psychiat.*, **121**, 45–51.

SEMANTIC DIFFERENTIAL TECHNIQUE

OSGOOD, C. E., SUCI, G. J., and TANNENBAUM, P. H. (1957) *The Measurement of Meaning*, Urbana, Ill.

OSGOOD, C. E. (1962) Studies on the generality of affective meaning systems, *Amer. Psychol.*, **17**, 10–28.

PERSONAL QUESTIONNAIRE TECHNIQUE

SHAPIRO, M. B. (1961) A method of measuring psychological changes specific to the individual psychiatric patient, *Brit. J. med. Psychol.*, **34**, 151–5.

PHILLIPS, J. P. N. (1968) A further type of personal questionnaire technique, *Bull. Brit. Psychol. Soc.*, **21**, 117 (abstract).

PHILLIPS, J. P. N. (1970) A new type of personal questionnaire technique, *Brit. J. soc. clin. Psychol.*, **9**, 241–56.

SHAPIRO, M. B. ed. (1971) *The Reduction of Mental Distress*, London.

INTERPERSONAL PERCEPTION METHOD

LAING, R. D., PHILLIPSON, H., and LEE, A. R. (1966) *Interpersonal Perception Method: a Theory and a Method of Research*, London.

SOME COMPUTER PROGRAMS AVAILABLE

For *semantic differential*, *repertory grid* and *personal questionnaire* data:

There is an MRC computer service run by Dr. P. Slater at the Institute of Psychiatry, London, offering a free computer service for clinical and research purposes. The several programs analyse data from the individual or group, and compare several grids from one person or one grid from several people. These programs are named INGRID, DELTA, and COIN.

The MRC has a program for the analysis of a bipolar implications grid, named FRAN II.

J. P. N. Phillips reports on a program for the analysis of a personal questionnaire in the *British Journal of Social and Clinical Psychology* (1968), **7**, 309–10, and indicates he can supply further information.

18

HOW TO WRITE A SCIENTIFIC PAPER

DENIS LEIGH

The primary aim of a scientific paper is to present in the simplest possible manner the results of a particular inquiry and the conclusions which stem from them. Originality, clarity, and brevity are the three essentials of a satisfactory paper. Unfortunately, apart from the difficulties inherent in being original, brief, and clear, and in writing understandable English, psychiatry poses its own difficulties. The very breadth of psychiatric research, embracing so many different subjects and disciplines, makes writing in this field confusing and difficult. The editorial policies of many journals are not made sufficiently explicit, leaving the would-be author in doubt as to how to write his paper, and what kind of a paper to write. Lastly, psychiatrists are probably amongst the most literate and long-winded members of the medical profession, and all too often confuse literary with scientific ability. To write an essay on, say, 'The Psychopathology of John Keats' demands a different approach to that which concerns us here, the writing of a scientific paper. It might be imagined that this is self-evident, but many papers are in fact a mixture of the literary, the philosophical, and the scientific, curiously reminiscent of the style prevailing in the late nineteenth century. The best scientific papers are terse and very brief; of necessity, they are few in number—most of us can only hope to be average. It is with the technique of writing the average scientific paper that the following pages are concerned.

There are some sixty journals in the world dealing with psychiatric topics; a handful only have an international scientific reputation. Before embarking on the actual writing of your paper, study the journals you consider suitable, and choose the journal to which you will submit your paper. The choice of journal may determine the choice of title, the style, the length, the organization, and whether or not to include illustrations, as well as that very important matter, the bibliography. It is unwise to write the paper first, and then to consider the journal to which it might be sent. Editors do not take kindly to manuscripts which do not conform to their 'directions to authors'. Alas, for the unfortunate authors, no uniform policy exists amongst the many different psychiatric journals. You must therefore study the journals with the following points in mind.

First and foremost, note the interests and background of the editorial staff. Editors are human and have their prejudices; they sometimes even produce a journal which conforms to their own particular biases. Do not impose upon an editor—second-rate papers submitted by friends of the editor, or simply because they have been delivered as lectures to an organization linked with a journal, may be at times a positive embarrassment. Do not get a colleague of greater prestige or status than yourself to submit your paper for you accompanied by a personal letter to the editor.

Secondly, scan the various journals, and choose a journal with whose style you feel familiar, which you respect, and—this is most important— which is within your range. It is always upsetting to have your article rejected, and you must choose the journal which will give you the best chance of seeing your paper in print.

Thirdly, always try to choose a journal published in your own country. This is not always possible since the only appropriate journal may be published abroad—in this case it is the subject matter which will determine the choice of your journal. But where there are several journals of the same character published in different countries, an editor will be rather suspicious when he receives papers from foreign sources—suspicious that the paper has already been rejected by the national journal.

Fourthly, and lastly, consult a more experienced colleague, and discuss with him the kind of journal for which you should write your paper. He may be more able to assess your chances than you are yourself.

The business of writing the paper then begins. Your results will already have been analysed and tabulated. and you will have compressed the information into readily assimilable tables and graphs.

A series of headings can then be drawn up and the first draft written in the style which comes most naturally. Do not refer to dictionaries, grammars, or technical works on writing at this stage. Get this first draft roughly typed, triple spaced, with wide margins (at least $1\frac{1}{2}$ inches: 37 mm) around the typescript. Then re-read the paper, correct typographical errors, and now begin to make use of the dictionaries. Do not use the same word repeatedly, choose the simplest, most appropriate, and most clearly definable word. Pay attention to punctuation at this stage, and above all, ruthlessly prune the text. Tables and graphs often mean a great deal of work for the typist or draughtsman, and great care must be taken in their preparation before embarking on their typing or drawing.

This is the time to hand over the manuscript to a colleague, preferably one who is not familiar with the work, to read and criticize it. The draft is then amended and should be put aside for a short time. Staleness must be avoided like the plague, and a break from work will make the final drafting a great deal easier and more decisive. In general do not be in a hurry to publish—it is better to reflect and ponder on your findings than to rush into print with a paper which you may later regret. However, most authors are anxious to communicate their views to the world at large and we may therefore pass on to deal with the detailed aspects of writing a paper.

ORGANIZATION

The paper is divided into the following sections: Title; Authorship; Introduction; Material and Methods; Results; Discussion; Summary. In certain foreign journals an abstract must be provided, usually in English, French, or German.

THE TITLE

Much thought must be given to the choice of a crisp yet maximally informative title. Remember that it will be the bibliographical clue to other workers, and that your work may be overlooked unless it is appropriately titled. Common faults are pretentiousness and banality. Phrases such as 'A Study of', 'A Critical Review', 'A Comprehensive Approach to the Problem of' are redundant and should not be used. From ten to fifteen words represent the outside length for a title. Obtain the opinion of your friends on this matter, and be prepared to alter your title several times, and if necessary to solicit editorial opinion when you submit the paper.

AUTHORSHIP

There is a widespread convention that the first author listed has been responsible for the major part of the research. Nevertheless, authors may opt to be listed in alphabetical order; both systems are acceptable. Journals differ in their policy, but the custom of omitting all degrees and titles is growing. Your paper will be judged by its content, not by your position, profession or degrees; a string of letters may mean something in one country, and nothing in another. It can be argued that it is worth knowing if an author is a psychologist, biochemist, or medical man and what is his status. But how does this affect the value of a piece of research? Only if the reader has little knowledge of the subject can these details possibly help.

When the study has a joint authorship some method of recognizing the locus of the authors must be used. Either a symbol, such as an asterisk, and a footnote reference can be used, or an author separation as follows:

Denis Leigh, Edward Marley,
The Institute of Psychiatry,
The University of London
and
R. M. Bruce Pearson,
King's College Hospital, London, S.E.5.

For such details consult the particular journal to which you have decided to send your paper.

INTRODUCTION

No heading is necessary and the author should launch straight into an account of the problem, the hypothesis he seeks to establish, why he has set up the hypothesis, and summarize the already available evidence on the subject. The introduction must be brief, and should not be a review of the literature. A sterile scholasticism must be avoided at all costs—far too many papers have an obsessional quality about them, and refer to every possible piece of previous work. Experience and knowledge of the subject alone can give the author the faculty of selecting what are the important relevant contributions.

MATERIALS AND METHODS

A clear account of the material and methods must be given—all of which can be printed in small type. The aim of this section is to enable the experiment to be repeated if necessary by other observers. Subjects, controls, experimental apparatus, and the methods of measurement should be described. Complicated apparatus may best be portrayed diagrammatically—photographs should not be used if at all possible. They are difficult to reproduce, expensive, and include too much irrelevant detail. There is a regrettable tendency in many psychological journals to use abbreviations such as S for subject and E for experimenter in this part of a paper. Equations of a pseudoscientific nature also make for difficulty in reading—the English language needs none of this to convey meaning economically and precisely. The metric system must be used at all times.

RESULTS

The results should be set out so that sufficient information is given to justify the conclusions; it is unnecessary to detail every individual finding. Statistical methods must be used whenever appropriate, and every attempt made to condense the material. Any statistical terminology must be clear, and should follow that employed in any up-to-date statistical textbook. Diagrammatic representation of the data can be used whenever this makes for condensation and precision, but should not be used unless absolutely necessary. The preparation of blocks is expensive and wasteful of space; in some journals the author may be charged for any diagrams in excess of a certain number. Four methods can be used to concentrate the volume of information: (1) tables; (2) graphs; (3) drawings; (4) photographs.

Tables. Tables represent the first step in the analysis of the experimental data. Much thought and reshaping should go into the production of the final table since tables cost more per page than text. Tables should be designed to fit the page size of the journal, and should not be too large. Instead of clarifying data, a large table will confuse the reader; therefore break tables up as much as possible. They should never be so long as to need a folding sheet—this is most expensive, and also inefficient as folding sheets are liable to tear easily.

In general there are two types of table: (1) those containing the original data, or data condensed from them; and (2) those illustrating certain relationships derived from the data. Do not try to demonstrate too many findings in one table, and yet do not make the table so simple that a line or two of print would be equally satisfactory. When drawing up the tables, use only accepted abbreviations, and see that every one is capable of being immediately understood. When symbols are used, a footnote to the table must give an adequate explanation of their significance. The style of tables, whether open or ruled, varies from journal to journal—consult the particular journal before you prepare your table. In all cases, however, tables must be numbered (arabic numerals) and a legend or title must be used to describe each one.

Graphs. The preparation of suitable graphs is a complicated business and details may be sought in any of the sources listed in the section of bibliography devoted to 'How to write a paper'. Graphs are particularly useful for demonstrating changes in, or relationships between, particular functions. They are an economical way of presenting data, for several curves may be drawn on the same graph.

In designing a graph the first point is to relate its size to the size of the printed page. You will often see graphs or other illustrations with a good deal of plain white surrounding them. This is bad planning and is rarely seen in the best American journals, where technical author efficiency is, on the whole, highest. If the graph had been drawn in correct proportion to page size, then two graphs might have been included in the same space. To do this, measure the full page width of the chosen journal, and decide whether your graph can be made to fit the whole, or half page. The actual size of your graph should be made about twice the linear size of the printed graph—the proportions are the essential feature. The diagram (FIG. 18.1) illustrates how a

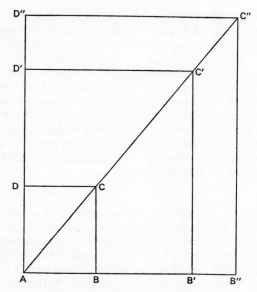

FIG. 18.1. Any rectangle constructed on the
diagonal will retain the same proportions as
the desired printed size of the figure.

figure may be drawn in proportion to the size of the printed page. The
rectangle ABCD is made to the exact size of the reproduction, the width
of the column of print, but the height is made slightly less than the page
height to allow space for the legend. By prolonging the diagonal AC
to any desired point, so can your original drawing be later reduced to
the correct page size.

Do not draw the graphs on paper larger than the sheets of typed
text—this is a rule applicable to all illustrations. If this is impossible,
photograph the illustration and send reduced glossy prints. Always
make exact copies of all illustrations, and for this purpose photography
is ideal.

In the preparation of graphs the following rules are generally acceptable:

1. The independent variable is plotted on the horizontal axis, as are
   units of time.
2. The dependent variable is plotted on the vertical axis.
3. The same scale of co-ordinates should be used in all your graphs.
4. Grid lines are not usually necessary.
5. Leave an ample (1½ inches; 37 mm) margin on each side of the
   lettering along each axis.

WMP

Drawings. Histograms and drawings are rarely necessary. Their main use is as illustrations for lectures, except when a piece of apparatus can be simply reduced to a diagram—for instance an electrical circuit.

Photographs. There are the most expensive of all illustrations and should be avoided unless you are reproducing histological preparations, radiographs, or clinical conditions. You will almost certainly be asked to pay for any colour reproductions. Submit high contrast, glossy prints. Do not write on the back with a ball-point pen. If photographs of patients are to be published, then the patients' written permission should be submitted with the photographs. All illustrative material should be suitably protected by hardboard covers.

DISCUSSION

In most papers the discussion is far too long, and too many references are included. Its purpose is to demonstrate in what way the study confirms or contradicts previous work in the field, how current theory has to be modified, and what are the implications of the results for future research. The topics in a discussion are often dealt with in the following order: 1. Technical points. 2. Tidy-up results. 3. Internal consistency of data. 4. Relationship to author's previous work. 5. Relationship to other work. 6. Suggestions for future experiments deriving from the present work.

SUMMARY

One of the most important parts of the paper is the summary. Here is the one part of your paper which is the most likely to be read, and on it, the reader may decide whether it is worth his while to devote precious time to reading your whole paper. It may be printed in abstract journals, and in a multilingual journal it will be translated into French and German. Devote particular care to your summary, which should be written in impeccable English. It can be prepared as follows. Go through your text and note each fresh step in your exposition, the results, and their relation to your own and previous hypotheses, and the conclusions you draw from the whole piece of work. Each phase can then be summarized in a single sentence—the total length of the summary should rarely exceed 100 words. Never use phrases such as 'The findings are discussed', 'The findings show', 'It seems reasonable to assume'.

When the summary is to be translated into another language, always arrange this yourself, and do not leave it to the editorial staff of the journal. The most comical translations are liable to be made by the staffs of foreign journals. Similarly, never allow your paper to be translated into another language without reserving the right of correcting the translation.

ACKNOWLEDGEMENTS

It is customary to render thanks to a whole range of individuals from professors down to laboratory assistants. My own view is that this is a deplorable formality—these individuals are there to help, and are paid to help. Acknowledgements clutter up the journals. If you have to do it, make it brief, and do not include too many people.

BIBLIOGRAPHY

Journals differ in their bibliographical demands, but some degree of uniformity is now being reached. The most widely used method is as follows: Author's name. Year Title. *Journal*, **Volume Number**, Page Numbers. For example:

COPPEN, A. J. (1958) Psychosomatic aspects of pre-eclamptic toxaemia, *J. Psychosom. Res.*, **2**, 241–65.

The use of a bibliography is to inform the reader of previous work in the field so that he can choose which papers might be worth reading—hence the desirability of including the titles of papers. The abbreviations should follow those laid down in the *World List of Scientific Periodicals* and great care should be taken to conform absolutely to these abbreviations. A glance at the bibliography will often tell the editor how experienced, how careful, and how critical is an author, and whether the paper has been rejected by another journal. It is most injudicious to send an editor a paper which does not conform bibliographically to the expressed editorial policy of his journal. When listing books the correct citation is as follows: Author's name. Date *Title*, Place of publication, Publisher, Pages.
For example:

SCHNECK, JEROME, M. (1960) *A History of Psychiatry*, Springfield, Ill. Charles C. Thomas, pp. ix, 196.

If reference is made to a particular part of the book, the page or pages must be cited, as in:

WOLF, S. G., JR., and WOLFF, H. G. (1943) *Human Gastric Function*, New York, Oxford University Press, pp. 145–8.

Do not try to be all-embracing in your bibliography. The day of the learned review is almost over; the Year Books which exist in almost every subject now subserve this function. If your work is so original as to be of major importance, very few papers will be relevant, and if extensive enough to warrant an exhaustive review of the literature, you should publish a monograph. In general, the best papers have the fewest references.

Always double space between every line, not only between each reference.

TYPING THE PAPER

The general typographical quality of British scientific papers is extremely poor in comparison with American papers. The near universal use of the electric typewriter in American institutions puts our secretaries at a great disadvantage. Similarly, the greater technical skill of the American secretary, the high quality of the materials used, such as the paper, the illustrations and graphs, puts most British papers to shame. Nevertheless, if the following points are borne in mind the editorial eyestrain and irritation will be greatly minimized:

1. Always use a machine having a clear type and a fresh, well-inked ribbon.
2. Carbon paper must be comparatively fresh so as to give clear, crisp copies. The practice of photocopying (dry process) is growing. All copies are then as legible as the top copy. Some journals will allow photocopies of diagrams.
3. White bond paper of a standard size (A4, 210×297 mm) and of first-class quality should be used for the top copy. For the remaining two copies a slightly thinner paper is recommended, but *not* an airmail-thin paper.
4. Always double space and leave margins of $1\frac{1}{4}$ inches (33 mm) on each side of the page, 2 inches (51 mm) at the top and 1 inch (25 mm) at the bottom. Let no doubts arise about paragraphs—many papers are typed in a curiously illiterate manner with regard to paragraphs.
5. Three copies of the paper must be produced. The top copy plus one carbon copy is sent to the journal, one being retained by the author for later proof correction.
6. Type all tables separately and insert into the text a legend showing where a table should be inserted, for example:

(Table 1 here)

Never type a table running along with the text. Similarly, footnotes should not be typewritten into the text, but should always be on separate sheets, carefully numbered. All tables and footnotes should be placed at the end of the paper.

7. Always carefully number the pages in the top right-hand corner of the page. Nothing is more annoying to an editor than to get an unnumbered manuscript.
8. Do not staple the pages; use a flat, square clip which can be easily detached. For bulky paper use a large, solid clip.
9. Carefully correct the typescript. Assume that mistakes have been made, check and recheck. Write corrections in the body of the manuscript—leave the margins for the editor, sub-editors, and printers. If a lengthy correction is necessary, to avoid re-typing paste the correction over the original type. Never use staples for this purpose. For details of how to correct typescript consult Trelease (1958).

TRANSPORTING THE PAPER

Many manuscripts from this country reach the editor in a deplorable condition—crumpled or even torn. See that the envelope is sufficiently strong, and that the manuscript is protected by a cardboard wrapping. If the paper is at all bulky, string it. Label the envelope clearly, and check the address to which the paper should be sent. Editors change, voluntarily and involuntarily, and so may their locations. Lastly, always check on the postage—editors cannot be expected to pay postage due. If they are kind enough to do so, your paper will already be starting with a prejudice against it. Always use first class or air mail postage.

THE EDITORIAL DECISION

Your letter to the Editor must be brief and formal. An acknowledgement should reach you by return post, and show clearly the date your paper has been received. All reputable scientific journals use assessors, and your paper will be read by a minimum of two assessors, as well as a member of the Editorial Board. Anonymity for the assessors is a prerequisite for what may prove at times an onerous task. The function of the Editor-in-Chief is to take the final decision regarding publication, having taken into consideration *inter alia* the opinions of his assessors, the paper itself, the needs of the journal, and the back-log of papers awaiting publication. This decision is then sent to the author. In those cases where the assessors may have suggested omissions or corrections, these are best accepted without demur; bickering is to be avoided at all costs, for the Editor's decision is final and other papers are jostling with yours for publication. Editorial policy varies considerably when informing the author that his paper has been rejected, ranging from a flat rejection to detailed explanation. It is important to realize that the

Editor is under no obligation to inform you of his reasons for the rejection of your paper. Great literary artists have all been familiar with rejection slips at some time in their careers; scientific work gives no mandate for protest against Editorial decisions.

PROOF CORRECTION

The paper has now been accepted and has been sent to the publishers. The final responsibility of the author is the correction of the proofs of his article. At some time varying between 6 and 12 weeks after acceptance of his paper, he should receive the proofs, together with his original manuscript. It is his duty to check on the accuracy of the printer's work and to make any corrections necessary. First, get a colleague to read out the manuscript slowly, including punctuations, and spelling any words which may have presented technical difficulty to the printer, and follow this reading on the proof. Pay particular attention to numbers and tables. When this first reading is completed put aside the proof for a time, and then read it again, this time noting if any phrases or sentences have been omitted or transposed. Lastly, go over the proof again checking particularly on the correctness of names, titles, institutions, bibliographical references, and tables. Bibliographical references should preferably be checked against the original articles wherever possible. Check all hyphenated words on the right-hand side of the sheet to assure yourself that the correct breaks have been used.

When correcting proofs the aim is to give your instructions simply to the printer—you are not a professional author and need not worry about not knowing the correct symbols. Lists of these can easily be obtained, however. Just write the correction in ink, in the margin, not between lines of print. Do not make radical changes in the proof—even altering or expunging a single word near the beginning of a paragraph may mean that the whole paragraph has to be reset. It cannot be emphasized too strongly that the proof is no more than a copy of your manuscript, that you are responsible for its accurate identity, and that no alterations, apart from the correction of the printer's errors, are justifiable. Many journals charge the expenses of alterations to the author, and this is an excellent rule.

The corrected proofs should be returned promptly to the printer, with or without your manuscript, depending on the rules of the journal concerned. Always retain a carefully corrected copy of the final stage of your paper, so that any mishaps or queries can be dealt with efficiently. Notify any change of address to the editor—and if there are several authors, decide which of you is going to be responsible for the correction of proofs, and make this clear to the publishers.

WRITING GOOD ENGLISH

The scientific paper is not a literary essay, nor should we expect scientists to be exquisite literary craftsmen. Good writers are born, not made; anyone familiar with the craft of literature also knows how much intense work, correction, and recorrection goes into the production of a play, novel, or other creative effort. Do not therefore be discouraged by articles, usually written by elderly professors deploring the present-day standards of literary merit in medical or scientific publications. Editors today do not concern themselves overmuch with literary merit, but they do expect that a paper should conform to certain rules of good writing. A glance at a page of typescript will tell the experienced editor whether the paper is likely to be well written or not.

PARAGRAPHS

The orderly flow of ideas is cardinal to the presentation of data. Each step in the argument requires a distinct emphasis, and for this the device of paragraphing is used. Paragraphs are often too long, and include several statements. On the other hand they should not be too short, for this makes reading difficult and jerky The transition from one paragraph to another must read easily so that the presentation flows along in an orderly way.

PUNCTUATION

Sentences should be short—complicated and cumbersome strings of words are unnecessary. The purpose of punctuation is to aid the sense of the writing, and serves much the same function as phrasing in music. Use your ear, rather than ponder over complicated rules. A full stop or period is used at the end of a complete statement, although a semicolon is sometimes used to give variety. Dashes can be used to indicate a pause between two parts of a sentence which might otherwise be wrongly read together. On the whole, authors either handle punctuation correctly, or are quite unable to master its purpose.

REPETITION

It is extraordinarily easy for the same word to occur time and time again, without the author's recognition. Always check your manuscript for the presence of these 'repeaters'; you may then consult one of your dictionaries, Fowler, or Roget's Thesaurus, for alternative choices. It may even be necessary to rephase a particular section completely, for some words are extremely difficult to replace. Words and phrases used too frequently include 'work', 'research', 'findings', 'found', 'study', 'consider', 'it can be', 'it is', 'it may be'. The amount of repetition usually directly relates to the general literary competence of the writer.

JARGON AND COLLOQUIALISMS

The word jargon is too often thrown at the head of the scientist to mean very much. In fact the word refers to a professional vocabulary, but has come to be a term 'applied contemptuously to the language of scholars, the terminology of a science or art' (OED). It is derived from the French—meaning the warbling of birds; chattering. When scientific or professional terms are correctly and clearly used, no objection can be made; it is only when there seems to be an excessive and unnecessary use of obscure terms that we are justified in using the word jargon. Do not therefore use unfamiliar words, do not coin words, and if a word in common usage can be employed, so much the better.

Colloquialisms should never be used. Your foreign readers cannot be expected to be familiar with them, and you are not, after all, conducting a conversation or delivering a lecture. Colloquialisms are particularly apt to creep into descriptions of laboratory work, for instance 'hook-up' or 'set-up'. Always check doubtful words in your dictionary.

TENSES

Lastly, the correct tense must be used. Past tenses are used in describing the experimental facts, whilst the present tense is used for the presentation of data. Alteration of tense is most confusing—as long as there is a systematic and consistent use of the present or past tense, few editors will be over-critical.

The books listed under 'How to write English' are invaluable aids to the writing of good simple English, and should be part of your own library.

REFERENCES

TRELEASE, S. F. (1958) *How to Write Scientific and Technical Papers*, Baltimore.
WORLD LIST OF SCIENTIFIC PERIODICALS (1900–1950) 3rd ed., London.

DICTIONARIES

ENGLISH, H. B., and ENGLISH, H. C. (1958) *A Comprehensive Dictionary of Psychological and Psychoanalytical Terms*, London.
THE BRITISH MEDICAL DICTIONARY (1961) London.
THE CONCISE OXFORD DICTIONARY OF CURRENT ENGLISH (1964) 5th ed., Oxford
HINSIE, L. E., and CAMPBELL, R. J. (1970) *Psychiatric Dictionary*, 4th ed., New York.
THE SHORTER OXFORD ENGLISH DICTIONARY (1959) 3rd ed., Oxford.

FURTHER READING

HOW TO WRITE A PAPER

ANON (1950) *General Notes on the Preparation of Scientific Papers*, London.

BRITISH STANDARD FOR PRINTERS' AND AUTHORS' PROOF CORRECTIONS (1945) British Standards Institution, London.

NUTTALL, G. H. F. (1940) Notes on the preparation of papers for publication, in *The Journal of Hygiene and Parasitology*, London.

PUBLICATION MANUAL OF THE AMERICAN PSYCHOLOGICAL ASSOCIATION (1957) Washington, D.C.

HOW TO WRITE ENGLISH

FOWLER, H. W. (1965) *A Dictionary of Modern English Usage*, 2nd ed., Oxford.

GOWERS, E. (1948) *Plain Words. A Guide to the Use of English*, London, H.M.S.O.

GOWERS, E. (1951) *A.B.C. of Plain Words*, London, H.M.S.O.

ROGET, P. M. (1963) *Thesaurus of English Words and Phrases*, London.

INDEX